Learning Imaging

Series Editors:

R. Ribes · A. Luna · P.R. Ros

María I. Martínez León · Luisa Ceres Ruiz
Juan E. Gutiérrez (Editors)

Learning Pediatric Imaging

100 Essential Cases

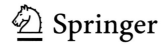 Springer

María I. Martínez León
Radiology Department
Pediatric Radiology Unit
Hospital Materno-Infantil del C.H.U. Carlos Haya
Arroyo de los Angeles
29011 Málaga
Spain

Luisa Ceres Ruiz
Radiology Department
Pediatric Radiology Unit. Chief
Hospital Materno-Infantil del C.H.U. Carlos Haya
Arroyo de los Angeles
29011 Málaga
Spain

Juan E. Gutiérrez
Health Science Center
University of Texas
Elmscourt
78230 San Antonio, TX
USA

ISBN 978-3-642-16891-8   e-ISBN 978-3-642-16892-5

DOI 10.1007/978-3-642-16892-5

Springer Heidelberg Dordrecht London New York

Library of Congress Control Number: 2011921251

Cover design: eStudioCalamar, Figueres/Berlin

Printed on acid-free paper

9 8 7 6 5 4 3 2 1

Springer is part of Springer Science+Business Media (www.springer.com)

Preface

The pediatric radiology field is a unique area of study; it deals with patients that are different to those of other radiological subspecialties. Their illnesses and ailments only belong to them, their behavior is different, and the way we approach them from the radiological point of view is very specific. They are unlike anything else. It might sound pretentious but I just intend to show how thrilled and enthusiastic I am about my field of work, pediatric radiology.

The authors have written this book to transmit their in-depth knowledge of the subject and to provide a comprehensive coverage for residents, general radiologists, or other pediatric radiologists. There is a wide range of diagnostic cases presented in this book, some of them can be diagnosed by simple radiography and others need multivoxel spectroscopy or functional imaging.

Learning Pediatric Imaging is a further volume of a series that started with *Learning Diagnostic Imaging*; here we intend to show how challenging, interesting, and rewarding pediatric radiology is.

Like a well known pediatric radiologist wrote: "This book is for all the sick children."

Málaga-Granada, Spain   María I. Martínez León

Contents

6 Tumoral Abdomen

Contributors

GUSTAVO ALBI RODRÍGUEZ
Radiology Department
Pediatric Radiology Unit
Hospital del Niño Jesús
Madrid
Spain

DIEGO ALCAIDE MARTÍN
Radiology Resident
Hospital Clínico Universitario
Virgen de la Victoria
Málaga
Spain

ANA ALONSO MURCIANO
Radiology Resident
Complejo Hospitalario Universitario
Carlos Haya
Málaga
Spain

IGNACIO ALONSO USABIAGA
Fetal Medicine Unit. Centro Gutenberg
Málaga
Spain

BEATRIZ ASENJO GARCÍA
Radiology Department
Neuroradiology Unit
Complejo Hospitalario
Universitario Carlos Haya
Málaga
Spain

BEATRIZ AVILA GAMARRA
Radiology Resident
Complejo Hospitalario
Universitario Carlos Haya
Málaga
Spain

IGNASI BARBER
Radiology Department
Pediatric Radiology Unit
Hospital Materno-Infantil Vall d´Hebron
Barcelona
Spain

MERCEDES BERNABÉ DURÁN
Radiology Resident
Complejo Hospitalario Universitario
Carlos Haya
Málaga
Spain

CRISTINA BRAVO BRAVO
Radiology Department
Pediatric Radiology Unit
Hospital Materno-Infantil
del C.H.U. Carlos Haya
Málaga
Spain

SUSANA CALLE RESTREPO
Pontifícia Universidad Javeriana
Bogotá
Colombia

ANA G. CARVAJAL REYES
Radiology Resident
Hospital Clínico Universitario
Virgen de la Victoria
Málaga
Spain

LUISA CERES RUIZ
Radiology Department
Pediatric Radiology Unit. Chief
Hospital Materno-Infantil del C.H.U Carlos Haya
Málaga
Spain

ANA COMA MUÑOZ
Radiology Department
Pediatric Radiology Unit
Hospital Materno-Infantil Vall d´Hebron
Barcelona
Spain

HÉCTOR CORTINA ORTS
Radiology Department
Pediatric Radiology Unit. Chief
Hospital La Fe
Valencia
Spain

ELISA CUARTERO MARTÍNEZ
Radiology Resident
Complejo Hospitalario Universitario
Carlos Haya
Málaga
Spain

Mª DOLORES DOMÍNGUEZ PINOS
Radiology Resident
Complejo Hospitalario Universitario
Carlos Haya
Málaga
Spain

ALEJANDRA DOROTEO LOBATO
Radiology Department
Hospital de la Axarquía
Málaga
Spain

Mª JESÚS ESTEBAN RICÓS
Radiology Department
Pediatric Radiology Unit
Hospital La Fe
Valencia
Spain

CARMEN GALLEGO HERRERO
Radiology Department
Pediatric Radiology Unit
Hospital Universitario 12 de Octubre
Madrid
Spain

ELENA GARCÍA ESPARZA
Radiology Department
Pediatric Radiology Unit
Hospital del Niño Jesús
Madrid
Spain

PILAR GARCÍA-PEÑA
Radiology Department
Pediatric Radiology Unit
Hospital Materno-Infantil Vall d´Hebron
Barcelona
Spain

PASCUAL GARCÍA-HERRERA TAILLEFER
Radiology Department
Pediatric Radiology Unit
Hospital Materno-Infantil del
C.H.U. Carlos Haya
Málaga
Spain

JORGE GARÍN FERREIRA
Radiology Department
Genitourinary Unit
Complejo Hospitalario Universitario
Carlos Haya
Málaga
Spain

EVA GÓMEZ ROSELLÓ
Radiology Department
Neuroradiology Unit
Hospital Jusep Trueta
Girona
Spain

JUAN E. GUTIÉRREZ
Health Science Center
University of Texas
Elmscourt
San Antonio, TX
USA

SARA M. KOENIG
University of Texas
Health Science Center
San Antonio
USA

Naiara Linares Martínez
Radiology Department
Hospital La Fe
Valencia
Spain

Miguel Angel López Pino
Radiology Department
Pediatric Radiology Unit
Hospital del Niño Jesús
Madrid
Spain

Roberto Llorens Salvador
Radiology Department
Pediatric Radiology Unit
Hospital la Fe
Valencia
Spain

Carlos Marín
Radiology Department
Pediatric Radiology Unit
Hospital General Universitario
Gregorio Marañón
Madrid
Spain

César Martín Martínez
Radiology Department
UDIAT Diagnostic Center
Corporació Sanitària Parc Taulí
Sabadell
Spain

María I. Martínez León
Radiology Department
Pediatric Radiology Unit
Hospital Materno-Infantil del C.H.U Carlos Haya
Málaga
Spain

L. Santiago Medina
Health Outcomes
Policy and Economics Center
Division of Neuroradiology and Brain Imaging
Miami Children's Hospital
Miami
FL, USA

Elena Méndez Donaire
Radiology Department
Clínica Radiológica Mario Gallegos
Málaga
Spain

Francisco Menor Serrano
Radiology Department
Pediatric Radiology Unit
Hospital La Fe
Valencia
Spain

Amparo Moreno Flores
Radiology Department
Pediatric Radiology Unit
Hospital La Fe
Valencia
Spain

Dolores Muro Velilla
Radiology Department
Pediatric Radiology Unit
Hospital La Fe
Valencia
Spain

María Isabel Padín Martín
Radiology Department
Thorax Radiology Unit
Complejo Hospitalario Universitario
Carlos Haya
Málaga
Spain

Lourdes Parra Ruiz
Radiology Department
Hospital Parque San Antonio
Málaga
Spain

Elena Pastor Pons
Radiology Department
Pediatric and Gynecologic Unit
Hospital Virgen de las Nieves
Granada
Spain

LAURA PELEGRÍ MARTÍNEZ
Radiology Department
Hospital La Fe
Valencia
Spain

VÍCTOR PÉREZ CANDELA
Radiology Department
Pediatric Radiology Unit. Chief
Hospital Universitario
Materno-Infantil de Canarias
Las Palmas de Gran Canaria
Spain

FRANCISCO PÉREZ NADAL
Radiology Department
Hospital La Serranía de Ronda
Málaga
Spain

SARA PICÓ ALIAGA
Radiology Department
Pediatric Radiology Unit
Hospital la Fe
Valencia
Spain

JUIO RAMBLA VILAR
Radiology Department
Hospital la Fe
Valencia
Spain

CAROLINA RAMÍREZ RIBELLES
Radiology Resident
Hospital la Fe
Valencia
Spain

ANTONIO RODRÍGUEZ FERNÁNDEZ
Nuclear Medicine Department
Hospital Universitario Virgen
de las Nieves
Granada
Spain

SONIA ROMERO CHAPARRO
Radiology Department
Hospital Parque San Antonio
Málaga
Spain

CINTA SANGÜESA NEBOT
Radiology Department
Pediatric Radiology Unit
Hospital La Fe
Valencia
Spain

CARLOS SANTIAGO RESTREPO
Chest Division
Health Center at San Antonio
San Antonio
TX, USA

CRISTINA SERRANO GARCÍA
Radiology Department
Pediatric Radiology Unit
Hospital Virgen de la Arrixaca
Murcia
Spain

SARA SIRVENT CERDÁ
Radiology Department
Pediatric Radiology Unit
Hospital del Niño Jesús
Madrid
Spain

INÉS SOLÍS MUÑIZ
Radiology Department
Pediatric Radiology Unit
Hospital del Niño Jesús
Madrid
Spain

JORGE A. SOTO
Department of Radiology
Boston Medical Center
Boston University
USA

CAROLINA TORRES ALÉS
Radiology Department
Hospital La Serranía de Ronda
Málaga
Spain

PABLO VALDÉS SOLÍS
Radiology Department Chief
Hospital de Marbella
Málaga
Spain

MARÍA VIDAL DENIS
Radiology Department
Complejo Hospitalario
Universitario Carlos Haya
Málaga
Spain

SILVIA VILLA SANTAMARÍA
Cedimed SA
Medellin
Colombia

BERNARDO WEIL LARA
Pathologist Department
Hospital Materno-Infantil del
C.H.U. Carlos Haya
Málaga
Spain

Contents

M.I. Martínez-León et al., *Learning Pediatric Imaging*, Learning Imaging,
DOI: 10.1007/978-3-642-16892-5_1, © Springer-Verlag Berlin Heidelberg 2011

Case 1.1
Pilocytic Astrocytoma

■

Beatriz Avila Gamarra and María I. Martínez León

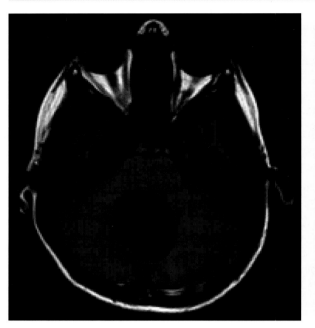

Fig. 1.1

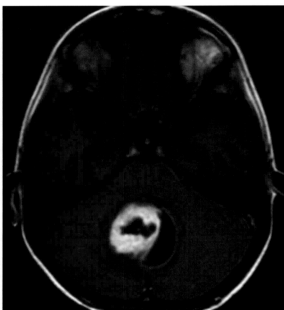

Fig. 1.2

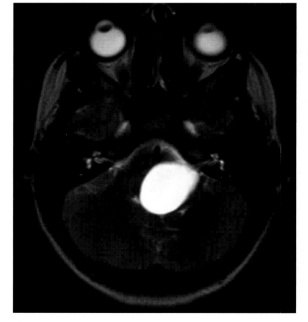

Fig. 1.3

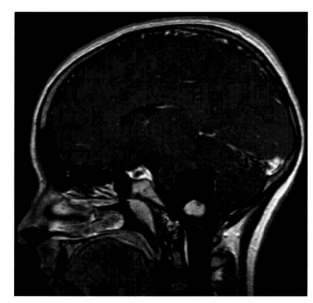

Fig. 1.4

Case 1.1a: An 8-year-old boy presents with headache and vomiting.
Case 1.1b: A 13-year-old girl presents with ataxia.

Pilocytic astrocytoma (PA) is the most common infratentorial brain tumor in children and frequently presents in the first and second decade of life. It is usually a slow-growing neoplasm and approximately 85% arise in the cerebellar vermis. The World Health Organization (WHO) classifies PA as a grade I central nervous system tumor.

Pilocytic astrocytomas are most commonly cystic masses with mural nodules. If supratentorial, its location is usually the optic nerve or chiasm (frequent in NF-1), as well as the cerebral hemispheres and thalamic region.

In CT images, the solid component of the lesion is isodense to the cerebral parenchyma and its cystic portion is hypodense. In T1-weighted MR images, PA is iso- or hypointense and in T2-weighted and FLAIR MR images, hyperintense. The cystic component of the mass tends to have a signal similar to CSF, although it may increase depending on the percentage of proteinaceous content of the fluid. More than 95% of these lesions have contrast enhancement. The most frequent presentation is a strong contrast uptake by the mural nodule (50%). Vasogenic edema adjacent to the tumor is rare. Spectroscopy studies have shown very low creatine concentrations, low myo-inositol, and low tCho concentrations consistent with their low cellularity. Lipids are slightly elevated and an increase in lactate has also been documented.

The first line of treatment for PA is surgical removal with a 5-year 90% survival rate after complete resection of the tumor. The prognosis is often less favorable for lesions affecting the optic tract or hypothalamic region treated with chemotherapy and radiotherapy.

Case 1.1a: The axial T1-weighted MR sequence with and without contrast shows a midline mass in the cerebellar vermis with a predominantly cystic component that surrounds a solid portion (Figs. 1.1 and 1.2). With contrast administration, there is strong enhancement that identifies a central necrotic zone. There is no evidence of edema. The lesion compresses the fourth ventricle causing supratentorial hydrocephaly (dilatation of temporal horns).

Figure 1.1 Pilocytic astrocytoma. Case 1.1a
Figure 1.2 Pilocytic astrocytoma. Case 1.1a

Case 1.1b: In MR, T2-weighted axial and a T1-weighted sagittal images with contrast show a brainstem tumor of similar characteristics: a cystic mass with an enhancing mural nodule (Figs. 1.3 and 1.4). In both examples, a slight mural contrast enhancement is seen.

Figure 1.3 Pilocytic astrocytoma. Case 1.1b
Figure 1.4 Pilocytic astrocytoma. Case 1.1b

Case 1.2
Pilomyxoid Astrocytoma
■

María I. Martínez León

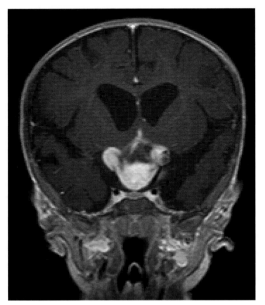

Fig. 1.5

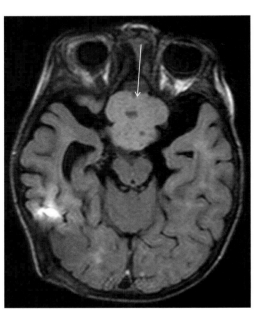

Fig. 1.6

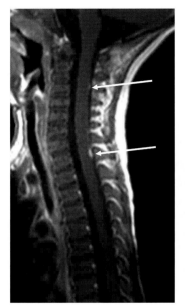

Fig. 1.7

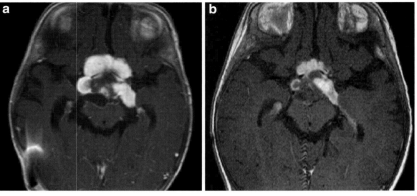

Fig. 1.8

An 8-month-old boy presents with findings consistent with intracranial hypertension.

Pilomyxoid astrocytoma (PMA) is a central nervous system tumor that was once believed to be a variant of pilocytic astrocytoma (PA) and has recently been described as a separate entity. This neoplasm has been shown to have a more aggressive progression and a greater tendency to disseminate through the CSF and to recur after treatment than PA. Furthermore, significant histological differences between these two tumors have granted PMA a WHO grade II classification. Originally described by Janisch as "childhood-onset diencephalic pilocytic astrocytoma," Tihan went on to name and describe the histopathologic characteristics of PMA in 1999. The grand majority of PMAs grow in the hypothalamic and chiasmatic regions and present in patients under 4 years of age. In images, this tumor usually presents as a solid mass without a necrotic or cystic component and with homogeneous contrast uptake.

As stated above, the histologic behavior of the PMA differentiates it from PA. The absence of Rosenthal fibers and eosinophilic granular bodies is characteristic of this neoplasm.

Given the increased tendency of the PMA to disseminate through CSF, radiologic findings indicative of dissemination warrant complete neuroaxis extension studies.

Spectroscopy studies suggest differences in metabolite concentrations between pilocytic and pilomyxoid astrocytomas. PMA has been shown to present a lower concentration of choline, creatine, and NAA, while PA tends to have elevated choline levels with a decrease of the other two metabolites. This is yet another finding that may aid in differentiating between these two tumors.

MR T1-weighted coronal image, rapid sequence with contrast, shows slight ventricular dilatation caused by a diencephalic tumor (final diagnosis was made by biopsy obtained by premamillary ventriculostomy) (Fig. 1.5). MR axial FLAIR image displays a predominantly homogenous solid mass (arrow) (Fig. 1.6). In a spinal cord study, sagital T1-weighted with Fat Saturation and contrast, two enhancing punctiform lesions on the spinal surface, consistent with leptomeningeal dissemination, can be identified (arrows) (Fig. 1.7). The T1-weighted axial MR image with contrast shows a significant enhancement and decrease in size after 6 months of treatment with chemotherapy (Fig. 1.8a, b).

Figure 1.5 Pilomyxoid astrocytoma
Figure 1.6 Pilomyxoid astrocytoma
Figure 1.7 Pilomyxoid astrocytoma
Figure 1.8 (**a, b**) Pilomyxoid astrocytoma

Case 1.3
Ependymoma
■
Elena García Esparza

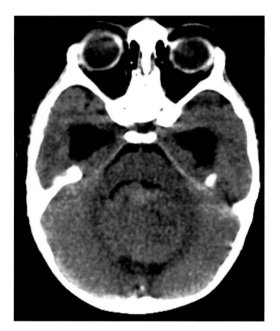

Fig. 1.9

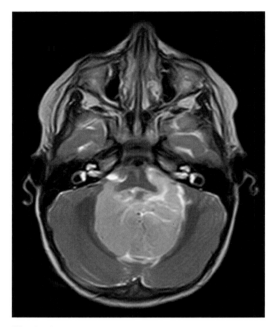

Fig. 1.10

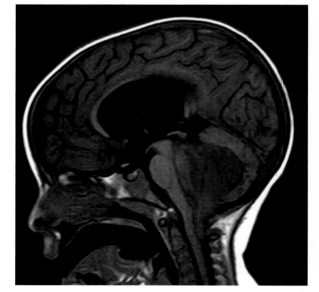

Fig. 1.11

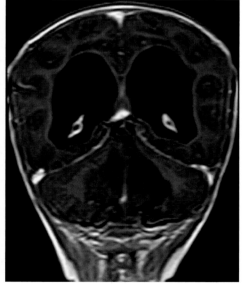

Fig. 1.12

A 14-month-old boy with a 2-week history of progressive vomiting. Weeks prior to admission, the patient had presented axial instability with incapability to walk and torticollis. There were no cranial nerve alterations upon examination.

Comments

The ependymoma constitutes approximately 10% of all intracranial tumors in children. Presentation is most frequent in children under 2 years and its incidence decreases with age. Ependymomas arise from the ependyma, which explains their relation to the ventricle walls and the spinal ependymal canal.

The ependymoma is not usually considered an aggressive tumor (WHO grade II). Nevertheless, it has been shown to have a high tendency to recur if a complete resection is not achieved, which is especially difficult if its localization is infratentorial or intraventricular. A less frequent, WHO grade III variant of the ependymoma has been described as malignant or anaplastic ependymoma.

In children, 90% of ependymomas are intracranial and 70% are found to grow in the posterior cranial fossa. The most common location is the interior of the fourth ventricle. Given its consistency and plasticity, the tumor tends to adapt to the shape of the ventricle and then extends through the foramen of Luschka and Magendie toward the pontocerebellar angle or cisterna magna, and through the foramen magnum to the cervical spinal canal.

Thirty percent of pediatric ependymomas have a supratentorial location and in this case, as opposed to infratentorial tumors, they tend to be extraventricular.

Because of the para or intraventricular location of these tumors, both grade II and grade III ependymomas have the ability to disseminate through the CSF, thus warranting extension studies of the spine with contrast.

Imaging Findings

The CT image shows a large posterior fossa mass in the interior of the fourth ventricle, with a similar density to that of the cerebral parenchyma, causing significant hydrocephaly (Fig. 1.9). The MR axial T2-weighted image shows how the ependymoma exits through the foramen of Luschka toward both pontocerebellar angles (Fig. 1.10). In the sagittal T1-weighted MR image extension of the tumor through the foramen magnum toward the spinal canal can be observed, as well as a displacement of the mesencephalic tectum superiorly (Fig. 1.11). The T1-weighted coronal MR image with contrast shows very slight enhancement (Fig. 1.12). Nevertheless, this is not its typical presentation since ependymomas usually have a more intense heterogeneous contrast uptake. Significant supratentorial hydrocephaly can also be identified.

Figure 1.9   Ependymoma
Figure 1.10 Ependymoma
Figure 1.11 Ependymoma
Figure 1.12 Ependymoma

Case 1.4

Infrequent Presentation of Medulloblastoma

Diego Alcaide Martín and María I. Martínez León

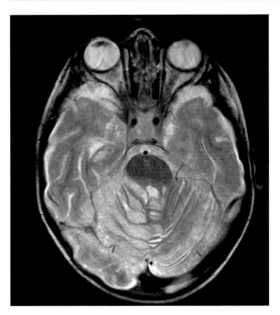

Fig. 1.13

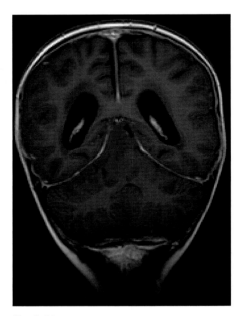

Fig. 1.14

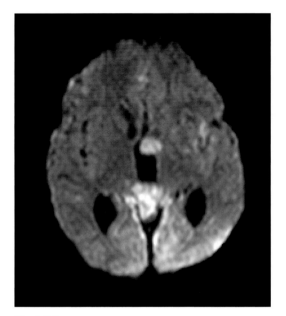

Fig. 1.15

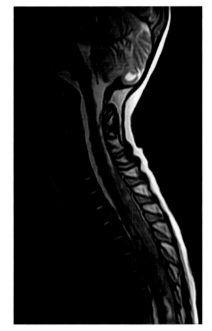

Fig. 1.16

A3-year-old boy with history of head trauma presents with progressive headache and irritability.

Medulloblastoma is an aggressive neuroepithelial neoplasm that presents more frequently in children and is classified by the WHO as a grade IV tumor. The medulloblastoma is both the most frequent malignant CNS tumor in children and the most common tumor found in the posterior fossa in this population. Its location is generally the cerebellum (95%), specifically the cerebellar vermis (75%) and less frequently the cerebellar hemispheres.

Clinical manifestations include headache, nausea, and vomiting. Central ataxia and spasticity are common signs when the mass affects the cerebellar vermis. On the other hand, peripheral ataxia and dysdiadochokinesia develop when the tumor is located in the cerebellar hemispheres.

Radiologically, medulloblastoma presents as a mass located in the cerebellar vermis that is characteristically hyperdense on contrast-enhanced CT, hypointense on T1-weighted MR images, and of variable intensity on T2-weighted MR images. Also, it typically shows contrast enhancement and diffusion restriction on DWI. In addition, hydrocephaly can be seen due to ventricular system compression.

CSF dissemination, generally to the spinal cord, is a relatively common finding (33%), On the other hand, satellite metastases are infrequent, yet when they occur are usually to the bone.

Differential diagnoses include ependymoma, pilocytic astrocytoma, lymphoma, Lhermitte–Duclos disease, and mestastases.

Treatment consists of a combination of surgery and radiotherapy (radiosensitive), with or without adjuvant chemotherapy. Currently, advances in diagnosis and management of medulloblastoma have increased its 5-year survival rate to approximately 70–80%.

An infrequent presentation of medulloblastoma is shown mimicking Lhermitte–Duclos disease. MR images reveal an infiltrative lesion of the cerebellar vermis and hemispheres (predominantly the right) extending toward the ventricles and the infra and supratentorial cisterns, deforming the cerebellar folds and mimicking a "striated cerebellum" (Fig. 1.13). There is no contrast enhancement (Fig. 1.14) and in DWI there is notable restriction to diffusion (Fig. 1.15) and ventricular dilatation. Neuroaxial extension studies reveal extramedular and intraspinal dissemination with masses that compress the spinal cord causing significant compromise (Fig. 1.16).

Figure 1.13 Infrequent presentation of medulloblastoma
Figure 1.14 Infrequent presentation of medulloblastoma
Figure 1.15 Infrequent presentation of medulloblastoma
Figure 1.16 Infrequent presentation of medulloblastoma

Case 1.5
Brainstem Tumors
■
Elena Méndez Donaire and María I. Martínez León

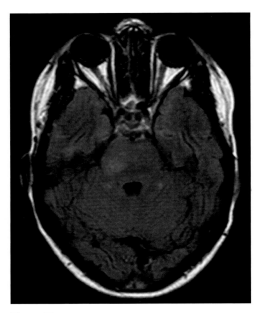

Fig. 1.17

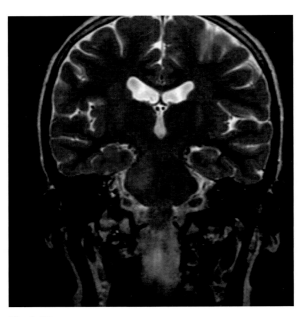

Fig. 1.18

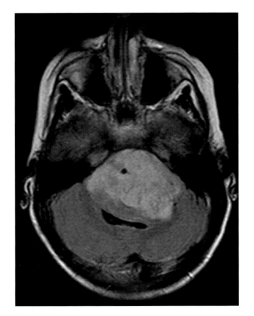

Fig. 1.19

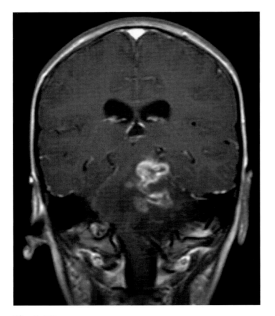

Fig. 1.20

Case 1.5a: An 8-year-old patient presents with history of headache.

Case 1.5b: A 6-year-old patient presents with hemiparesis and headache.

Brainstem tumors (BT) comprise approximately 10–20% of all central nervous system tumors in the pediatric population. Diagnosis is usually made between 7 and 9 years of age and there is no gender predilection.

These tumors include those that affect the midbrain, pons, medulla oblongata, and superior cervical spine. The diffuse glioma is the most frequent of the BT and has the worst prognosis. On the other hand, the focal lesions are a minority and have a better prognosis. The clinical presentation and behavior of BT depend on the location and the growth pattern they present. Special attention must be paid to obtain a thorough clinical history because signs and symptoms of these tumors can be insidious and difficult to identify. BT can also be found in the context of neurofibromatosis type I, although pilocytic astrocytoma is the most frequent tumor to arise in this syndrome.

With MRI, BT can be further classified into subgroups, which in turn entail different treatment plans and prognosis. The Barkovich classification system takes into account the following parameters: location (midbrain, pons, and medulla oblongata), focality (diffuse or focalized), direction and extension of tumoral growth, mass size, exophytic growth in relation to the brainstem, associated hemorrhage and/or necrosis, and evidence of secondary hydrocephaly.

The treatment of BT depends on the location and growth pattern of the tumor. In focalized lesions, surgical resection is the first line of treatment. On the other hand, the treatment of choice in diffuse BT is radiotherapy and/or chemotherapy.

Case 1.5a: Axial FLAIR and coronal T2-weighted MR images show a localized mass in the right hemi-pons with poorly delineated margins, which causes minimal deformity of the structure with enlargement that does not obliterate the adjacent cistern (Figs. 1.17 and 1.18). This mass does not enhance with administration of contrast (image not shown). Final diagnosis of high-grade glioma was made.

Figure 1.17 Brainstem tumor
Figure 1.18 Brainstem tumor

Case 1.5b: Axial FLAIR and coronal T1-weighted plus contrast MR images show a tumor that compromises both pons and medulla oblongata, with diffuse extension surrounding the basilar artery in 360º, IV ventricular compression with secondary hydrocephalous. A poor, heterogeneous contrast enhancement can be seen (Figs. 1.19 and 1.20). Final diagnosis of diffuse glioma was made.

Figure 1.19 Brainstem tumor
Figure 1.20 Brainstem tumor

Case 1.6
Choroid Plexus Tumors
■

María I. Martínez León

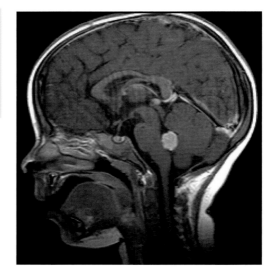

Fig. 1.22

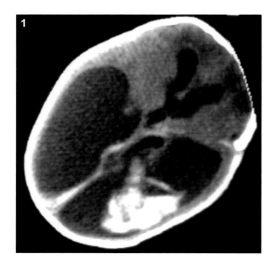

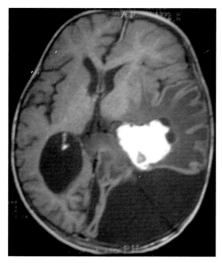

Fig. 1.21

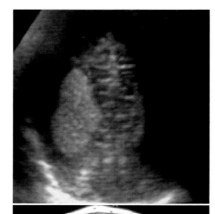

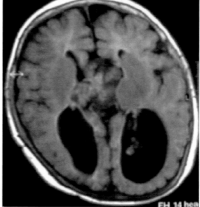

Fig. 1.23

Fig. 1.24

Choroid plexus tumors are infrequent intraventricular neoplasms that arise from the epithelium of the choroid plexus. These can be classified as papillomas or carcinomas, papillomas being much more common. While papillomas have been documented in adults, carcinomas are almost exclusively seen in children less than 2 years of age. The vast majority arise in the atrium of the lateral ventricles and those found in the fourth ventricle are more common in adults. The clinical manifestations are often caused by an increase in intracranial pressure secondary to hydrocephaly from alterations in the dynamic of CSF, namely, hyperproduction of CSF by the tumor, flow obstruction by the mass and decreased drainage secondary to recurrent subarachnoid hemorrhage, and accumulation of proteinaceous material produced by the neoplasm itself. A few cases have been described in Li–Fraumeni Syndrome and Aicardi Syndrome. Furthermore, an association has also been shown between plexus hypertrophy and neurocutaneous syndromes such as Sturge–Weber Syndrome.

Imaging studies for choroid plexus papillomas usually show solid, predominantly heterogeneous intraventricular tumors with lobulated "cauliflower" morphology and a significant contrast enhancement. Over 24% have calcifications and, as mentioned previously, hydrocephaly is a common finding. On the other hand, choroid plexus carcinomas present greater signal heterogeneity (necrosis, hemorrhage, cysts) with extraventricular extension to the adjacent parenchyma and periventricular white matter edema. Papillomas are classified as a WHO grade I tumor while carcinomas are classified as grade III.

Surgery is curative for papillomas and tends to resolve the secondary hydrocephaly. Presurgical embolization of intratumoral and supplying arteries, in an attempt to reduce blood flow and facilitate resection, has been described. Radical surgery in carcinomas is difficult due to the extent of vascularization and local tissue invasion. Therefore, adjuvant therapy is needed to adequately manage this tumor. Consequently, carcinomas have a poorer 5-year survival rate.

Comments

An old CT with contrast shows a typical choroid plexus papilloma in the atrium of the left lateral ventricle, associated hydrocephalus (Fig. 1.21). Sagittal T1-weighted MR image with contrast shows a papilloma of the fourth ventricle (Fig. 1.22). Choroid plexus carcinoma with local invasion, edema, and hydrocephaly (Fig. 1.23). Metachronic papillomas in Aicardi Syndrome – transfontanellar sonography of a choroid plexus papilloma in the right atrium, and a second tumor, which grew in the third ventricle 2 years after surgical resection of the first, flair MRI sequence (Fig. 1.24).

Imaging Findings

Figure 1.21 Choroid plexus tumors
Figure 1.22 Choroid plexus tumors
Figure 1.23 Choroid plexus tumors
Figure 1.24 Choroid plexus tumors

Case 1.7
Atypical Teratoid/Rhabdoid Tumor of the CNS
■
Ana G. Carvajal Reyes and María I. Martínez León

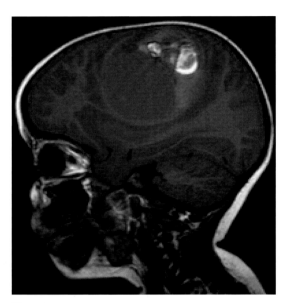

Fig. 1.25

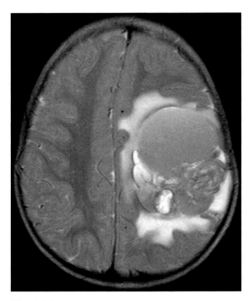

Fig. 1.26

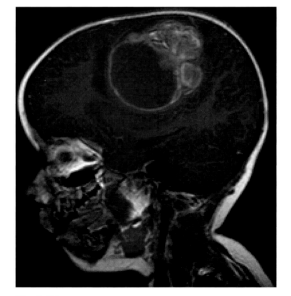

Fig. 1.27

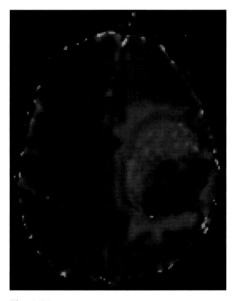

Fig. 1.28

A 20-month-old girl presents with 1-month history of decreased strength and impaired movement of the right upper extremity. During the past week, the patient has shown lower right extremity paresis.

Malignant rhabdoid tumors are neoplasms of embryonic origin that may occur in various locations, of which the CNS and kidney are most common. In the CNS, the most frequent type is the atypical teratoid/rhabdoid tumor (AT/RT). They are formed partially or entirely by rhabdoid cells, areas similar to PNET and mesenchymal tissue or malignant epithelium. Genetic studies have described the presence of anomalies in the long arm of chromosome 22, namely, deletion of the 22q11.2 region, which results in the inactivation of the INI1/SMARCB1 gene.

AT/RT of the CNS is an extremely aggressive and rare neoplasm, occurring more frequently in children under the age of 2. It can appear in any location of the CNS, the most frequent one being the cerebellum (60%). They have an increased tendency to disseminate to the leptomeninges. The clinical presentation depends on the age of the patient and the location of the mass. AT/RT is classified as WHO grade IV tumor. The true incidence of AT/RT is unknown due to the fact that it is often misdiagnosed as medulloblastoma because of their histopathological similarities.

Imaging findings are unspecific, but they tend to be large masses with calcifications, hemorrhage, necrosis, and CSF dissemination. Differential diagnoses include medulloblastoma, PNET, ependymoma, choroid plexus carcinoma, and high-grade astrocytoma. Immunohistochemical techniques and genetic analysis allow for a precise pathological diagnosis.

MRI shows both a large, intra-axial solid and cystic tumor located in the left parietal lobe with significant mass effect and associated vasogenic edema. The T1-weighted sagittal MR image shows heterogeneous signal intensity with hyperintense areas indicative of hemorrhage (Fig. 1.25). The T2-weighted axial MR image shows large, hyperintense cystic and necrotic areas and associated intermediate signal corresponding to its solid portion (Fig. 1.26). With the administration of contrast the solid portion of the mass displays an important, heterogeneous uptake, while its cystic component presents peripheral rim enhancement (Fig. 1.27). Diffusion-weighted images show a notable restriction by the solid component of the mass, appearing as hypointense on the ADC map (Fig. 1.28).

Figure 1.25 Atypical teratoid/rhabdoid tumor of the CNS
Figure 1.26 Atypical teratoid/rhabdoid tumor of the CNS
Figure 1.27 Atypical teratoid/rhabdoid tumor of the CNS
Figure 1.28 Atypical teratoid/rhabdoid tumor of the CNS

Case 1.8
Glioblastoma
■
Beatriz Asenjo García

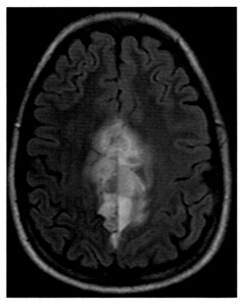

Fig. 1.29

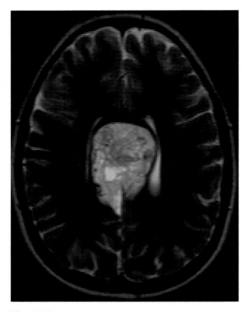

Fig. 1.30

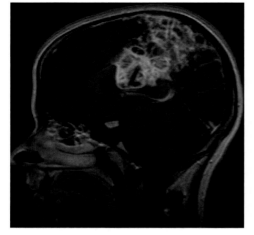

Fig. 1.31

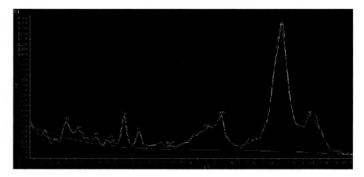

Fig. 1.32

A 13-year-old girl presents with sudden functional impairment of the right lower limb associated with a 1-week history of bilateral temporal headache.

Comments

High-grade glioblastomas in pediatrics comprise a heterogeneous group of tumors with different locations and histological characteristics. They may affect children in a wide range of ages. These tumors arise most frequently in the supratentorial region and brainstem and are uncommon in the cerebellum and spinal cord. Incidence is significantly less in children than in adults. While gliomas represent 50% of all pediatric CNS tumors, only 6–12% are supratentorial high-grade gliomas and 3–9% are high-grade diffuse astrocytomas of the brainstem.

The glioblastoma can present with a wide variety of clinical manifestations. At diagnosis, patients show symptoms related to the affected area of the brain, including seizures and signs of intracranial hypertension. Radiologically, the most common finding is a heterogeneous lesion located in the supratentorial white matter with associated vasogenic edema and mass effect.

The first line of treatment for high-grade gliomas in children older than 3 years combines surgery, radiotherapy, and chemotherapy. Surgery is the first line of management of these tumors and a strong correlation exists between the location of the mass and the grade of resection. For tumors located in the midline, surgical removal is often less successful than for those that affect the cerebral cortex. Experience removing these masses in patients under 3 years of age is scarce due to their low incidence.

Imaging Findings

The axial FLAIR and T2-weighted MR images show a parasagittal, hyperintense, solid, infiltrative lesion with ill-defined margins that affects both white and gray matter at either side of the interhemispheric midline (Figs. 1.29 and 1.30). The T1-weighted sagittal MR image with contrast displays a lesion with heterogeneous enhancement, areas of necrosis, and signs of invasion of the corpus callosum (Fig. 1.31). Univoxel spectroscopy with short echo time located in the mass shows a lipid peak and a decrease of the remaining metabolites (Fig. 1.32). This pattern is one of the most frequent among glioblastomas, in which the increase in lipids is indicative of intratumoral necrosis.

Figure 1.29 Glioblastoma
Figure 1.30 Glioblastoma
Figure 1.31 Glioblastoma
Figure 1.32 Glioblastoma

Case 1.9
Rhabdomyosarcoma
■
Miguel Angel López Pino

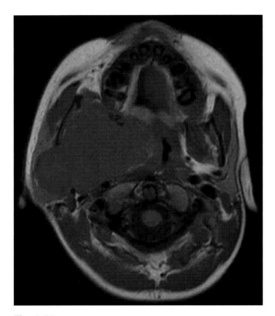

Fig. 1.33

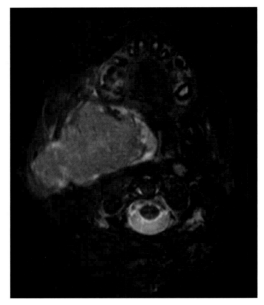

Fig. 1.34

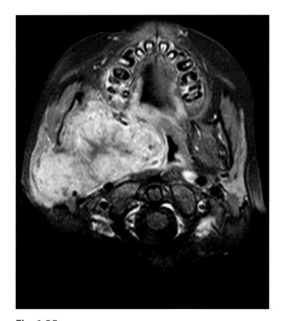

Fig. 1.35

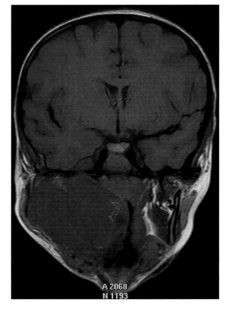

Fig. 1.36

A 6-year-old boy presents with right cervical mass, significant dysphagia, and trismus.

Rhabdomyosarcomas are malignant tumors that arise from primitive muscular cells. They are the most common malignant soft-tissue neoplasms present in childhood and are especially frequent during the first decade of life (70% of cases in children under 12 years of age). The most common location is the head and neck (more than 40% of cases). Nevertheless, they may appear anywhere in the body, including the urinary tract, retroperitoneum, and extremities, among others. Three histological variants have been described: pleomorphic, alveolar, and embryonic. While tumors located in the orbit are usually embryonic, those arising from the extremities, more typical in adolescents, are frequently alveolar. The pleomorphic variant is less frequent and usually occurs in adults.

Although most cases are found to be sporadic, certain conditions have been shown to increase the risk of tumor development, including: congenital cerebral anomalies, neurofibromatosis, nephroblastoma, and retinoblastoma. An association has also been described between a mutation of the p53 suppressor gene and the development of rhabdomyosarcoma. Furthermore, these tumors have been shown to arise secondary to radiotherapy for concomitant neoplasms.

Rhabdomyosarcoma must be considered as a differential diagnosis for any soft-tissue mass of malignant characteristics that appears in childhood. They present variable contrast uptake and an estimated 25% show associated bone destruction. Nevertheless, there are no specific imaging findings and rhabdomyosarcomas may, on occasion, simulate benign lesions such as hemangiomas. The treatment of choice is usually a combination of surgery and chemotherapy.

The MRI shows a mass of the right parapharyngeal space with extension to the parotid and carotid space and associated protrusion of the pharyngeal mucosa. The axial T1-weighted MR image displays a predominantly hypointense lesion that decreases the lumen of the oropharynx (Fig. 1.33). In the T2-weighted fat-suppressed MR image, ill-defined margins and invasion to the parotid gland and pterigoid muscles can be observed (Fig. 1.34). Administration of contrast on a T1-weighted image displays an intense, heterogeneous enhancement (Fig. 1.35). The coronal T1-weighted MR image shows extension to the skull base, through the foramen ovale and with a slight intracranial component due to perineural dissemination through V3 (Fig. 1.36).

Figure 1.33 Rhabdomyosarcoma
Figure 1.34 Rhabdomyosarcoma
Figure 1.35 Rhabdomyosarcoma
Figure 1.36 Rhabdomyosarcoma

Case 1.10
Pineoblastoma
■

María Vidal Denis and María I. Martínez León

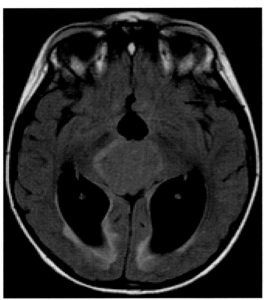

Fig. 1.37

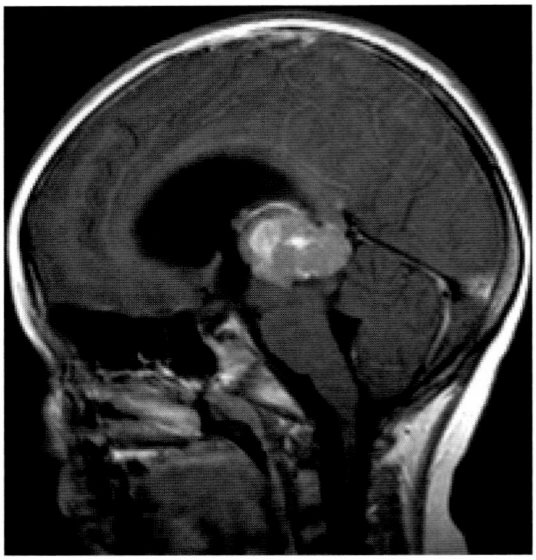

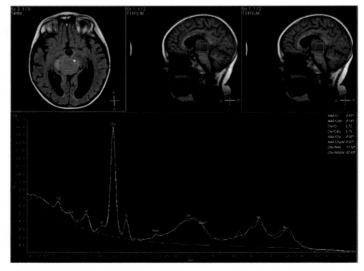

Fig. 1.38

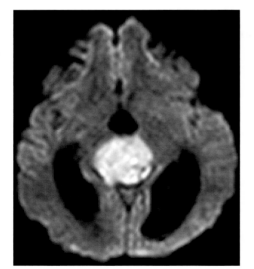

Fig. 1.39

Fig. 1.40

A 5-year-old girl presents with headache and visual impairment.

The pinealoblastoma is a malignant neoplasm that arises from the pineal region and is the least frequent type of tumor to develop in this gland. They usually present in children under the age of 10 and have no predilection for gender.

Histologically, pinealoblastomas are composed of undifferentiated, immature cells with small cytoplasms. These features cause the tumor's characteristic restriction to diffusion, very similar to other tumors of neuroepithelial tissue such as medulloblastoma.

The WHO classifies the pinealoblastomas as a grade IV tumor, and they have a high tendency to disseminate trough the CSF (extension studies are indicated) and to invade adjacent structures.

The clinical manifestations of the pinealoblastoma are typical of its location. A triad of symptoms has been described, which include: obstruction of the Sylvian aqueduct (supratentorial hydrocephaly, papilledema and headache), functional alterations of the roof of the mesencephalon (causing Parinaud Syndrome, anisocoria, superiorly deviated gaze, and convergence paresis), and endocrine changes.

A rare variant of this neoplasm is the trilateral retinoblastoma, which consists of a coexistence of pinealoblastoma and bilateral retinoblastoma. This is usually a hereditary syndrome and, therefore, all patients with bilateral retinoblastoma should undergo cerebral imaging studies.

The pinealoblastoma presents as a mass located in the pineal region of the brain and causes dilatation of the third ventricle and both lateral ventricles (with transependymal migration of CSF). On T1-weighted MR images they appear isointense, and on T2-weighted and FLAIR MR images (Fig. 1.37) they appear hyperintense, with significant contrast enhancement (Fig. 1.38) and without areas of necrosis or hemorrhage. Given the tumor's cellularity, the pinealoblastoma presents a significant restriction to diffusion (Fig. 1.39). With the univoxel spectroscopy study, the lesion displays a high peak of choline, with a choline to creatine ratio greater than 2 and an absence of normal neurons, demonstrated by a significant decrease in NAA, indicative of malignancy (Fig. 1.40).

Figure 1.37 Pinealoblastoma
Figure 1.38 Pinealoblastoma
Figure 1.39 Pinealoblastoma
Figure 1.40 Pinealoblastoma

Further Reading

Books

Atlas SW (2004) RM cabeza y columna. Marban, Madrid

Barkovich AJ (1994) Pediatric neuroimaging. Lippincott – Raven, St. Louis, MO

Barkovich AJ (2000) Pediatric neuroimaging, 3rd edn. Lippincott Williams & Wilkins, Philadelphia, PA

Kleihues P, Cavernee WK (2000) Pathology and genetics. Tumours of the nervous system. Ed IARCP WHO, Lyon, pp 83–93

Kransdorf M, Murphey M (2008) Imaging of soft tissue tumors. Lippincott Williams & Wilkins. Capítulo 8

Louis DN, Oggki H, Wiestler OD et al (eds) (2007a) World Health Organization classification of tumours. Pathology and genetics of tumours of the nervous system. IARC, Lyon, France

Osborn AG (1994) Astrocytomas and other glial neoplasms. In: Osborn AG (ed) Diagnostic neuroradiology. Mosby, St. Louis, MO, pp 529–578

Osborn AG (1996) Neuroradiología diagnóstica. Hardbound, ISBN: 84-8174-119-1,1996. Ed: Elsevier

Osborn AG (2004) Diagnostic imaging: brain. Amirsys, Salt Lake City, UT

Osborn et al. (2004) Diagnostic imaging: brain. Amirsys, Salt Lake City, UT, pp I–6–52

Web Links

http://www.pedrad.info/

http://www.pilomyxoid.com

http://www.emedicine.medscape.com/article/277621-overview

http://www.uptodate.com/home/index.html

www.pediatricradiology.com

www.auntminnie.com, Choroid plexus papilloma. Case of the day: one-year-old girl with increasing head circumference. 2003, July 10

www.ajnr.org

www.TheOncologist.com

http://www.nci.nih.gov/cancertopics/types/childrhabdomyosarcoma/

http://emedicine.medscape.com/article/249945-overview

Articles

Allen SD, Moskovic EC, Fisher C, Thomas JM (2007) Adult rhabdomyosarcoma: cross-sectional imaging findings including histopathologic correlation. AJR Am J Roentgenol 189:371–377

Arslanoglu A, Cirak B, Horska A et al (2003) MR Imaging characteristics of pilomyxoid astrocytomas. AJNR Am J Neuroradiol 24:1906–1908

Arslanoglu A, Aygun N, Tekhtani D, Aronson L, Cohen K, Burger PC et al (2004) Imaging findings of CNS atypical teratoid/rhabdoid tumors. AJNR Am J Neuroradiol 25(3):476–480

Barkovich AJ, Krischer J, Kun LE, Packer R, Zimmerman RA, Freemman CR, Wara WM, Albright L, Allen JC, Hoffman HJ (1990) Brain stem gliomas: a classification system based on magnetic resonance imaging. Pediatr Neurosurg 16:73–83

Beni-Adani L, Gomori M, Spektor S, Constantini S (2000) Cyst wall enhancement in pilocytic astrocytoma: neoplastic or reactive phenomena. Pediatr Neurosurg 32:234–239

Berger C, Thiesse P, Lellouch-Tubiana A, Kalifa Ch, Pierre-Kahn A, Bouffet E (1998) Choroid plexus carcinomas in childhood: clinical features and prognostic factors. Neurosurgery 42:470–475

Bonneville F, Savatovsky J, Chiras J (2007) Imaging of cerebellopontine angle lesions: an update. Part 1: enhancing extra-axial lesions. Eur Radiol 17:2472–2482

Bourgouin PM, Tampieri D, Grahovac SZ, Leger C, Del Carpio R, Melançon D (1992) CT and MR imaging findings in adults with cerebellar medulloblastoma: comparison with findings in children. AJR Am J Roentgenol 159:609–612

Brat DJ, Scheithauer BW, Fuller GN, Tihan T (2007) Newly codified glial neoplasms of the 2007 WHO classification of tumours of the central nervous system: angiocentric glioma, pilomyxoid astrocytoma and pituicytoma. Brain Pathol 17:319–324

Broniscer A, Gajjar A (2004) Supratentorial high-grade astrocytoma and diffuse brainstem glioma: two challenges for the pediatric oncologist. Oncologist 9:197–206

Ceppa EP, Bouffet E, Griebel R, Robinson Cj, Tihan T (2007) The pilomyxoid astrocytoma and its relationship to pilocytic astrocytoma: report of a case and critical review of the entity. J Neurooncol 81:191–196

Chang YW, Yoon HK, Shin HJ, Roh HG, Cho JM (2003) MR imaging of glioblastoma in children: usefulness of diffusion/perfusion-weight MRI and MR spectroscopy. Pediatr Radiol 33:836–842

Chen KS, Hung PC, Wang HS, Jung SM, Ng SH (2002) Medulloblastoma or cerebellar dysplastic gangliocytoma (Lhermitte-Duclos disease)? Pediatr Neurol 27:404–406

Chikai K, Ohnishi A, Kato T et al (2004) Clinico-pathological features of pilomyxoid astrocytoma of the optic pathway. Acta Neuropathol 108:109–114

Cho B, Wang K, Nam D, Kim D, Jung H, Kim H (1998) Pineal tumors: experiencie with 48 cases over 10 years. Childs Nerv Syst 14:53–58

Cirak B, Horská A, Barker PB, Burger PC, Carson BS, Avellino AM (2005) Proton magnetic resonance spectroscopic imaging in pediatric pilomyxoid astrocytoma. Childs Nerv Syst 21:404–409

Cuccia V, Rodríguez F, Palma F, Zuccaro G (2006) Pinealoblastomas in children. Childs Nerv Syst 22:577–585

Daltro P, Cruz CH, Do A, Nogueira R, Porto MTC (2008) Medulloblastoma. In: Ribes R, Luna A, Ros PR (eds) Learning diagnostic imaging. Springer, New York, pp 220–221

Dang T, Vassilyadi M, Michaud J, Jimenez C, Ventureyra EC (2003) Atypical teratoid/rhabdoid tumors. Childs Nerv Syst 19(4):244–248

Desai KI, Nadkarni TD, Muzumdar DP, Goel A (2001) Prognostic factors for cerebellar astrocytomas in children: a study of 102 cases. Pediatr Neurosurg 35:311–317

Due-Tonnessen B, Helseth E, Skullerud K, Lindar T (2001) Choroid plexus tumors in children and young adults: report of 16 consecutive cases. Childs Nerv Syst 17:252–256

Epstein F (1985) A staging system for brain stem gliomas. Cancer 56:1804–1806

Evans A, Ganatra R, Morris SJ (2001) Imaging features of primary malignant rhabdoid tumour of the brain. Pediatr Radiol 31(9):631–633

Fenton LZ, Foreman NK (2003) Atypical teratoid/rhabdoid tumor of the central nervous system in children: an atypical series and review. Pediatr Radiol 33(8):554–558

Fernandez C, Figarella-Branger D, Girard N, Bouvier-Labit C, Gouvernet J, Paredes A et al (2003) Pilocytic astrocytomas in children: prognostic factors-a retrospective study of 80 cases. Neurosurgery 53:544–553

Fischbein NJ, Prados MD, Wara W (1996) Radiologic clasification of brain stem tumors: correlation of magnetic resonance imaging appearence with clinical outcome. Pediatr Neurosurg 24:9–23

Fisher PG, Breiter SN (2000) A clinicopathologic reappraisal of brain stem tumor classification. Cancer 89:1569–1576

Fulham MJ, Melisi JW, Nishimiya J, Dwyer AJ, Di Chiro G (1993) Neuroimaging of juvenile pilocytic astrocytomas: an enigma. Radiology 189:221–225

Gallucci M, Catalucci A, Scheithauer BW, Forbes GS (2000) Spontaneous involution of pilocytic astrocytoma in a patient without neurofibromatosis type 1: case report. Radiology 214:223–226

Gasparetto EL, Cruz LC Jr, Doring TM, Araújo B, Dantas MA, Chimelli L et al (2008) Difusión-weighted MR images and pinealoblastoma: diagnosis and follw-up. Arq Neuropsiquiatr 66:64–68

Herzog CE, Stewart JM, Blakely ML (2003) Pediatric soft tissue sarcomas. Surg Oncol Clin N Am 12:419–447

Hicks J, Flaitz C (2002) Rhabdomyosarcoma of the head and neck in children. Oral Oncol 38:450

Holsinger FC, Weeks BH, Hicks MJ, Friedman EM (2002) Contemporary concepts in the management of pediatric rhabdomyosarcoma. Curr Opin Otolaryngol Head Neck Surg 10:91–96

Hwang H, Egnaczyk GF, Ballard E, Dunn RS, Holland SK, Ball WS Jr (1998) Proton MR spectroscopic characteristics of pediatric pilocytic astrocytomas. AJNR Am J Neuroradiol 19:535–540

Jallo GI, Bisher-Rohrbaugh A, Freed D (2004) Brainstem gliomas. Childs Nerv Syst 20:143–153

Janisch W, Schreiber D, Martin H, Gerlach H (1985) Diencephalic pilocytic astrocytoma wiht clinical onset in infancy. Biological behaviour and pathomorphological findings in 11 children. Zentralbl Allg Pathol 130:31–43

Johnsen DE, Woodruff WW, Allen IS, Cera PJ, Funkhouser GR, Coleman LL (1991) MR imaging of the sellar and yuxtasellar regions. Radiographics 11:727–758

Joubert A, Sanint Pierre G, Fauchon F, Privat K, Bouffet E, Ruchoux MM et al (2000) Pineal parenchymal tumors: a correlation of histological features with prognosis in 66 cases. Brain Pathol 10:49–60

Kaplan AM, Albright AL, Zimmerman RA (1996) Brainstem gliomas in children. Pediatr Neurosurg 24:185–192

Khanani MF, Hawkins C, Shroff M et al (2006) Pilomyxoid astrocytoma in a patient with neurofibromatosis. Pediatr Blood Cancer 46:377–380

Koeller KK, Rushing EJ (2004) From the archives of the AFIP: Pilocytic astrocitoma: radiologic-pathologic correlation. Radiographics 24:1693–1708

Koeller KK, Sandberg GD (2002a) From the archives of the afip: cerebral intraventricular neoplasms: radiologic-pathologic correlation. Radiographics 22:1473–1505

Koeller KK, Sandberg GD (2002b) Cerebral intraventricular neoplasms: radiologic-pathologic correlation. RadioGraphics 22:1473–1505

Koeller KK, Sandberg GD (2002c) From the archives of the AFIP: cerebral intraventriclar neoplasms: radiologic-pathologic correlation. Radiographics 22:1473–1505

Koller KK, Rushing EJ (2003) Medulloblastomas: a comprehensive review with radiologic-pathologic correlation. Radiographics 23:1613–1637

Komotar RJ, Mocco J, Jones JE et al (2005) Pilomyxoid astrocytoma: diagnosis, prognosis, and management. Neurosurg Focus 18(6A):E7

Koral K, Gargan L, Bowers DC, Gimi B, Timmons CF, Weprin B et al (2008) Imaging characteristics of atypical teratoid-rhabdoid tumor in children compared with medulloblastoma. AJR Am J Roentgenol 190(3):809–814

Kordes U, Gesk S, Fruhwald MC, Graf N, Leuschner I, Hasselblatt M et al (2010) Clinical and molecular features in patients with atypical teratoid rhabdoid tumor or malignant rhabdoid tumor. Genes Chromosom Cancer 49(2):176–181

Louis DN, Hiroko O, Wiestler OD et al (2007b) The 2007 WHO classification of tumours of the central nervous system. Acta Neuropathol 114:97–109

Louis DN, Ohgaki H, Wiestler OD et al (2007c) The 2007 WHO classification of tumours of the central nervous system. Acta Neuropathol 114:97–109

Majós C (2005) Espectroscopia por resonancia magnética de protón en el diagnóstico de tumores cerebrales. Radiología 47:1–12

Majós C, Alonso J, Aguilera C et al (2003) Proton magnetic resonance spectroscopy (1 H MRS) of human brain tumours: assessment of differences between tumour types and its applicability in brain tumour categorization. Eur Radiol 13:582–591

Mason WP, Maestro RD, Eisenstat D (2007) Canadian recommendations for the treatment of glioblastoma multiforme. Curr Oncol 14:110–117

McCarville MB, Spunt SL, Pappo AS (2001) Rhabdomyosarcoma in pediatric patients: the good, the bad, and the unusual. AJR Am J Roentgenol 176:1563–1569

McEvoy AW, Harding BN, Phipps KP, Ellison DW, Elsmore AJ, Thompson D et al (2000) Management of choroid plexus tumours in children: 20 years experience at a single neurosurgical centre. Pediatr Neurosurg 32:192–199

Mermuys K, Jeuris W, Vanhoenacker PK, Van Hoe L, D'Haenens P (2005) Best cases from the AFIP: supratentorial ependymoma. Radiographics 25:486–490

Meyers SP, Kemp SS, Tarr RW (1992) MR imaging features of medulloblastomas. AJR Am J Roentgenol 158:859–865

Meyers SP, Khademian ZP, Biegel JA, Chuang SH, Korones DN, Zimmerman RA (2006) Primary intracranial atypical teratoid/rhabdoid tumors of infancy and childhood: MRI features and patient outcomes. AJNR Am J Neuroradiol 27(5):962–971

Miller CR, Perry A (2007) Glioblastoma: morphologic and molecular genetic diversity. Arch Pathol Lab Med 131:397–406

Moghrabi A, Kerby T, Tien RD (1995) Pronostic value of contrast-enhanced magnetic resonance imaging in brainstem gliomas. Pediatr Neurosurg 23:293–298

Moll A, Imhof S, Schouten-can A, Meeter A (2002) Screening for pinealoblastoma in patients with retinoblastoma. Arch Ophtalmol 120:1774

Mueller DP, Moore SA, Sato Y, Yuh WT (1992) MRI spectrum of medulloblastoma. Clin Imaging 16:250–255

Nagib MG, O'Fallon MT (2000) Lateral ventricle choroid plexus papilloma in childhood: management and complications. Surg Neurol 54:366–372

Nishi M, Hatae Y (2004) Epidemiology of malignant neoplasms in soft tissue during childhood. J Exp Clin Cancer Res 23: 437–440

Oi S, Matsuzawa K, Choi J et al (1998) Identical characteristics of the patient populations with pineal region tumors in Japan and in Korea and therapeutic modalities. Childs Nerv Syst 14:36–40

Packer RJ, Siegel KR, Sutton LN, Litmann P, Bruce DA, Schut L (1985) Leptomeningeal dissemination of primary central nervous system tumors of childhood. Ann Neurol 18: 217–221

Parham DM (2001) Pathologic classification of rhabdomyosarcomas and correlations with molecular studies. Mod Pathol 14:506–514

Parmar H, Hawkins C, Bouffet E, Rutka J, Shroff M (2006) Imaging findings in primary intracranial atypical teratoid/rhabdoid tumors. Pediatr Radiol 36(2):126–132

Pollack IF (1994) Brain tumors in children. N Engl J Med 331:1500–1507

Prince MR, Chew FS (1991) Ependymoma of the fourth ventricle. AJR Am J Roentgenol 157:1278

Provenzale JM, Weber AL, Klintworth GK, McLendonn RE (1995) Radiologic-pathologic correlation. Bilateral retinoblastoma with coexistent pinealoblastoma (trilateral retinoblastoma). AJNR Am J Neuroradiol 16:157–165

Recinos PF, Sciubba MD, Jallo GI (2007) Brainstem tumors: where are we today? Pediatr Neurosurg 43:192–200

Reddy AT (2005) Atypical teratoid/rhabdoid tumors of the central nervous system. J Neurooncol 75(3):309–313

Rees J, Smirniotopoulos J, Jones R et al (1996) Glioblastoma multiforme: radiologic-pathologic correlation. Radiographics 16:1413–1438

Reni M, Gatta G, Mazza E, Vecht C (2007) Ependymoma. Crit Rev Oncol Hematol 63:81–89

Rubin G, Michowitz S, Horev G (1998) Pediatric brain stem gliomas: an update. Childs Nerv Syst 14:167–173

Rumboldt Z, Camacho DL, Lake D, Welsh CT, Castillo M (2006a) Apparent diffusion coefficients for differentiation of cerebellar tumors in children. AJNR Am J Neuroradiol 27:1362–1369

Rumboldt Z, Camacho DL, Lake D, Welsh CT, Castillo M (2006b) Apparent diffusion coefficients for differentiation of cerebellar tumors in children. AJNR Am J Neuroradiol 27(6):1362–1369

Sarkar C, Sharma MC, Gaikwad S, Sharma C, Singh VP (1999) Choroid plexus papilloma: a clinicopathological study of 23 cases. Surg Neurol 114:902–905

Shinoda J, Kawaguchi M, Matsuhisa T, Deguchi K, Sakai N (1998) Choroid plexus carcinoma in infants: report of two cases and review of the literature. Acta Neurochir 140:557–563

Smith AB, Rushing EJ, Smirniotopoulos JG (2010) From the archives of the AFIP: lesions of the pineal region: radiologic-pathologic correlation. Radiographics 30:2001–2020

Spoto GP, Press GA, Hesselink JR, Solomon M (1990) Intracranial ependymoma and subependymoma: MR manifestations. AJNR Am J Neuroradiol 11:83–91

Stein-Wexler R (2009) MR imaging of soft tissue masses in children. Magn Reson Imaging Clin N Am 17:489–507

Strong JA, Hatten HP, Brown MT, Debatin JF, Friedman HS, Oakes WJ et al (1993) Pilocytic astrocytoma: correlation between the initial imaging features and clinical aggressiveness. AJR Am J Roentgenol 161:369–372

Stupp R, Mason WP, Van Den Bent J (2005) Radiotherapy plus concomitant and adyuvant temozolomide for glioblastoma. N Engl J Med 352:987–996

Sung L, Anderson JR, Arndt C, Raney RB, Meyer WH, Pappo AS (2004) Neurofibromatosis in children with Rhabdomyosarcoma: a report from the Intergroup Rhabdomyosarcoma study IV. J Pediatr 144:666–668

Taggard DA, Menezes AH (2000) Three choroid plexus papillomas in a patient with Aicardi síndrome. A case report. Pediatr Neurosurg 33:219–223

Tihan T, Fisher PG, Kepner JL et al (1999) Pediatric astrocytomas with monomorphous pilomyxoid features and a less favorable outcome. J Neuropathol Exp Neurol 58: 1061–1068

Tortori-Donati P, Fondelli MP, Cama A, Garrè ML, Rossi A, Andreussi L (1995) Ependymomas of the posterior cranial fossa: CT and MRI findings. Neuroradiology 37:238–243

Van Rijn RR, Wilde JC, Bras J, Oldenburger F, McHugh KM, Merks JH (2008) Imaging findings in noncraniofacial childhood rhabdomyosarcoma. Pediatr Radiol 38:617–634

Vazquez E, Castellote A, Mayolas N, Carreras E, Peiro JL, Enríquez G (2009) Congenital tumours involving the head, neck and central nervous system. Pediatr Radiol 39:1158–1172

Warmuth-Metz M, Bison B, Dannemann-Stern E, Kortmann R, Rutkowski S, Pietsch T (2008) CT and MR imaging in atypical teratoid/rhabdoid tumors of the central nervous system. Neuroradiology 50(5):447–452

Won Kwon J, Kim I (2006) Paediatric brain-stem gliomas: MRI, FDG- PET and histological grading correlation. Pediatr Radiol 36:959–964

Yoshida M, Fushiki S, Takeuchi Y, Takanashi M, Imamura T, Shikata T et al (1998) Diffuse bilateral thalamic astrocytomas as examined serially by MRI. Childs Nerv Syst 14: 384–388

Yuasa H, Tokito S, Tokunaga M (1993) Primary carcinoma of the choroid plexus in Li-Fraumeni syndrome: case report. Neurosurgery 32:131–134

Yuh EL, Barkovich AJ, Gupta N (2009) Imaging of ependymomas: MRI and CT. Childs Nerv Syst 25:1203–1213

Zattara-Cannoni H, Gambarelli D, Lena G, Dufour H, Choux M, Grisoli F et al (1998) Are juvenile pilocytic astrocytomas benign tumors? A cytogenetic study in 24 cases. Cancer Genet Cytogenet 104:157–160

Zee CS, Segall H, Apuzzo M, Destian S, Colletti P, Ahmadi J et al (1991) MR imaging of pineal region neoplasms. J Comput Assist Tomogr 15:56–63

Zimmerman RA, Bilaniuk LT, Pahlajani H (1978) Spectrum of medulloblastomas demonstrated by computed tomography. Radiology 126:137–141

Zuccaro G, Sosa F, Cuccia V, Lubieniecky F, Monges J (1999) Lateral ventricle tumors in children: a serie of 54 cases. Childs Nerv Syst 15:774–785

Contents

M.I. Martínez-León et al., *Learning Pediatric Imaging*, Learning Imaging,
DOI: 10.1007/978-3-642-16892-5_2, © Springer-Verlag Berlin Heidelberg 2011

Case 2.1
Nasal Chondromesenchymal Hamartoma
■

L. Santiago Medina and Sara M. Koenig

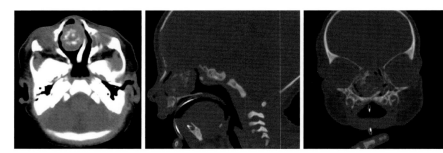

Fig. 2.1

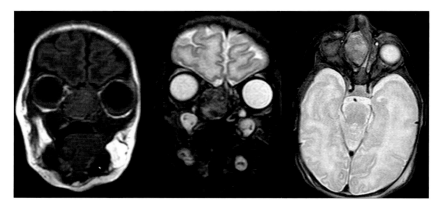

Fig. 2.2

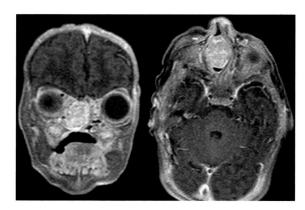

Fig. 2.3

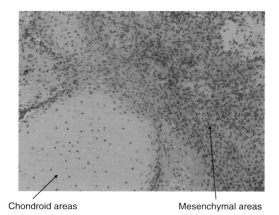

Chondroid areas   Mesenchymal areas

Fig. 2.4

A 3-day-old neonate develops cyanosis during feeding. MRI reveals a large mass in the sinonasal region, calcifications, and erosion of adjacent bony structures.

Comments

Nasal chondromesenchymal hamartoma is very rare and benign ossifying fibromyxoid tumor, and it most commonly presents during infancy as a congenital condition, although it may present later in childhood. It is must be distinguished from other masses such as a dermoid teratoma, nasal glioma, and estheseioneuroblastoma as well as other chondroid, angiomatous, or lipomatous hamartomas. A hamartoma is a tumor-like formation that originates from excessive growth of tissues native to the site of origin, unlike a teratoma known to be caused by excessive growth of pleuripotential cells foreign to the site of origin. Additional presenting symptoms of nasal chondromesenchymal hamartomas include deficits or impairment of eye movement (unilaterally), asymmetry of the face, asymmetric maxillary swelling, difficulty or inability to breathe nasally, and protruding nasal polyps.

Histologically, a chondromesenchymal hamartoma consists of proliferative lobules of cartilage with contiguous spindle cells and myxoid areas of mesenchymal tissue, as well as extensive RER and Golgi complexes and microfilamentous bundles within the cells.

Treatment typically involves complete resection of the aberrant tissue. In this case, a septoplasty and right middle turbinectomy were also performed. Recurrence is common after an incomplete resection, but the tumor typically remains as a microscopic residual tumor. No adjuvant therapy is necessary.

Image Findings

Axial, sagittal, and coronal CT images show irregular broad-based mass located in the anterior and medial nasal fossa on the right with multiple calcifications, mass effect to the surrounding structures, and deviating the nasal septum to the left (Fig. 2.1a–c). Coronal T1-weighted and coronal and axial Fat Sat (FS) T2-weighted MR images demonstrate the mass being iso- to hypointense in a T1-weighted MR image and slightly hyperintense in a T2-weighted image with well-defined margins and calcifications better defined on CT. No apparent extension to the brain or orbits (Fig. 2.2a–c). T1-weighted FS coronal and axial images with contrast show homogeneous and intense contrast enhancement with adequate border delineation of the lesion without intracranial or intraconal extension (Fig. 2.3a, b). Biopsy specimen pathology slide confirmed the diagnosis (Fig. 2.4).

Figure 2.1
Figure 2.2
Figure 2.3
Figure 2.4

Acknowledgment   Acknowledgment to Dr. Raj Palani for their help on the preparation of this case.

Case 2.2
Pleomorphic Xanthoastrocytoma
■
Francisco Menor Serrano and María Jesús Esteban Ricós

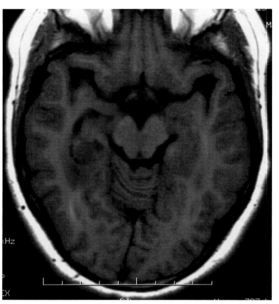

Fig. 2.5

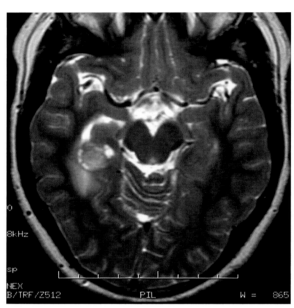

Fig. 2.6

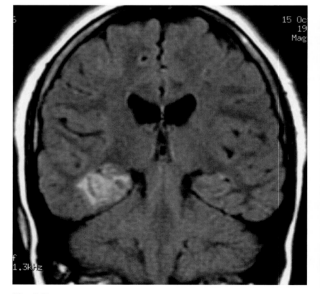

Fig. 2.7

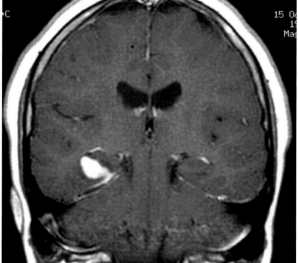

Fig. 2.8

An 11-year-old boy presents with sudden-onset focal left arm seizure.

Pleomorphic xanthoastrocytoma (PXA) is a rare, superficially located tumor arising from subpial astrocytes and often showing extensive involvement of the leptomeninges. Kepes et al. coined the term PXA to describe this tumor in 1979 and it was added to the WHO classification in 1993 as a grade II tumor. PXA is associated with a higher frequency of recurrence, anaplastic transformation, and death in comparison with other low-grade gliomas. Extent of primary resection is a significant factor in the prediction of recurrence-free survival. Response to chemo- and radiotherapy is uncertain. Isolated cases with widespread neuro-axis dissemination at diagnosis and some observations of PXA forming part of both ganglioglioma and dysembryoplastic neuroepithelial tumor have been reported. PXA is rarely diagnosed in infants, being discovered most commonly in adolescents and young adults. The most common single location of PXA is the temporal lobe (50%) and affected patients commonly present with seizures. PXA is uncommon in the basal ganglia, cerebellum, and spinal cord.

The classical, although nonspecific, appearance of PXA is a well-circumscribed superficial temporal solid-cystic mass. Solid components usually exhibit iso-attenuation in relation to gray matter on CT, iso or slightly hypo-intensity on T1-weighted images, iso or mildly hyper-intensity on T2-weighted images, and hyperintensity on FLAIR images and significant contrast enhancement. Calcification is variable and hemorrhage is rare. Large or small cysts are present in about 50% of cases. Surrounding vasogenic edema is usually minimal or absent. Leptomeningeal contrast enhancement is a distinctive finding, seen in more than two thirds of MRI studies.

Axial SE T1-weighted (Fig. 2.5) and T2-weighted MR images (Fig. 2.6) show a right, predominantly solid temporal lobe mass with small peripheral cysts surrounded by edema. The solid component is slightly hypointense on T1-weighted MRI and mildly hyperintense on T2-weighted MR images compared to gray matter. On coronal FLAIR MR images, the tumor exhibits greater hyperintensity, being difficult to make it out from surrounding vasogenic edema; note the small peripheral cysts being hyperintense in comparison to the ventricles (Fig. 2.7). Coronal post-contrast image demonstrates intense contrast enhancement of both the solid tumoral component and adjacent leptomeninges (Fig. 2.8. Reprinted with permission of Editorial Médica Panamericana; Menor F. Imagen en Oncología 2009).

Figure 2.5
Figure 2.6
Figure 2.7
Figure 2.8

Case 2.3
Desmoplastic Infantile Ganglioglioma
■
María I. Martínez León

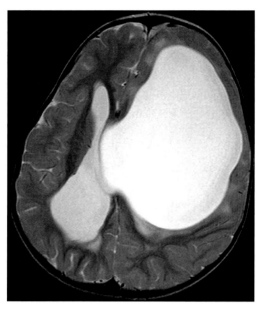

Fig. 2.9

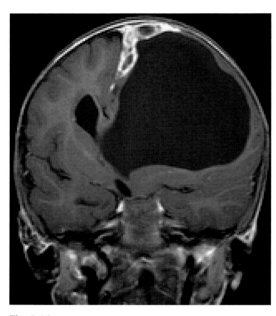

Fig. 2.10

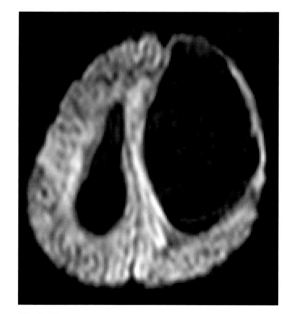

Fig. 2.11

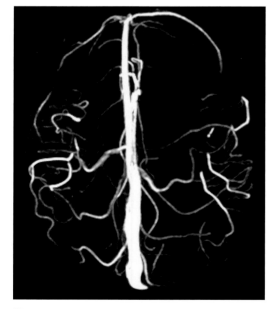

Fig. 2.12

A 27-month-old boy presents with a single epileptic seizure episode. On physical examination, the infant had a protruding forehead on the left side.

Desmoplastic Infantile Ganglioglioma (DIG) is a rare, benign intracranial neoplasm of early childhood with involvement of the superficial cerebral cortex and leptomeninges. They are usually large, predominantly cystic tumors located in the frontal or parietal lobes. DIGs are classified as a benign WHO grade I tumor of infancy and consist of an uncommon variety of ganglioglioma that occur exclusively in infants. Seizures are the most common clinical symptom. Also, a rapidly enlarging head size may be seen.

With CT, a heterogeneous mass containing both a solid and cystic component is identified. With MR T1-weighted imaging, the solid portion of the tumor is isointense relative to normal brain parenchyma and demonstrates significant contrast enhancement. The cystic component has a low signal intensity on T1-weighted MR images and a high signal intensity on T2-weighted MR images. MR spectroscopy shows a lower NAA/creatine ratio, a higher choline/creatine ratio, and no significant change in myoinositol/creatinine ratio. This study may aid in narrowing down the diagnosis.

The differential diagnoses, based on the neuroimaging findings, are primarily, cystic supratentorial astrocytomas, and secondly, high-grade astrocytomas, PNETs, and ependymomas. If the leptomeningeal component of the tumor is large, meningioma and meningeal sarcoma are other possible considerations.

Total resection of the tumor may be curative, eliminating the need for chemotherapy or radiation.

Axial T2-weighted MR image revealed a large supratentorial, predominantly cystic tumor in the left cerebral hemisphere, displacing midline structures to the right. Additionally, the left lateral ventricle is effaced and displaced (Fig. 2.9). Coronal T1-weighted MR image with contrast shows a large cystic component with strong enhancement of a solid mural portion. Contrast enhancement is not seen in the walls of the cyst and the solid component is widely attached to the dura (arrow) (Fig. 2.10). MR diffusion-weighted imaging shows no restriction of the solid or cystic components (Fig. 2.11). MR venography was done before surgical intervention to highlight the absence of longitudinal superior sinus involvement (Fig. 2.12). Tumor was completely resected with surgery and the histological diagnosis was DIG. No recurrence was documented on follow-up examinations.

Figure 2.9
Figure 2.10
Figure 2.11
Figure 2.12

Case 2.4

Dysembryoplastic Neuroepithelial Tumor of the Septum Pellucidum (DNET SP)

■

María I. Martínez León and Bernardo Weil Lara

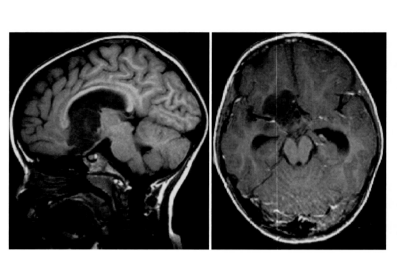

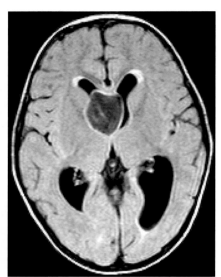

Fig. 2.13

Fig. 2.14

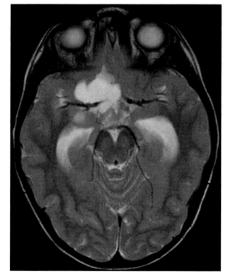

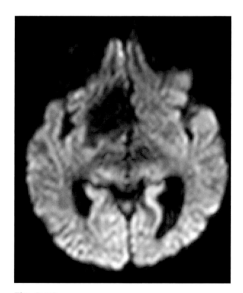

Fig. 2.15

Fig. 2.16

A 3-year-old girl presents with headache.

DNET SP are low-grade neoplasms arising at the midline, in the region of the septum pellucidum, with many of the histological features of the DNET. Imaging shows tumors extending into the lateral ventricles from the septal region and obstructing the foramen of Monro causing varying degrees of hydrocephalus. The lesions are lobular, well-delineated, internally septated, hypointense to gray matter on T1-weighted MR images, and hyperintense on T2-weighted MR images. There is usually no mass effect nor is there edema. Diffusion is not restricted and ADC map is high (may be attributable to the presence of large extracellular spaces and their low cellularity). DNET SP is usually non-enhancing or shows only minimal peripheral contrast uptake.

This neoplasm presents with the histological features of DNET, including the "specific glioneuronal element," a histopathological hallmark characterized by axon bundles that form columns lined by small oligodendroglial-like cells.

First line of treatment is surgical resection and adjuvant chemotherapy or radiotherapy is not commonly needed.

On the basis of both neuroimaging and histopathology, DNET-like lesions should be considered as a differential diagnosis of midline, intraventricular tumors in children and young adults. Differentiating these tumors from more aggressive neoplasms is essential because of the benign evolution DNET SP.

There is a mass located in the anterior recesses of the third ventricle. Sagittal T1-weighted MR images without contrast and axial, T1-weighted MR images with contrast show its location with caudal extension to the suprachiasmatic recess and cranial extension to the intraventricular midline. Signal intensity is slightly increased in relation to CSF in T1-weighted MR images and there is no enhancement with contrast (Fig. 2.13 a, b). A slightly high signal similar to CSF can be appreciated on FLAIR sequences (Fig. 2.14), along with secondary ventricular dilatation due to obstruction of the foramen of Monro. T2-weighted MR image shows a signal similar to that of the CSF. Note that the vessels are encased by the tumor without alteration (Fig. 2.15). No restriction on DWI is identified (Fig. 2.16). According to the location, signal intensity, and behavioral pattern, the findings are indicative of DNET SP. There is histological confirmation of the radiological diagnosis.

Figure 2.13
Figure 2.14
Figure 2.15
Figure 2.16

Case 2.5
CNS Langerhans Cell Histiocytosis
■
Diego Alcaide Martín and María I. Martínez León

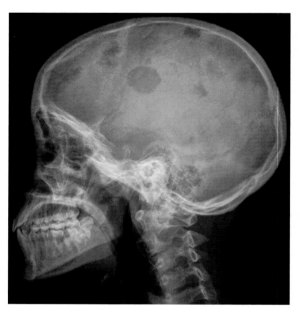

Fig. 2.17

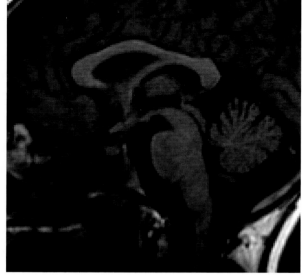

Fig. 2.18

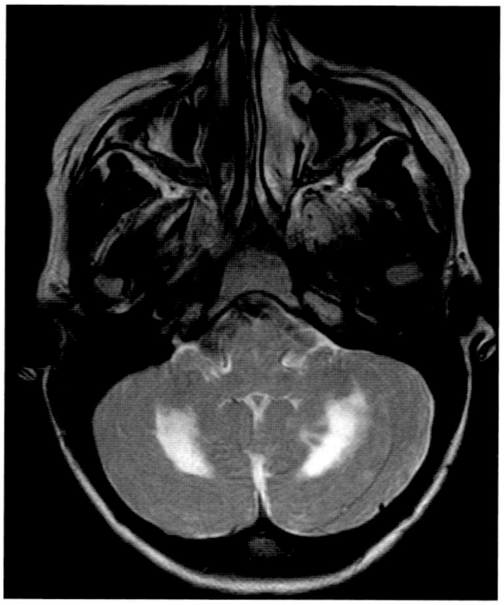

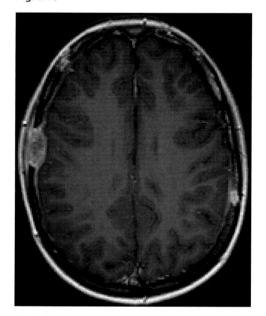

Fig. 2.19

Fig. 2.20

A 15-year-old patient was sent to the endocrinology department for assessment of diabetes insipidus.

Langerhans cell histiocytosis (LCH) is a rare condition that especially affects children and displays a wide variety of clinical manifestations. The most common features are bone lesions. There is limited knowledge about extra-osseous affectations of LCH. Examples of targeted systems include skin (55%) and the CNS (35%).

Approximately 25–35% of children with LCH, especially those who show multisystem manifestations, have CNS involvement. Two patterns have been described: granuloma formation and degenerative changes.

Granulomas can develop anywhere in the CNS, the most frequent location being the hypothalamic–hypophysary axis. MRI shows a loss of normal T1 signal from the neurohypophysis due to a decrease in storage of vasopressin, which leads to diabetes insipidus, a distinctive characteristic of the condition. MRI also displays an abnormal thickening and increased contrast enhancement of the hypophysis due to histiocytic infiltration.

Degenerative changes tend to occur in the cerebellum, especially in the dentate nuclei in a bilateral, symmetrical manner. Less often, the basal ganglia and brainstem are affected. These lesions cause inflammatory diffuse axonal damage, which leads to demyelination and, ultimately, atrophy. MRI shows hypointense lesions in T1-weighted MR images and iso or hyperintense lesions in T2-weighted MR images, which enhance with contrast proportionally to their degree of activity.

Lateral radiographs of the skull show multiple geographic lytic lesions of the bone with well-defined, non-sclerosed margins (Fig. 2.17). The MR T1-weighted image shows loss of the normal high signal from the neurohypophysis (Fig. 2.18). Bilateral, symmetric lesions of the white matter that are hypointense in T1-weighted images (not shown) and hyperintense in T2-weighted images characterize the cerebellar involvement (Fig. 2.19). After administering contrast, the hypophysis shows a normal uptake (not seen here) and the lytic lesions show a significant enhancement (Fig. 2.20). On the other hand, the cerebellar lesions do not present contrast uptake, which signifies demyelination and gliosis.

Figure 2.17
Figure 2.18
Figure 2.19
Figure 2.20

Case 2.6

Hemangioma of Infancy

■

Cristina Bravo Bravo and Pascual García-Herrera Taillefer

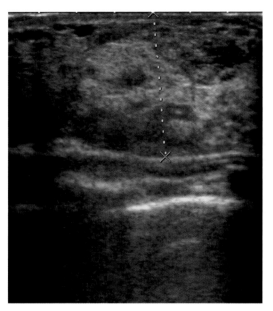

Fig. 2.21

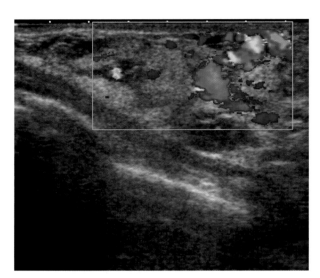

Fig. 2.22

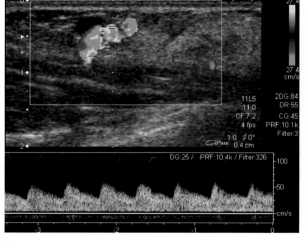

Fig. 2.23

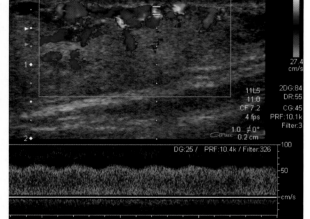

Fig. 2.24

A 2-month-old girl presents with a rapidly growing bluish tumor on the right mammary gland that had appeared at approximately 2–3 weeks of age.

Hemangiomas are the most common soft-tissue tumors of infancy. They are usually absent at birth and appear between the second and sixth week of life. Hemangiomas show a characteristic clinical evolution: a phase of rapid proliferation (3–9 months) followed by a period of relative stability and finally, a phase of slow involution (18 months up to 10 years of age). Most are diagnosed clinically and do not require further diagnostic studies or treatment. The GLU-T1 immunohistochemical marker serves to differentiate the hemangioma of infancy from congenital hemangiomas and vascular malformations. Ultrasound and MRI are indicated in atypical cases and in lesions that are large in size in order to evaluate the extent of compromise and its relation with neighboring structures. Furthermore, imaging may aid in assessing associated abnormalities such as lumbar hemangiomas, spinal dysraphisms, segmented facial hemangiomas, PHACE syndrome, multiple cutaneous hemangiomas, and diffuse neonatal hemangiomatosis.

Sonographically, these tumors are well-delineated, lobulated, and show variable echogenicity. On gray scale, US vascular structures are not usually identified; although, on occasion, peripheral supplying arteries can be seen. Doppler US reveals high vessel density with high systolic arterial velocities and a low resistance pattern. There is little or no evidence of arteriovenous shunting, and veins show a monophasic pattern. Diagnostic criteria for hemangiomas of infancy include the presence of five or more blood vessels by square centimeters of area and displacement of the systolic frequency by 2 kHz or more. During the involutive phase, the size of the lesion and the number of vessels decrease, but arterial velocities remain unchanged.

Possible differential diagnoses include vascular malformations and other soft-tissue tumors. If a lesion does not meet the diagnostic criteria for hemangioma, a biopsy must be taken.

Ultrasound shows a predominantly echogenic mass with heterogeneous echo-structure and peripheral blood vessels (Fig. 2.21). Color Doppler shows a high vessel density with occasional areas of turbulent blood flow (Fig. 2.22). Spectral Doppler (Fig. 2.23) displays a low-resistance vascular pattern with high systolic velocities and a pulsatile venous flow due to small arteriovenous fistulas (Fig. 2.24). These findings are consistent with a hemangioma of infancy in a proliferative phase.

Figure 2.21
Figure 2.22
Figure 2.23
Figure 2.24

Case 2.7
Vascular Lesion of the Face

Sara M. Koenig and Juan E. Gutiérrez

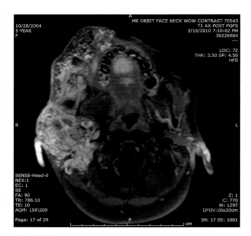

Fig. 2.26

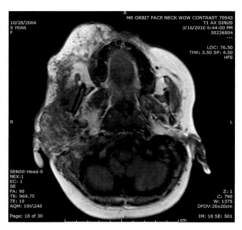

Fig. 2.25

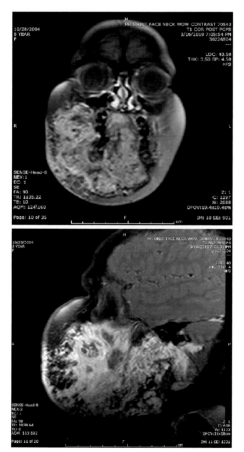

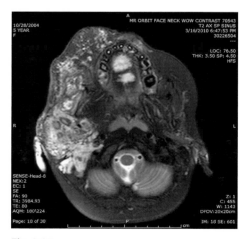

Fig. 2.27

Fig. 2.28

A 5-year-old female presents with a left-sided facial vascular malformation and history of prior surgical interventions.

Capillary hemangiomas and venous malformations are each typically benign lesions of vascular channels. Hemangiomas are benign endothelial cell neoplasms that commonly occur in children, especially under the age of 12 months. A red-colored lesion with a lobulated appearance appears on the skin, from which rapid growth may occur within the first 12 months of life. Angiography reveals a capillary lesion with well-demarcated dense opacification throughout, and with substantial blood flow arising from dilated arteries and dilated venous drainage. These benign lesions are typically harmless and only pose a cosmetic defect that typically stabilizes within a year of age and, in some cases, regress within a few years. In some circumstances, hemangiomas may cause functional impairment that requires aggressive treatment. Functional impairments may include impairment of vision development, feeding patterns, or language due to location on the eyelid, lips, or inside the mouth. Other defects may include hemorrhage or airway defects due to obstruction. Treatment typically consists of surgical resection, laser coagulation, or embolization, whereas endovascular interventions are only used in extreme cases that involve thrombocytopenia and bleeding diathesis.

Arteriovenous malformations vary from hemangiomas in that they are a benign growth of vascular channels with little and poorly dermarcated opacification during angiography. Direct percutenous injection of contrast typically optimizes opacification for imaging. Arteriovenous and venous malformations are typically treated conservatively, although complications such as hemorrhage, infiltration, or osseous involvement may require surgical resection or endovascular treatments.

Axial unenhanced T1-w (Fig. 2.25), enhanced T1-w (Fig. 2.26), axial T2-w (Fig. 2.27) and coronal and sagittal T2-w (Fig. 2.28) MR images exhibit the large, complex lesion with cystic components and avid enhancement involving the right side of the face (and posterolateral aspect of the neck ending at the right posterior triangle of the neck). This mass involves the oral cavity, masticator compartment, parotid space, and submental regions. The imaging characteristics of this lesion are compatible with a large venous malformation.

Figure 2.25
Figure 2.26
Figure 2.27
Figure 2.28

Case 2.8
Retinoblastoma

Juan E. Gutiérrez and Sara M. Koenig

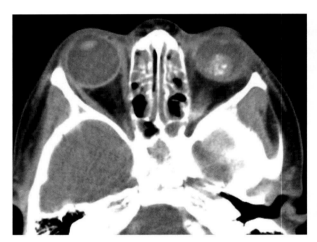

Fig. 2.29

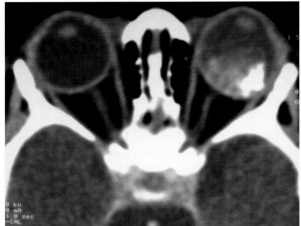

Fig. 2.30

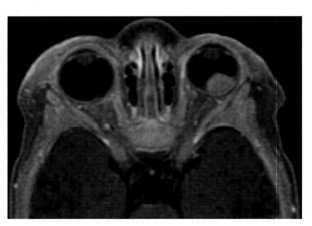

Fig. 2.31

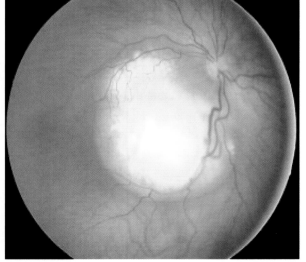

Fig. 2.32

A 14-month old male presents with an abnormal fundoscopic exam. His mother has a history of bilateral retinoblastoma. Calcifications appear in the soft tissue of the left eye.

Retinoblastoma (RB) is the most common intraocular malignancy in children. Of all retinoblastoma cases 70–80% are in infants less than 2 years old, and these tumors arise from retinal tissue. The most common presentation of retinoblastoma is leukocoria in early childhood, or a whitening of the retina seen on fundoscopic exam.

The most common mutation associated with RB is in the RB1 tumor suppressor gene on chromosome 13 controlling progression of the cell cycle, and greater than 200 mutations have been found. Most cases are sporadic; however, 10% are heritable as an autosomal dominant disease. Hereditary RB is often bilateral (rather than unilateral), and among all cases of retinoblastoma approximately 30% are bilateral and 30% multifocal. "Trilateral RB" occurs in approximately 4–7% of individuals with bilateral retinoblastoma, where a small cell intracranial tumor concurrently develops. These individuals often present at an earlier age than those with unilateral or sporadic retinoblastoma, have a higher likelihood of hereditary retinoblastoma, may develop additional tumors in the pineal, suprasellar, or fourth ventricular regions, and have a poor prognosis.

Imaging studies triangle usually starts with US. On CT scan revealing a high-density mass with calcifications arising from the retina, although margins may vary from well delineated to very unclear. Calcification within these tumors is considered a primary factor in the radiological diagnosis of RB. Retinal detachment is often seen due to the local mass effect of the tumor, and extension of the tumor often follows the optic nerve or the lymphatics of the orbit. MRI should be used in patients with suspected intracranial spread of the tumor or with bilateral retinoblastoma, and increased attention should be given to areas mentioned above: the pineal, suprasellar, and fourth ventricular regions. MR images are more sensitive to the spread of the tumor along the optic nerve and, with contrast, illustrate a well-enhanced intraocular mass. Unenhanced T1-and T2-weighted MRI show a mass at approximately the same intensity as normal gray matter.

CT without and with contrast, show of the left orbit revealing retinal high density enhancing mass with calcifications (Figs. 2.29 and 2.30). MRI axial Fat-Sat post-contrast image reveals left retinal detachment due to a solid mass with homogenous enhancement (Fig. 2.31). Fundoscopic appearance of the lesion (Fig. 2.32).

Figure 2.29
Figure 2.30
Figure 2.31
Figure 2.32

Case 2.9
Tuberous Sclerosis
■

Ana Alonso Murciano and María I. Martínez León

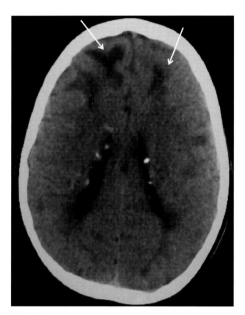

Fig. 2.33

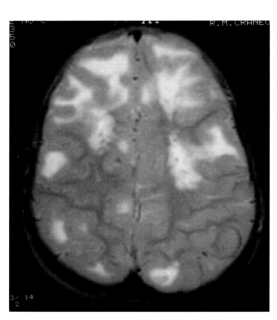

Fig. 2.34

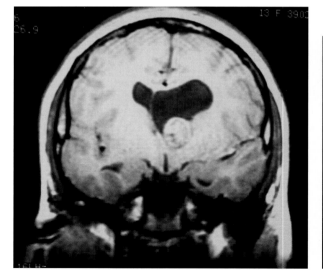

Fig. 2.35

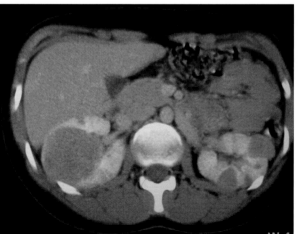

Fig. 2.36

Young boy presents with known congenital syndrome and uncontrolled seizures.

Tuberous Sclerosis (TS) is an autosomal dominant neurocutaneous syndrome characterized by the presence of benign congenital tumors in multiple organs. The diagnosis is usually established on the basis of major and minor diagnostic criteria applied to physical or radiological findings. The classical triad of epilepsy, mental retardation, and sebaceous adenoma is rare. TS is caused by a mutation of two tumor-suppressing genes known as TSC1 and TSC2. Mutation in TSC2 tends to result in a more severe form of the disease and a higher number of cortical tubers (CTs). Neurological involvement is seen in 95–100% of cases and includes CTs, subependymal nodules (SNs), subependymal giant-cell astrocytomas (SGCAs), and white matter abnormalities. Other common manifestations are renal angiomyolipomas (AMLs) (55–75% of cases) and cardiac rabdomyomas (50–65% of cases).

1. CTs are characterized by the presence of dysmorphic neurons and large astrocytes. Patients with more than six CTs present with a greater difficulty to control seizures.
2. SNs and SGCAs represent hamartomatous changes in subependymal tissue. SNs are frequently calcified. SGCAs are typically located in the foramen of Monro and have a benign course. Nevertheless, due to their location, they may cause obstructive hydrocephalus.
3. White matter alterations include superficial white matter abnormalities associated with cortical tubers, radial white matter bands, and cyst-like lesions.
4. Cardiac rabdomyomas are benign striated muscle tumors that are commonly located in the ventricular septum and may be single or multiple. Most of them do not cause clinical manifestations and spontaneous regression may occur.
5. AMLs are characterized by variable amounts of abnormal vessels and immature smooth-muscle and fat cells. In patients with TS, AMLs usually develops at a younger age and tends to be larger in size, bilateral, and multiple.

CT without contrast shows calcified subependymal nodules and frontal bilateral cortical tubers (arrows) (Fig. 2.33). Axial T2-weighted MR image depicts multiple cortical tubers and white matter abnormalities (Fig. 2.34). Coronal FLAIR MR image displays a left subependymal giant cell astrocytoma (Fig. 2.35). CT with contrast shows bilateral renal angiomyolipomas (Fig. 2.36).

Figure 2.33
Figure 2.34
Figure 2.35
Figure 2.36

Case 2.10
Neurofibromatosis Type 1
■

Inés Solís Muñiz

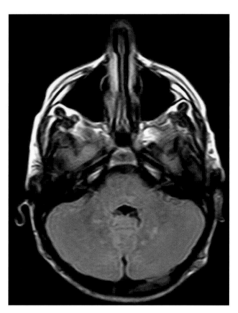

Fig. 2.37

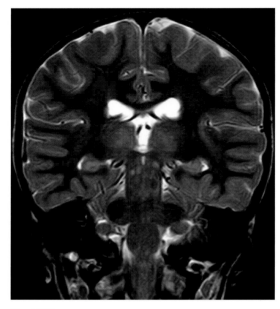

Fig. 2.38

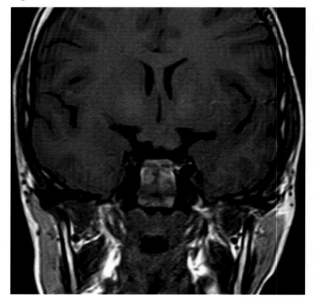

Fig. 2.39

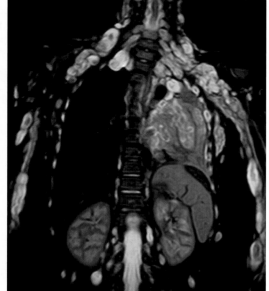

Fig. 2.40

A 12-year-old boy with known neurofibromatosis type 1 presents with multiple *café-au-lait* spots, visual disturbances, mild mental retardation, and scoliosis.

Neurofibromatosis type I (NF-1), formerly known as von Recklinghausen disease, is a relatively common (1/3,000 live births) autosomal dominant genetic disorder classified as a neurocutaneous syndrome or phakomatosis. Diagnosis is usually established in childhood based on a series of well-known major and minor criteria.

Apart from the dermatological manifestations of the condition (*café-au-lait* spots, axillary freckles, Lisch nodules of the iris), neurological abnormalities such as myelin vacuolization (40–90%), and optic tract (30%) and cerebral (1–3%) gliomas can also be identified. Dermal neurofibromas are seen in 90% of cases and plexiform neurofibromas in approximately 30% of patients. While neurofibromas are usually considered benign nerve-sheath tumors, the plexiform variation has shown malignant transformation in up to 10% of cases. Other abnormalities include bone dysplasia (5%) and scoliosis. Patients with NF-1 also have a higher risk of developing genetically related tumors such as rhabdomyosarcomas and neuroblastomas. Close monitoring is required due to their increased tendency to develop both benign and malignant neoplasms.

Imaging studies, specifically MRI, play an important role in the detection, extension assessment, and follow-up of the aforementioned neurological and non-neurological manifestations of the disease.

Surgical resection of symptomatic tumors is currently the first line of treatment.

Axial FLAIR (Fig. 2.37) and coronal T2-weighted (Fig. 2.38) MR images show multiple focal hyperintense lesions of the cerebellar white matter, brainstem, and bilateral thalami. No mass effect or contrast enhancement is observed. These findings are consistent with myelin vacuolization. Coronal T1-weighted MR image shows a predominantly left-sided volume increase of the optic chiasm consistent with glioma (Fig. 2.39). Coronal STIR MR image of the thorax and superior abdomen exhibits a large number of paravertebral, intercostal, and bilateral subcutaneous tumors. Additionally, a large mass can be seen on the left hemithorax with hyperintense lobulations and a central, target-like loss of signal, typical of neurofibromas (Fig. 2.40).

Figure 2.37
Figure 2.38
Figure 2.39
Figure 2.40

Further Reading

Books

Barnes L, Eveson JW, Reichart P, Sidransky D (2005) World Health Organization Classification of Tumors: Pathology and genetics of head and neck tumors. Lyon, IARC. p 53

Barkovich AJ (2000) Pediatric neuroimaging, 3rd edn. Lippincott Williams & Wilkins, Philadelphia, pp 494–496

Barkovich AJ (2005) Intracraneal, orbital, and neck masses of childhood. In: Pediatric neuroimaging, 4th ed. Lippincott Williams & Wilkins, Philadelphia, pp 506–658

Barkovich AJ (2005b) Pediatric Neuroimaging. Lippincott Williams & Wilkins, Philadeplphia

Barkovich AJ (2005c) Pediatric neuroimaging, 4th edn. Lippincott William & Wilkins, Philadelphia, pp 440–459

Groosman and Yousem. Neurorradiología. Ed. Marban 2007

Gutiérrez JE, Restrepo R, Soto JA (eds) (2004) Radiology and diagnostic imaging, 2nd ed, CIB Collection

Louis DN, Oggki H, Wiestler OD, et al (eds) (2007) World Health Organization Classification of tumours. Pathology and genetics of tumours of the nervous system. IARC, Lyon

Scott A (2004) Magnetic resonance imaging of the brain and spine, 3rd edn. Lippincott Williams & Wilkins, Philadelphia, pp 1340–1342

Siegel MJ (2004) Masas de partes blandas. In: Siegel MJ (ed) Ecografía Pediátrica, 2nd ed. pp 651–652

Web Links

http://www.childrenshospital.org/az/Site979/mainpageS979P0.html

http://www.searchmedica.com/search.html?q=pleomorphic%20xanthoastrocytoma

www.radiographics.org

http://journals.lww.com/ajsp/pages/default.aspx

http://scielo.isciii.es/scielo.php

www.issva.org (International Society for the Study of Vascular Anomalies)

http://www.mayoclinic.org/intracranial-venous-malformations/

http://www.cancer.gov/cancertopics/types/retinoblastoma. Retinoblastoma. United States National Cancer Institute

www.tuberous-sclerosis.org

http://emedicine.medscape.com/article/950151-overview

Articles

Alexiou GA, Stefanaki K, Sfakianos G, Prodromou N (2008) Desmoplastic infantile ganglioglioma: a report of 2 cases and a review of the literature. Pediatr Neurosurg 44(5):422–425

Alkan A, Sigirci A, Kutlu R et al (2005) Neurofibromatosis type 1: diffusion weighted imaging findings of brain. Eur J Radiol 56:229–234

Aoki S, Barkovich JA, Nishimura K et al (1989) Neurofibromatosis types 1 and 2: Cranial MR findings. Radiology 172:527–534

Bächli H, Avoledo P, Gratzl O, Tolnay M (2003) Therapeutic strategies and management of desmoplastic infantile ganglioglioma: two case reports and literature overview. Chikds Nerv Syst 19(5-.6):359–366

Bagley LJ, Hurst RW, Zimmerman RA, Shields JA, Shields CL, Potter P (2002) Imaging in the trilateral retinoblastoma syndrome. Pediatr Neurol 38(2):166–170

Baisden BL, Brat DJ, Mekhem ER, Rosenblum MK, King AP, Burger PC (2001) Dysembryoplastic neuroepithelial tumor-like neoplasm of the septum pellucidum: a lesion often misdiagnosed as glioma. Report of ten cases. Am J Surg Pathol 25:494–499

Balaji R, Ramachandran K (2009) Imaging of desmoplastic infantile ganglioglioma: a spectroscopic viewpoint. Childs Nerv Syst 25(4):497–501

Baron Y, Barkovich AJ (1999) MR imaging of tuberous sclerosis in neonates and young infants. AJNR 20:907–916

Bilginer B, Sÿlemezoglu F, Cila A, Akalan N (2009) Intraventricular dysembrioplastic neuroepithelial tumor-like neoplasm with disseminated spinal tumor. Turk Neurosurg 19:69–72

Biswas J, Mani B, Mahesh PS, Patwardhan D, Kumar KS, Badrinath SS (2000) Retinoblastoma in adults: report of three cases and review of the literature. Surv Opthalmol 44(5):409–414

Boukobza M, Enjolras O et al (1996) Cerebral developmental anomalies associated with head and neck venous malformations. Am J Neuroradiol 17:897–994

Brisse HJ et al (2001) Sonographic, CT, and MR imaging findings in diffuse infiltrative retinoblastoma: report of two cases with histologic comparison. Am J Neuroradiol 22:4 49–504

Brisse HJ et al (2007) Relevance of CT and MRI in retinoblastoma for the diagnosis of poastlaminar invasion with normal size optic nerve: a retrospective study of 150 patients with histological comparison. Pediatr Radiol 37:649–656

Brouwer PA et al (2009) Dynamic 320-section ct angiography in cranial arteriovenous shunting lesions. Am J Neuroradiol 31:767–770

Catalpete O, Marshall P, Smith TW (2009) Dysembryoplastic neuroepithelial tumor located in pericallosal and intraventricular area in a child. J Neurosurg Pediatr 3:456–460

Cervera-Pierot P, Varlet P, Chodkiewicz JP (1997) Daumas-DuportC. Dysembryoplastic neuroepithelial tumors located in the caudate nucleus area: report of four cases. Neurosurgery 40:1065–1070

Crespo-Rodríguez AM, Smirniotopoulos JG, Rushing EJ (2007) MR and CT imaging of 24 pleomorphic xanthoastrocytomas (PXA) and a review of the literature. Neuroradiology 49:307–315

Crino PB, Nathanson KL, Henske EP (2006) The tuberous sclerosis complex. N Engl J Med 355:1345–1356

Dariusch H et al (2008) Cerebral arteriovenous malformation: Spetzler–Martin classification at subsecond temporal-resolution four-dimensional MR angiography compared with that of DSA. Radiology 246:205–213

DiMario FJ Jr (2004) Brain abnormalities in tuberous sclerosis complex. J Child Neurol 1989:650–657

DiPaolo DP, Zimmerman RA, Rorke LB, Zackai EH, Bilaniuk LT, Yachnis AT (1995) Neurofibromatosis type 1: pathological substrate of high-signal intensity foci in the brain. Radiology 195:721–724

Donnelly LF, Adams DM, Bisset GS (2000) Vascular malformation and hemangiomas: a practical approach in a multidisciplinary clinic. AJR 174:597–608

Drolet BA, Esterly NB, Frieden IJ (1999) Hemangiomas in children. N Engl J Med 341:1173–1181

Dubois J, Garel L (1999) Imaging and therapeutic approach of hemangiomas and vascular malformations in the pediatric age group. Pediatr Radiol 29:879–893

Dubois J et al (1998) Soft-tissue hemangiomas in infants and children: diagnosis using Doppler sonography. AJR 171:247–252

Dubois J, Garel L, David M, Powell J (2002) Vascular soft-tissue tumors in infancy: distinguishing features on Doppler sonography. AJR 178:1541–1545

Dunnick NR (2000) The radiological Society of North America 85th scientific assembly and annual meeting: image interpretation session: 1999. Radiographics 20:257–278

Evans JC, Curtis J (2000) The radiological appearances of tuberous sclerosis. Br J Radiol 73:91–98

Finelli DA, Shurin SB, Bardenstein DS (1995) Trilateral retinoblastoma: two variations. Am J Neuroradiol 16:166–170

Finistis S et al (2009) Nasal Chondromesenchymal hamartoma in a child. Cardiovasc Intervent Radiol 32:593–597

Fishman SJ, Mulliken JB (1993) Hemangiomas and vascular malformations of infancy and childhood. Pediatr Clin N Am 40(6):1177–1200

Fordham LA, Chung CJ, Donelly LF (2000) Imaging of congenital vascular and lymphatic anomalies of the head and neck. Neuroimaging Clin N Am 10:117–136

Fortman BJ, Kuszyk BS, Urban BA (2001) Neurofibromatosis type 1: a diagnostic mimicker at CT. Radiographics 21:601–612

Fujisawa H, Marukawa K, Hasegawa M, Tohma Y, Hayashi Y, Uchiyama N (2002) Genetic differences between neurocytoma and dysembryoplastic neuroepithelial tumor and oligodendroglial tumors. J Neurosurg 97:1350–1355

Galluzzi P, Hadjistilianou T et al (2009) Is CT still useful in the study protocol of retinoblastoma? Am J Neuroradiol 30:1760–1765

Ganesan K, Desai Sm, Udwadia-Hegde A (2006) Non-infantile variant of desmoplastic ganglioglioma: a report of 2 cases. Pediatr Radiol 36(6):541–545

Geibprasert S et al (2010) Radiologic assessment of brain arteriovenous malformations: what clinicians need to know. Radiographics 30:483–501

Gorincour G, Kokta V, Rypens F, Garel J, Powell J, Dubois J (2005) Imaging characteristics of two subtypes of congenital hemangiomas: rapidly involuting congenital hemangiomas and non-involuting congenital hemangiomas. Pediatr Radiol 35:1178–1185

Goyal CM, Armstrong D (2002) Venous vascular malformations in pediatric patients: comparison of results of alcohol sclerotherapy with proposed MR imaging classification. Radiology 223:639–644

Grois N, Prayer D, Prosch H, Minkov M, Potschger U, Gadner H (2004) Course and clinical impact of magnetic resonance imaging findings in diabetes insipidus associated with Langerhans cell histiocytosis. Pediatr Blood Cancer 43:59–65

Grois N, Prayer D, Prosch H, Lassmann H (2005) Neuropathology of CNS disease in Langerhans cell histiocytosis. CNS LCH Co-operative Group. Brain 128:829–838

Guesmi H, Houtteville JP, Courthéoux P, Derlon JM, Chapon F (1999) Dysembryoplastic neuroepithelial tumors. Report of 8 cases including two with unusual localization. Neurochirurgie 45:190–200

Harter DH, Omeis I, Forman S, Braun A (2006) Endoscopic resection of an intraventricular dysembryoplastic neuroepithelial tumor of the septum pellucidum. Pediatr Neurosurg 42:105–107

Hoving EW, Kros JM, Groninger E, den Dunnen WF (2008) Desmoplastic infantile ganglioglioma with a malignant course. J Neurosurg Pediatr 1(1):95–98

Hoyosa M, Naito H, Nihei K (1999) Neurological prognosis correlated with variations over time in the number of subependymal nodules in tuberous sclerosis. Brain Dev 21:544–547

Hsueh C, Hsueh S, Crussi FG et al (2001) Nasal chondomesenchymal hamartoma in children. Arch Pathol Lab Med 125(3):400–403

Ishizawa K, Terao S, Kobayashi K, Yoshida K, Hirose T (2007) A neuroepithelial tumor showing combined histological features of dysembryoplastic neuroepithelial tumor and pleomorphic xanthoastrocytoma – a case report and review of the literature. Clin Neuropathol 26:169–175

James SH, Halliday WC, Branson HM (2010) Trilateral retinoblastoma. Radiographics 30:833–837

Johnson C et al (2006) Nasal chondromesenchymal hamartoma: radiographic and histopathologic analysis of a rare pediatric tumor. Pediatr Radiol 37:101–104

Kang Jun, Young Ok Hong, Gung Hwan Ahn, Young Min Kim, Hee Jeong Cha, Hye-Jeong Choi (2007) Nasal chondromesenchymal hamartoma: a case report. Korean J Path 41:258–62

Kato K, Reiko I, Yukichi T, Masamichi H, Kennichi S (Jan 2002) Nasal chondromesenchymal hamartoma of infancy: the first Japanese case report. Pathol Int 49(8):731–736

Kepes JJ, Rubinstein LJ, Eng LF (1979) Pleomorphic xanthoastrocytoma: a distinctive meningocerebral glioma of young subjects with relatively favorable prognosis. A study of 12 cases. Cancer 44:1839–1852

Kim EY, Choi JU, Kim TS, Kim DI, Kim KY (1995) Huge Langerhans cell histiocytosis granuloma of choroids plexus in a child with Hand-Schüller-Christian disease. J Neurosurg 83:1080–1084

Kim B, Park SH, Min HS, Rhee JS, Wang KC (2004) Nasal chondromesenchymal hamartoma of infancy clinically mimicking meningoencephalocele. Pediatr Neurosurg 40(3):136–140

Kim JE et al (2009) Nasal chondromesenchymal hamartoma: CT and MR imaging findings. Korean J Radiol 10(4):216–419

Koeller KK, Henry JM (2001) From the archives of the AFIP: superficial gliomas: radiologic-pathologic correlation. Radiographics 21:1533–1556

Lee BB, Bergan JJ (2002) Advanced management fo congenital vascular malformations: a multidisciplinary approach. Cardiovasc Surg 10(6):523–533

Legiehn GM, Heran MK (2009) Venous malformations: classification, development, diagnosis, and interventional radiologic management. Radiol Clin N Am 46:545–597

Ak L, Robson WL (2007) Tuberous sclerosis complex: a review. J Pediatr Health Care 21:108–114

Lellouch-Tubiana KS, Kulkarni AV A, Sainte-Rose C (2006) Pleomorphic xanthoastrocytoma of the cerebellopontine angle in a child. Childs Nerv Syst 22:1479–1482

Levy AD, Patel N, Dow N, Abbott RM, Miettinen M, Sobin LH (2005) From the Archives of the AFIP. Abdominal neoplasms in patients with neurofibromatosis type 1: radiologic-pathologic correlation. RadioGraphics 25:455–480

Lopes Ferraz Filho JR, Munis MP, Soares Souza A, Sanches RA, Goloni-Bertollo EM, Pavarino-Bertelli EC (2008) Unidentified bright objects on brain MRI in children as a diagnostic criterion for neurofibromatosis type 1. Pediatr Radiol 38:305–310

Maghnie M, Aricò M, Villa A, Genovese E, Beluffi G, Severi F (1992) MR of the hypothalamic-pituitary axis in Langerhans cell histiocytosis. AJNR 13:1365–1371

Maher CO, White JB, Scheithauer BW, Raffel C (2008) Recurrence of dysembryoplastic neuroepithelial tumor following resection. Pediatr Neurosurg 44:333–336

Marton E, Feletti A, Orvieto E, Longatti P (2007) Malignant progression in pleomorphic xanthoastrocytoma: personal experience and review of the literature. J Neurol Sci 252:144–153

Mautner VF, Hartmann M, Kluwe L, Friedrich RE, Fünsterer C (2006) MRI growth pattern of plexiform neurofibromas in patients with neurofibromatosis type 1. Neuroradiology 48:160–165

McDermott MB, Bonder BT, Dehner LP (1998) Nasal chondromesenchymal hamartoma: an upper respiratory tract analogue of the chest wall mesenchymal hamartoma. Am J Surg Pathol 22(4):425–433

Menor F, Martí-Bonmatí L, Mulas F, Poyatos C, Cortina H (1992) Neuroimaging in tuberous sclerosis: a clinicoradiological evaluation in pediatric patients. Pediatric Radiol 22(7):485–489

Menor F, Marti-Bonmati L, Arana E, Poyatos C, Cortina H (1998) Neurofibromatosis type 1 in children: MR imaging and follow-up studies of central nervous system findings. Eur J Radiol 26:121–131

Metry DW, Hebert AA (2000) Benign cutaneous vascular tumors of infancy. when to worry, what to do. Arch Dermatol 136:905–914

Moon HH et al (1999) Craniofacial arteriovenous malformation: preoperative embolization with direct puncture and injrection of n-butyl cyanoacrylate. Radiology 211:661–666

Mulliken JB, Glowacki J (1982) Hemangiomas and vascular malformations in infants and children: a classification based on endothelial characteristics. Plasr Reconstr Surg 69:412–420

Murdo Sk Mc Jr, Moore SG, Brant-Zawadzki M, Berg BO, Koch T, Newton TH et al (1987) Mr imaging of intracranial tuberous sclerosis. AJR 148:791–796

Nakagawa T, Sakamoto T, Ito J (2009) Nasal chondromesenchymal hamartoma in an adolescent. Int J Pediatr Otorhinolaryngol 4:111–113

Narayanan V (2003) Tuberous sclerosis complex: genetics to pathogenesis. Pediatr Neurol 29:404–409

Norman ES, Bergman S, Trupiano JK (2004) Nasal chondromesenchymal hamartoma: report of a case and review of the literature. Pediatr Dev Pathol 7(5):517–520

Okazaki T, Kageji T, Matsuzaki K, Horiguchi H, Hirose T, Watanabe H et al (2009) Primary anaplastic pleomorphic xanthoastrocytoma with widespread neuroaxis dissemination at diagnosis – a pediatric case report and review of the literature. J Neurooncol 94:431–437

Passone E, Pizzolitto S, D'Agostini S, Skrap M, Gardiman MP, Nocerino A et al (2006) Non-anaplastic pleomorphic xantoastrocythoma with neuroradiological evidence of leptomeningeal dissemination. Childs Nerv Syst 22:614–618

Patiel HJ, Burrows PE, Kozakewich HP, Zurakowski D, Mulliken J (2000) Soft-tissue vascular anomalies: utility of US for diagnosis. Radiology 214:747–754

Petropoulou K, Whiteman ML, Altman NR, Bruce J, Morrison G (1995) CT and MR of pleomorphic xanthoastrocytoma: unusual biologic behavior. J Comput Assist Tomogr 19:860–865

Poe LB, Dubowy RL, Hochhauser L, Collins GH, Crosley CJ, Kanzer MD et al (1994) Demyelinating and gliotic cerebellar lesions in Langerhans cell histiocytosis. AJNR 15:1921–1928

Prayer D, Grois N, Prosch H, Gadner H, Barkovich AJ (2004) MR imaging presentation of intracranial disease associated with Langerhans cell histiocytosis. AJNR 25:880–891

Provenzale JM, Gururangan S, Klintworth G (2004) Trilateral retinoblastoma: clinical and radiologic progression. AJR 183:505–511

Robson CD (2010) Imaging of head and neck neoplasms in children. Pediatr Radiol 40:499–509

Rodjan F, Graaf P et al (2010) Brain abnormalities on MR imaging in patients with retinoblastoma. Am J Neuroradiol 31:237–245

Rosenfield NS, Abrahams J, Komp D (1990) Brain MRI in patients with Langerhans cell histiocytosis: findings and enhancement with Gd-DTPA. Pediatr Radiol 20:433–436

Saito T, Sugiyama K, Yamasaki F, Tominaga A, Kusisu K, Takeshima Y (2008) Familial occurrence of dysembryoplastic neuroepithelial tumor-like neoplasm of the septum pellucidum: case report. Neurosurgery 63:370–372

Sevick RJ, Barkovich AJ, Edwards MS et al (1992) Evolution of white matter lesions in neurofibromatosis type 1: MR findings. AJR 159:171–175

Shin JH, Lee HK, Khang SK, Kim DW, Jeong AK, Ahn KJ et al (2002) Neuronal tumors of the central nervous system: radiologic findings and pathologic correlation. Radiographics 22:1177–1189

Smidt S, Eich G, Hanquinet S, Tschäppeler H, Waibel P, Gudinchet F (2004) Extra-osseous involvement of Langerhans' cell histiocytosis in children. Pediatr Radiol 34:313–321

Smidt S, Eich G, Geoffray A, Hanquinet S, Waibel P, Wolf R et al (2008) Extraosseus Langerhans cell histiocytosis in children. Radiographics 28:707–726

Spence J, Krings T et al (2010) Percutaneous sclerotherapy for facial venous malformations: subjective clinical and objective MR imaging follow-up results. Am J Neuroradiology 31:955–960

Strottmann JM, Ginsberg LE, Stanton C (1995) Langerhans cell histiocytosis involving the corpus callosum and cerebellum: gadolinium-enhanced MRI. Neuroradiology 37:289–292

Sugita Y, Irie K, Ohshima K, Hitotsumatsu T, Sato O, Arimura K (2009) Pleomorphic xanthoastrocytoma as a component of temporal lobe cystic ganglioglioma: a case report. Brain Tumor Pathol 26:31–36

Takeshima H, Kawahara Y, Hirano H, Obara S, Niiro M, Kuratsu J (2003) Postoperative regression of desmoplastic infantile gangliogliomas: report of two cases. Neurosurgery 53(4):979–983

Tamburrini G, Colosimo C Jr, Giangaspero F, Riccardi R, Di Rocco C (2003) Desmoplastic infantile ganglioglioma. Childs Nerv Syst 19(5–6):292–297

Umeoka S, Koyama T, Miki Y, Akai M, Tsutsui K, Togashi K (2004) Pictorial review of tuberous sclerosis in various organs. Radiographics; Sept 4, on line

Yamasaki F, Kurisy K, Satoh K, Arita K, Sugiyama K, Ohtaki M (2005) Apparent diffusion coefficient of human brain tumors at MR imaging. Radiology 235:985–991

Zacharia TT, Jaramillo D, Poussaint TY, Korf B (2005) MR imaging of abdominopelvic involvement in neurofibromatosis type 1: a review of 43 patients. Pediatr Radiol 35:317–322

Non-tumoral Neurology

Contents

M.I. Martínez-León et al., *Learning Pediatric Imaging*, Learning Imaging,
DOI: 10.1007/978-3-642-16892-5_3, © Springer-Verlag Berlin Heidelberg 2011

Case 3.1

Acute Disseminated Encephalomyelitis
■
Elisa Cuartero Martínez and María I. Martínez León

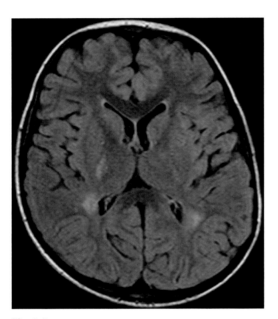

Fig. 3.1

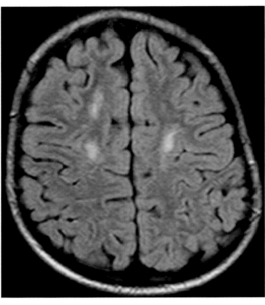

Fig. 3.2

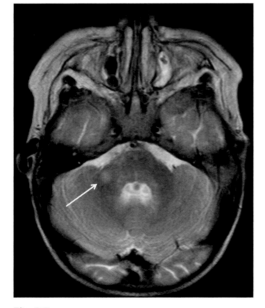

Fig. 3.3

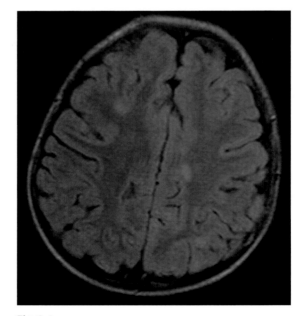

Fig. 3.4

Case 3.1a: A 3-year-old boy presents with fever and altered mental status that develops after a case of chickenpox.

Case 3.1b: A 2-year-old boy presents with fever and headache.

Case 3.1c: A 3-year-old boy presents with headache and 10-day history of nocturnal vomiting. Normal CT and CSF pressure are detected.

Acute disseminated encephalomyelitis (ADEM) is an autoimmune inflammatory and demyelinating disease of the CNS. Although the mechanism by which demyelination occurs is unclear, several theories have been suggested. In approximately 50–75% of cases, symptoms arise 4–15 days after an upper respiratory tract infection or after vaccination.

Comments

Clinically, multiple symptoms arise depending on the location of the CNS lesions. Occasionally, a prodromal period of fever, headache, nausea, vomiting, and altered mental status precede the remaining neurological manifestations. Although ADEM is typically monophasic, clinical recurrences occur in approximately 30% of cases and they develop more commonly in children under 10 years of age. Short- and long-term prognosis is usually favorable, yet in approximately 20% of patients neurologic sequelae persist.

T2-weighted and FLAIR MR images tend to show bilateral, irregular, ill-defined, and asymmetric lesions that are indicative of inflammation and demyelination of the subcortical white matter. A latency period of 2–35 days may exist between the onset of symptoms and the appearance of findings on MR.

The main differential diagnosis is multiple sclerosis, an aggressive, chronic illness with a poorer prognosis. An initial episode of multiple sclerosis can be almost indistinguishable from ADEM. Clinical, radiological, and serological CSF markers may be almost identical in both conditions. Treatment with corticosteroids and/or plasmapheresis is directed at suppressing the immune response toward the infectious agent or vaccine.

Case 3.1a: Axial FLAIR MR image shows hyperintense lesions on the posterior limb of the right interior capsule and the periventricular occipital white matter (Fig. 3.1). On a higher axial FLAIR MR image, hyperintense lesions of the bilateral semioval centers can be observed (Fig. 3.2).

Imaging Findings

Figure 3.1
Figure 3.2

Case 3.1b: Axial T2-weighted MR image displays a hyperintense lesion of the right cerebellar peduncle (arrow) (Fig. 3.3).

Figure 3.3 Case 3.1c: Axial FLAIR MR image exhibits hyperintense lesions of the cortico-subcortical white matter (Fig. 3.4).

Figure 3.4

Case 3.2
Multiple Sclerosis
■

Beatriz Asenjo García

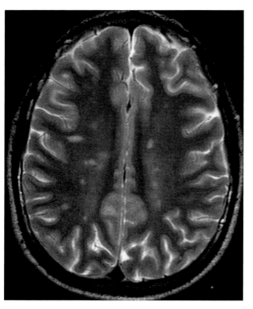

Fig. 3.5

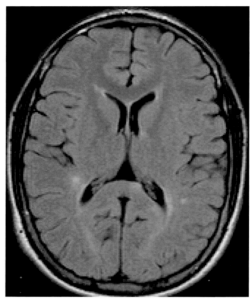

Fig. 3.6

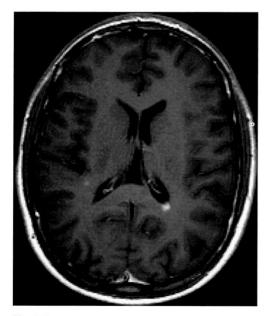

Fig. 3.7

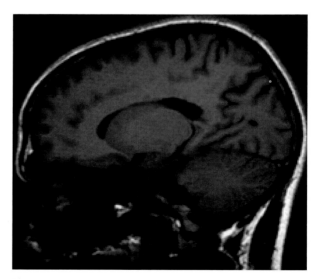

Fig. 3.8

A 13-year-old boy presents with paresthesia of the left side of the body.

Multiple sclerosis (MS) is a condition that is generally considered to be autoimmune in nature. It usually presents during young adulthood and is infrequent during childhood. Two types of presentation have been described: infantile (children under the age of 10) and juvenile (patients 10–15 years of age). The infantile form of the disease is a relapsing–remitting subtype that tends to resolve at puberty. On the other hand, the juvenile form of MS is more aggressive, has frequent relapses and up to 16% presents a chronically progressive clinical evolution.

MS presents with a single symptom in more than 50% of cases. Optic neuritis, ataxia, and paresis are common clinical manifestations at diagnosis. During childhood, differential diagnoses include metabolic illnesses, leukodystrophies, and especially disseminated acute encephalitis.

A diagnosis of MS is based on a series of clinical, radiologic, and laboratory findings. T1- and T2-weighted MR images with and without contrast are the conventional sequences used to detect and monitor demyelinating lesions. The appearance of new lesions, the enlargement of preexisting ones, or the presence of contrast enhancement determine the level of activity of the condition. Moreover, the severity of MS is related to the volume of the lesions themselves and the degree of cerebral atrophy. The most common diagnostic laboratory tool is the analysis of oligoclonal IgG bands in cerebrospinal fluid.

Currently, corticosteroid treatment is used to resolve active clinical crises. Management of MS with interferon beta-1a appears to reduce the continued activity of the disease and lowers the incidence of recurrences in patients with the relapsing–remitting form of MS. Nevertheless, the use of this drug in the pediatric population has many restrictions.

Axial T2-weighted and FLAIR MR images show multiple hyperintense, well-defined lesions located in the bilateral semioval centers and in the periatrial white matter (Figs. 3.5 and 3.6). Two of the lesions have enhancement on the T1-weighted MR image with contrast (Fig. 3.7). The post contrast T1-weighted sagittal MR image shows numerous, non-enhancing, hypointense lesions on the corpus callosum, termed "black holes" (Fig. 3.8). The presence of these lesions is consistent with diffuse axonal damage and therefore helps to determine the degree of disability.

Figure 3.5
Figure 3.6
Figure 3.7
Figure 3.8

Case 3.3
Posterior Reversible Encephalopathy Syndrome
Miguel Angel López Pino

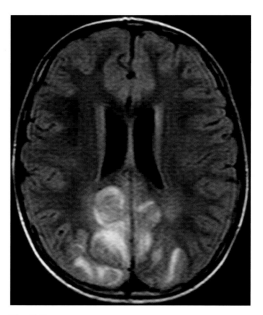

Fig. 3.9

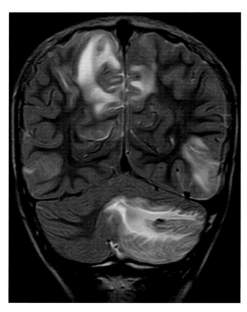

Fig. 3.10

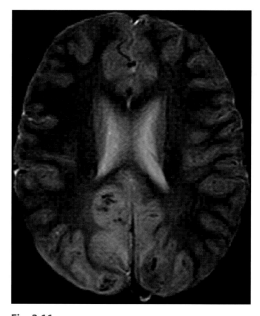

Fig. 3.11

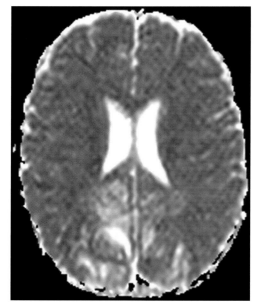

Fig. 3.12

A 5-year-old boy with a diagnosis of B-cell acute lymphocytic leukemia currently in chemotherapy presents with a partial seizure and a decreased level of consciousness. Upon examination, high blood pressure is detected.

Posterior reversible encephalopathy syndrome (PRES) is a clinical and radiologic entity that has received multiple names including posterior reversible leukoencephalopathy, posterior reversible edema syndrome, and hyperperfusion encephalopathy. None of these terms completely encompass the condition since it is not always reversible nor is it always located posteriorly.

Clinical manifestations include headache, visual disturbances, altered levels of consciousness, and epileptic seizures. A common cause is high blood pressure (HPB). Furthermore, an association has been described between chemotherapy (especially with cyclosporine A), bone marrow transplants, hematological diseases, eclampsia, autoimmune disorders, and the presence of PRES.

The pathogenesis consists of cerebral autoregulatory defects and endothelial damage that lead to a disturbance of the blood-brain barrier (BBB) with secondary leakage of fluid to the extracellular space. When HPB ensues, causing vasospasm, the posterior region on the brain becomes more vulnerable, given its poorer sympathetic innervation.

On MRI, T2-weighted and FLAIR images show a predominantly posterior, bilateral, hyperintense, cortico-subcortical signal with ADC elevation consistent with vasogenic edema. Cerebellar and brainstem involvement is not uncommon. Microhemorrhagic foci may be present and contrast enhancement is generally minimal or absent.

The clinical evolution of PRES is heterogeneous. Although usually benign, this condition is not always reversible and imaging findings may not normalize, especially in patients with comorbidities.

FLAIR MR image shows symmetric, bilateral, predominantly posterior (parietal and occipital) cortico-subcortical signal hyperintensity (Fig. 3.9). Cerebellar involvement with both white and gray matter lesions can also be observed (Fig. 3.10). Occasional low-signal foci consistent with hemosiderin from microhemorrhages can be seen on gradient-echo imaging (Fig. 3.11). Diffusion-weighted MR images do not show restriction and ADC maps depict an increased diffusion coefficient due to vasogenic edema (Fig. 3.12). No abnormal contrast enhancement is observed (not shown).

Figure 3.9
Figure 3.10
Figure 3.11
Figure 3.12

Case 3.4
Focal Cortical Dysplasia
■

Mercedes Bernabé Durán and María I. Martínez León

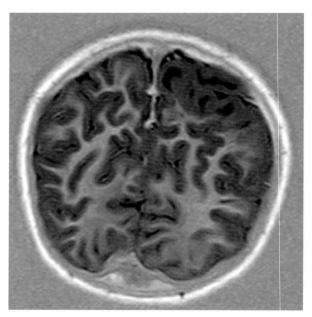

Fig. 3.13

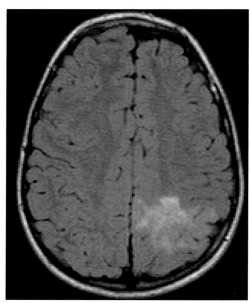

Fig. 3.14

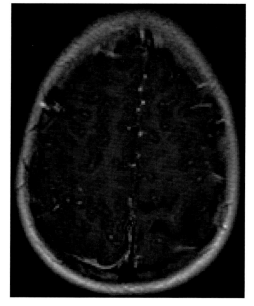

Fig. 3.15

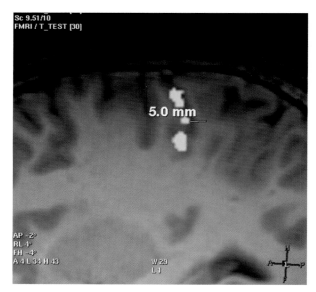

Fig. 3.16

A 10-year-old girl presents with long-term seizures unresponsive to treatment.

Focal Cortical Dysplasia (FCD) was first described by Taylor in 1971. FCD is a defect that occurs during the process of neuronal proliferation in early stages of brain development. The condition Taylor described is characterized by a destructurization of the cellular architecture of the cerebral cortex.

The main clinical manifestations of FCD are epileptic seizures that begin in the first decade of life and do not respond to medical treatment. This condition may or may not be accompanied by different degrees of mental retardation.

The ideal imaging study for diagnosis is MRI. FCD presents as a localized area of cortical thickening associated with lack of definition between white and gray matter. In addition, varying degrees of macrogyria and/or abnormal widening of sulci can also be identified. FCD signal is hyperintense in T1-weighted, T2-weighted, and FLAIR MRI sequences.

Patients may benefit from definitive surgical treatment aided by functional MRI studies that make the preservation of essential brain structures during resection possible.

The first differential diagnosis that must be considered is glioma, although they tend to have a larger size and are often associated with mass effect, edema, and gliosis. Additionally, while gliomas tend to enhance with contrast administration, FCD does not.

Spectroscopy of FCD shows an increase in the NAA/Creatine ratio; on the other hand, the Choline/Creatine ratio increases more in neoplasms. In diffusion-weighted sequences, the ADC in gliomas is significantly greater than in cortical defects such as FCD.

T1-weighted inversion-recovery coronal MR image with thin slices shows an area of left posterior parietal cortical thickening (Fig. 3.13). T2-weighted FLAIR MRI displays a signal increase associated with some degree of gliosis and loss of differentiation between white and gray matter without any secondary mass effect (Fig. 3.14). T1-weighted MRI with contrast shows an absence of contrast uptake (Fig. 3.15). Sagittal T1-weighted functional MR image shows an eloquent area of the brain, which directs motor function of the right hand (yellow) 5 mm from the FCD lesion (Fig. 3.16) (Courtesy of Dr. Jorge Gómez).

Figure 3.13
Figure 3.14
Figure 3.15
Figure 3.16

Case 3.5
CNS Takayasu Arteritis
■
María I. Martínez León and Jorge Garín Ferreira

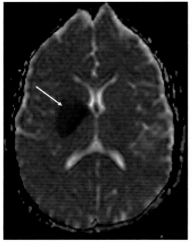

Fig. 3.17

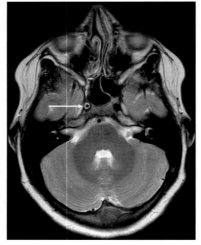

Fig. 3.18

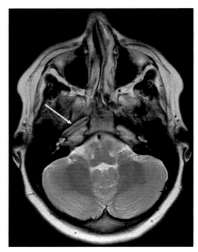

Fig. 3.19

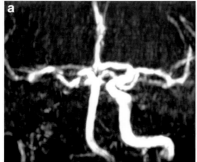
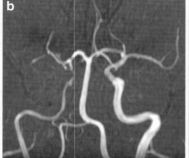
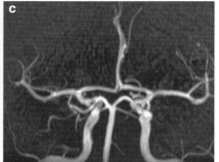

Fig. 3.20

An 11-year-old girl presents with left hemiparesis and facial paralysis secondary to acute stroke.

Takayasu arteritis (TA) is an idiopathic inflammatory vascular disorder primarily involving medium and large caliber arteries. This inflammatory granulomatous disease involves the tunica media and adventitia of vessel walls and thus results in luminal abnormalities (stenosis, occlusion, and aneurysm formation). Wall thickening and contrast enhancement can be seen early in the disease, while arterial stenosis, occlusions, and aneurysms appear later on.

Diagnosis is made based on clinical, laboratory, and radiologic data. The American College of Reumathology requires three of the following six criteria for diagnosis to be made: extremity claudication, age 40 or younger at onset, decreased brachial artery pulse, blood pressure difference greater than 10 mmHg, bruit over the subclavian artery and abnormal arteriogram.

MRI and ultrasound are two noninvasive techniques that allow for vasculature assessment. Both techniques are useful for early diagnosis because of their ability to evaluate vessel wall thickness rather than just luminal narrowing or dilatation.

High-dose corticosteroids are effective for treating TA.

Neurological involvement is reported in only a minority of patients and neurological symptoms as the first manifestation of disease is uncommon. The subclavian and common carotid arteries are the most frequently affected in CNS TA. Despite severe vascular involvement, the neurological prognosis of the disease with appropriate treatment is favorable.

ADC map image shows acute ischemic stroke of the territory of the perforating branches of the right middle cerebral artery (arrow) (Fig. 3.17). Axial T2-weighted MR image exhibits concentric wall thickening of the cavernous (Fig. 3.18) and petrous (Fig. 3.19) segments of the right internal carotid artery (arrows). Angiography of the circle of Willis without contrast with 3D reconstruction (with motion artifact) shows the absence of signal flow in the right internal carotid artery (Fig. 3.20a). Continued improvement was seen at 3 and 9 months of follow-up (Fig. 3.20b, c).

Figure 3.17
Figure 3.18
Figure 3.19
Figure 3.20a, b, c

Case 3.6
Premamilar Ventriculostomy
■
M. Dolores Domínguez Pinos and María I. Martínez León

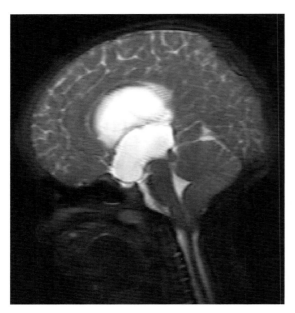

Fig. 3.21

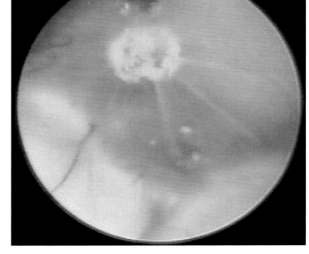

Fig. 3.22

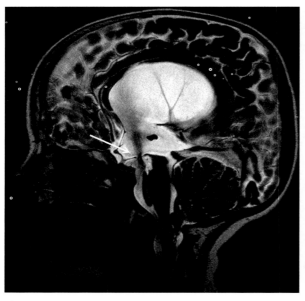

Fig. 3.23

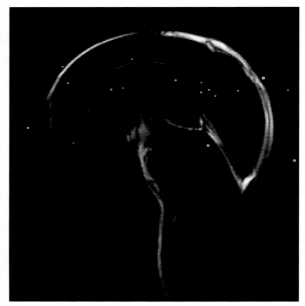

Fig. 3.24

Case 3.6a: Hydrocephalus due to myelomeningocele in a 6-year-old boy who needs premamilar ventriculostomy (PV) for cerebrospinal fluid (CSF) drainage.

Case 3.6b: A 3-year-old boy with cerebellar astrocytoma and secondary obstructive hydrocephalus.

Comments

High levels of CSF in ventricular system needs alternative pathways of drainage, classically ventriculoperitoneal derivations solve this problem. Nowadays, ventricular endoscopy allows ventriculocisternothomy for treatment of hydrocephalus.

The most frequent third ventriculostomy is premamilar that offers significant advantages: combines a minimal invasive approach with good visual control of the field of view, and low risk of vascular or neural damage. The perforation point is located at the midpoint of the height of the triangle formed by the base of the mamillary bodies and the apex of the infunfibular recess.

The radiological criteria for success can be:

1. Reduction in ventricular size ranging from 10% to 50% can be observed in the first week, even if the ventricles remain large.
2. Periventricular bright on T2, if present before operation, can disappear.
3. CSF flow artifact must be visible in midline on sagittal T2.
4. The floor of the third ventricle, if bulging downward in the preoperative images, must be straight on postoperative images.
5. Atrial diverticula and pseudocystic dilatation of the suprapineal recess, if present preoperatively, must disappear or decrease significantly.
6. Pericerebral sulci, if not visible before operation, must reappear or increase in size.

Imaging Findings

Case 3.6a: Preoperative sagittal T2 view of third ventricle showing triventricular hydrocephalus with suprachiasmatic recess dilated, the floor of the third ventricle is deformed and bulges into the prepontine cistern (Fig. 3.21). Endoscopic view of the floor of the third ventricle immediately after monopolar coagulation in PV (image yielded by Dr. Mosqueira from Neurosurgery Department of Carlos Haya Hospital) (Fig. 3.22). After 2 years, sagital T2 is showing ventriculostomomy persistence, floid void artifact is visible through the floor of the third ventricle (arrow) (Fig. 3.23).

Figure 3.21
Figure 3.22
Figure 3.23

Case 3.6b: Phase-contrast cine MRI showing functional third ventriculostomy (Fig. 3.24).

Figure 3.24

Case 3.7

Bilateral Cystic Microphthalmia (Bilateral Cystic Eye)

Lourdes Parra Ruiz and María I. Martínez León

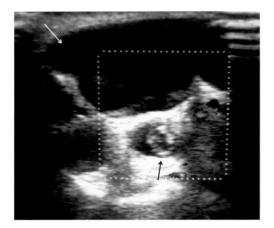

Fig. 3.25

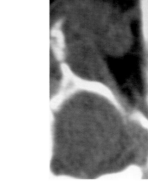

Fig. 3.26

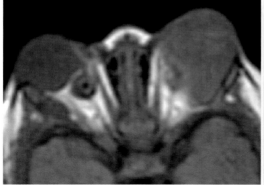

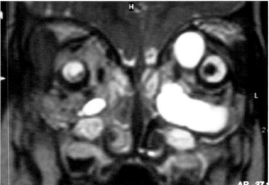

Fig. 3.27

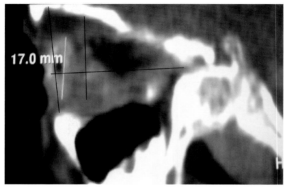

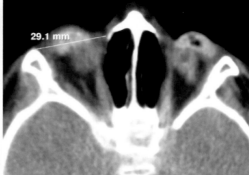

Fig. 3.28

Newborn presents with bluish mass that distends both inferior eyelids without visualization of the ocular globe upon examination.

Comments

Congenital unilateral or bilateral anophtalmia is a rare malformation. There are three classifications for this condition: primary, secondary, and consecutive/degenerative (bilateral 75%, unilateral 25%) anophthalmia. The terms anophthalmia and bilateral microphthalmia are used interchangeably due to the difficulty to differentiate between them clinically. Degenerative anophthalmia or severe cystic microphthalmia is due to disturbances during week 4–8 of fetal age, causing degeneration of the optic vesicle. Clinical manifestations include rudimentary optic nerves, small orbit size, and an absent or small ocular globe. On the other hand, primary or secondary anophthalmia is caused by the arrest of development between the 1st and 4th week of fetal age with subsequent complete optic tract and orbit aplasia, due to an absence of neuroectodermal tissue.

Neuroimaging studies are indicated in cystic microphthalmia in order to assess for further malformations (corpus callosum dysgenesis, visual cortex polymicrogyria, absence of the optic chiasm or posterior optic tract hypoplasia). Ipsilateral craniofacial malformations should be evaluated in unilateral anophthalmia. Hereditary cases have been reported and associations have been described between congenital rubella, maternal vitamin A deficiency and consanguinity and the presence of this malformation.

Opportune treatment is key to the functional and esthetic prognosis of these patients. Frequent follow-up and ocular prosthetics that increase in size according to facial development allow the orbit to expand in order to receive a definitive prosthesis at adulthood. Maintaining the ocular cysts inside the orbit allows for a more effective way of stimulating orbital development than prosthetic implants. Therefore, these remnants, although not functional, should be kept in place for the longest amount of time possible.

Imaging Findings

Ultrasound: multiple intraorbital cysts (white arrow) with cystic degeneration of the microphthalmic ocular globe and a malformed and hyperechogenic lens (black arrow) (Fig. 3.25). Axial CT shows extraconal space cysts, asymmetrical ocular globes that measure <1 cm, and a calcified lens (Fig. 3.26). Axial T1-weighted, coronal T2-weighted MR images show microphthalmia, intraconal cysts, optic nerve atrophy, and preservation of muscular structures (Fig. 3.27). Sagittal and axial CT images show the measurement of the anteroposterior, craniocaudal, and transverse dimensions of both orbits (Fig. 3.28).

Figure 3.25
Figure 3.26
Figure 3.27
Figure 3.28

Case 3.8
Tuberculous Meningitis
■

Miguel Angel López Pino

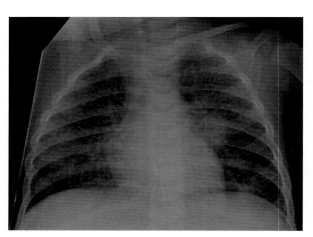

Fig. 3.29

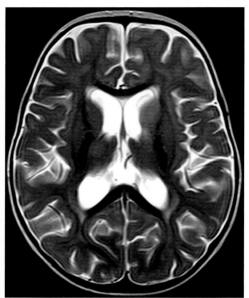

Fig.3.30

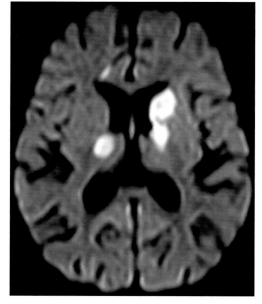

Fig. 3.31

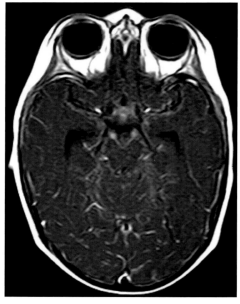

Fig. 3.32

A 10-month-old girl presents with fever, headache, vomiting, malaise, and anisocoria. CSF obtained by lumbar puncture showed pleocytosis, hyperproteinorrachia, and decreased glucose levels.

CNS involvement by tuberculosis (TB) is one of the relatively common (10%) extrapulmonary manifestations of this infectious disease. Clinical presentation may vary widely, thus making diagnosis difficult. There are three classifications for this condition: meningeal TB, intracranial tuberculoma, and spinal tuberculous arachnoiditis.

Meningeal TB occurs as a complication of post-primary infection in children. Up to one third of these patients present findings consistent with miliary TB on plain chest radiographs. The presence of tuberculous proteins in the subarachnoid space causes an intense inflammatory reaction (proliferative arachnoiditis), generally located in the basal cisterns. MR is superior to CT for establishing diagnosis. With FLAIR MR images, meningeal thickening, and presence of exudate in the suprasellar cisterns and perimesencephalic region can be seen. A significant contrast enhancement occurs and may extend to the cranial nerves and penetrating blood vessels. Associated vasculitis occurs in approximately 11% of cases and may cause thrombosis and ischemic changes in the basal ganglia, cerebral cortex, pons, and cerebellum. This inflammatory process causes communicating hydrocephalus in 50–75% of patients. In up to 5–10% of cases tuberculomas are also present.

Diagnosis is usually difficult and a timely detection is key to establishing a favorable prognosis. Analysis of CSF by lumbar puncture is essential to the patient's work-up. With neuroimaging studies, findings of basal meningeal contrast uptake with associated hydrocephalus are highly suggestive of TB meningitis.

An anteroposterior chest radiograph shows bilateral, perihilar, parenchymatous infiltrates, and a micronodular miliary pattern (Fig. 3.29). The axial FSE T2-weighted MR image shows subtle, bilateral foci of increased signal located in the basal ganglia, thalami, and white matter (Fig. 3.30). Additionally, a slight dilatation of the ventricles can be seen without signs of transependymal resorption. These lesions show restriction on DWI, which suggests cytotoxic edema in relation to acute ischemic lesions (vasculitic phenomena) (Fig. 3.31). The axial T1-weighted MR image with contrast shows diffuse meningeal enhancement, especially of the basal region (Fig. 3.32). Furthermore, significant contrast uptake is seen of the interpeduncular cistern and the perivascular region surrounding the middle cerebral arteries.

Figure 3.29
Figure 3.30
Figure 3.31
Figure 3.32

Case 3.9
Spinal Epidural Abscess
■

Víctor Pérez Candela

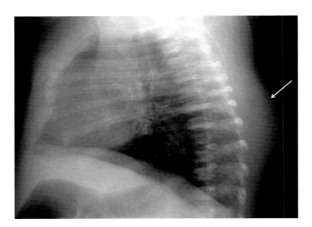

Fig. 3.33

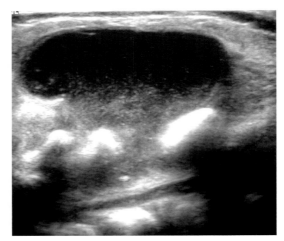

Fig. 3.34

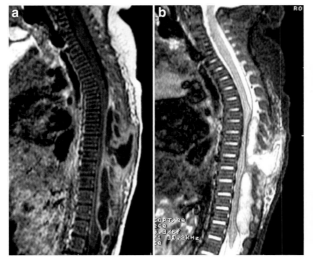

Fig. 3.35

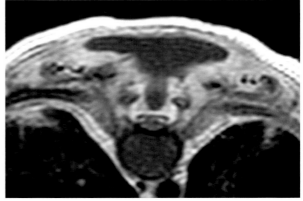

Fig. 3.36

A 32-day-old girl presents with a 5-day history of appearance of a 5 cm, midline mass located on the dorsal region on the back, which had increased progressively in size. Upon examination the mass had a soft consistency, no local inflammatory signs were observed and the patient presented paraparesis with slight flexion to pain stimuli.

Comments

Epidural abscesses are more frequent in older children and young adults rather than in infants and babies. Although many different microorganisms can cause epidural abscesses, *Staphylococcus aureus* is the most frequently implicated bacteria.

The most common clinical presentation includes fever, backache, and associated neurological deficit. Nevertheless, not all children present with an obvious mass as the girl in the case example did.

The disease-causing pathogens can present either a hematogenous dissemination or a direct extension to the spinal epidural space generating the formation of an abscess. The epidural space is wider at the dorsal lumbar region of the spine where the spinal cord is narrower. Epidural abscesses usually form at the dorsal aspect instead of the ventral side. This tendency is due to the fact that strong connective tissue filaments attach the dura to osseous structures ventrally while at the dorsal aspect the space contains adipose tissue.

In the specific case mentioned above, *S. aureus* was cultivated from the contents of the abscess. The suspected origin of the infection was thought to be the heel prick conducted to screen for metabolic abnormalities in newborns. A decompressive laminectomy was carried out to drain the abscess and the patient also received a 5-week IV antibiotic regimen. The girl's recovery was excellent and she presented no neurologic sequelae.

Imaging Findings

Lateral chest radiograph shows a soft-tissue increase at the dorsal portion of the back (arrow) (Fig. 3.33). Ultrasound displays the cystic nature of the mass with echogenicity suggestive of pus that extends to the spinal canal through the adjacent spinous processes (Fig. 3.34). The T1-weighted MR image with contrast shows a hypointense epidural abscess with peripheral enhancement, which compresses the spinal cord anteriorly and extends from T4 to L1 (Fig. 3.35a). On the T2-weighted sagittal MR image the lesion appears hyperintense and the dura is seen as a hypointense line that divides the abscess from the CSF (Fig. 3.35b). The axial T1-weighted MR image shows the subcutaneous extension of the abscess (Fig. 3.36).

Figure 3.33
Figure 3.34
Figure 3.35a, b
Figure 3.36

Case 3.10

Mitochondrial Myopathy, Encephalopathy, Lactic Acidosis, and Stroke (MELAS) Syndrome

L. Santiago Medina and Sara M. Koenig

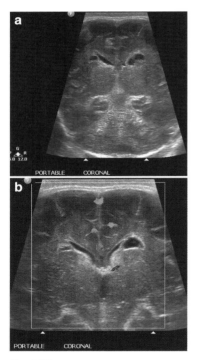

Fig. 3.37

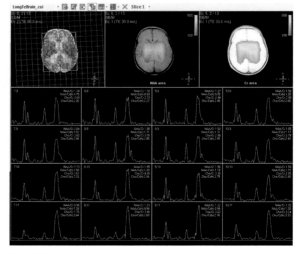

Fig. 3.38

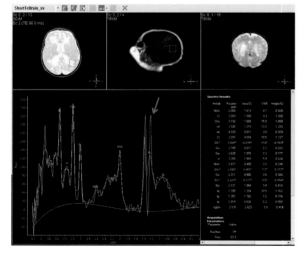

Fig. 3.39

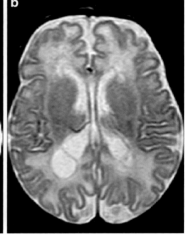

Fig. 3.40

A 7-day-old infant presents with respiratory distress. Clinical findings included pulmonary hypertension, cardiomyopathy, and respiratory failure.

Comments

MELAS refers to a group of mitochondrial disorders known to cause episodes of nausea, vomiting, headache, and reversible or irreversible stroke-like events. Onset is typically between 4 and 15 years of age, presenting most commonly in the second decade and uncommonly during infancy. At least six mutations are associated with MELAS syndrome, with the tRNA^{Leu} gene mutation, or the m3243 A-to-G point mutation, present in approximately 80% of cases. Other mutations may include mitochondrial DNA deletions.

Most patients present with lactic acidosis of both the serum and the CSF. During infancy, developmental delay, failure to thrive, stroke-like episodes, and seizures are very common. Also, cardiomyopathy is very common in MELAS, causing respiratory distress and shortness of breath. The cause of stroke-like episodes is unknown although it is thought to be related to the deficiency of functional mitochondria in the smooth muscle cells of arteries causing reduced cerebral blood flow.

Diagnosis is reached through imaging studies and mitochondrial DNA mutation analysis serving as a confirmatory test. Imaging studies during the acute phase indicate swelling and T1 and T2 prolongation of affected portions of the CNS, most prominently in the parietal lobe, occipital lobe, and basal ganglia. Between acute and chronic stages, adversely affected areas may disappear and then reappear during later imaging studies. The pattern created by these lesions is often random and does not follow a vascular distribution, thus ruling out infarct or embolism. MRS indicates increased lactate levels throughout the brain, elevated glucose, and reduced NAA, glutamate, and creatine.

Imaging Findings

Transcranial sonography (Fig. 3.37a, b), T1w-T2w MR images (Fig. 3.38a, b) that show changes on white matter with malacia secondary to chronic vascular events. MRS in MELAS indicates that lactate is very high, which is common due to dysfunctional mitochondria causing the cells to revert to glycolysis with an increase in lactate (Fig. 3.39). MRS also illustrates decreases in *N*-acetyl aspartate (NAA) and creatine (Cr) levels (Fig. 3.40).

Figure 3.37
Figure 3.38
Figure 3.39
Figure 3.40

Acknowledgment   Acknowledgment to Dr. Raj Palani for his help on the preparation of this case.

Further Reading

Books

Atlas SW (2004) RM de cabeza y columna. Ed. Marban, Madrid

Barkovich JA (2005) Pediatric neuroimaging. Lippincott Williams & Wilkins, Philadelphia, PA

Cinalli G, Maixner WJ, Sainte-Rose C (ed) (2005) Pediatric hydrocephalus, vol 27. Springer, Milan pp 397–405

Harrison (2010) Principios de medicina interna. 17º edición, vol II. Ed. Interamericana McGraw-Hill, p 2308

Ketonen LM, Hiwatashi A, Sidhu R, Westesson P-L (2005) Pediatric brain and spine. An atlas of MRI and spectroscopy, vol 4. Springer, New York, pp 160–161

Mann I (1957) Abnormalities affecting the eye as a whole. In: Mann I (ed) Developmental abnormalities of the eye. Lippincott, Philadelphia, PA, pp 60–66

Mukherji CM (1996) Imaging of the pediatric head, neck and spine. Lippincott-Raven, Philadelphia, PA, 17.12,698

Osborn A et al (2004a) Diagnostic imaging: Brain. AMIRSYS, Salt Lake City, UT

Osborn A et al (2004) Diagnostic imaging: brain. Amirsys, Salt Lake City, UT, 10: I-10-24

Raine CS (2000) Esclerosis múltiple. Bases clínicas y patogénicas. ISBN: 84-7714-186-X, 2000. Editores Médicos S.A

Web Link

http://emedicine.medscape.com/article/1147044-overview
www.esclerosismultiple.com
http://www.uptodate.com/home/index.html
www.ajnr.org
http://emedicine.medscape.com/article/1146574-overview
http://www.hydroassoc.org
http://www.scribd.com/doc/2437580
http://www.uptodate.com/home/index.html
http://www.pennstatehershey.org/healthinfo/hie/
http://www.umdf.org/site/c.otJVJ7MMIqE/b.5692881/k.4B7B/ Types_of_Mitochondrial_Disease.htm#MELAS/

Articles

Abdel Razek et al (2009) Disorders of cortical formation: MR imaging features. AJNR Am J Neuroradiol 30:4–11

Ahn KJ, You WJ, Jeong SL, Lee JW, Kim BS, Lee JH et al (2004) Atypical manifestations of reversible posterior leukoencephalopathy syndrome: findings on diffusion imaging and ADC mapping. Neuroradiology 46:978–983

Albernaz VS, Castillo M, Hudgins PA, Mukherji SK (1997) Imaging findings in patients with clinical anophtalmos. AJNR Am J Neuroradiol 18:555–561

Alehan F, Erol I, Agildere AM, Ozcay F, Baskin E, Cengiz N et al (2007) Posterior leukoencephalopathy syndrome in children and adolescents. J Child Neurol 22:406–413

Arend WP, Michel BA, Bloch DA, Hunder GG, Calabrese LH, Edworthy SM et al (1990) The American College of Rheumatology 1990 criteria for the classification of Takayasu arteritis. Arthritis Rheum 33:1129–1134

Auletta J, John CC (2001) Spinal epidural abscesses in children: A 15 year experience and review of the literature. Clin Infect Dis 32:9–16

Bair-Merrit M, Chung C, Collier A (2000) Spinal epidural abscess in a young child. Pediatrics 106(3):E39

Bakshi R, Thompson AJ, Rocca MA, Pelletier D, Dousset V, Barkhof F et al (2008) MRI in multiple sclerosis: current status and future prospects. Lancet Neurol 7:615–625

Bargalló N, Olondo L, García AI, Capurro S, Caral L, Rumia J (2005) Functional analysis of third ventriculostomy patency by quantification of CSF stroke volume by using cine phase-contrast MR imaging. AJNR Am J Neuroradiol 26:2514–2521

Bernaerts A, Vanhoenacker FM, Parizel PM, Van Goethem JW, Van Altena R, Laridon A et al (2003) Tuberculosis of the central nervous system: overview of neuroradiological findings. Eur Radiol 13:1876–1890

Bilaniuk LT, Farber M (1992) Imaging of developmental anomalies of the eye and the orbit. AJNR Am J Neuroradiol 13:793–804

Bilginer B, Oguz KK, Akalan N (2009) Endoscopic third ventriculostomy for malfunction in previously shunted infants. Childs Nerv Syst 25:683–688

Blumberg HM, Burman WJ, Chaisson RE, Daley CL, Etkind SC, Friedman LN et al (2003) American Thoracic Society/Centers for Disease Control and Prevention/Infectious Diseases Society of America: treatment of tuberculosis. Am J Respir Crit Care Med 167:603–662

Bronen RA, Vives KP, Kim JH, Fulbright RK, Spencer SS, Spencer DD (1997) Focal cortical dysplasia of Taylor, ballon cell subtype: MR differentiation from low grade tumors. AJNR Am J Neuroradiol 18:1141–1151

Callen DJ, Shroff MM, Branson HM, Li DK, Lotze T, Banwell DS (2009) Role of MRI in the differentiation of ADEM from MS in children. Neurology 72:968–973

Casey SO, Sampaio RC, Michel E, Truwit CL (2000) Posterior reversible encephalopathy syndrome: utility of fluid-attenuated inversion recovery MR imaging in the detection of cortical and subcortical lesions. AJNR Am J Neuroradiol 21:1199–1206

Chan KH, Cheung RT, Fong CY et al (2003) Clinical releance of hydrocephalus as a presenting feature of tuberculous meningitis. QJM 96:643–648

Chan KH, Cheung RT, Lee R, Mak W, Ho SL (2005) Cerebral infarcts complicating tuberculous meningitis. Cerebrovasc Dis 19:391–395

Chaudhry IA, Arat YO, Shamsi FA, Boniuk M (2004) Congenital microphthalmos with orbital cysts: distinct diagnostic features and management. Ophthal Plast Reconstr Surg 20:452–457

Chavhan GB, Babyn PS, Jankharia BG, Cheng Hai-Ling M, Shroff MM (2008) Steady-state MR imaging sequences: physics, classification, and clinical applications. Radiographics 28: 1147–1160

Chen WC, Wang JL, Wang JT, Chen YC, Chang SC (2008) Spinal epidural abscess due to Staphylococcus aureus: clinical manifestations and outcomes. J Microbiol Immunol Infect 41:215–221

Colliot O et al (2006) Individual voxel-based analysis of gray matter in focal cortical dysplasia. Neuroimage 29:162–171

Colombo N et al (2003) Focal cortical dysplasias: MR imaging, histopathologic and clinical correlations in surgically treated patients with epilepsy. AJNR Am J Neuroradiol 24:724–733

Covarrubias DJ, Luetmer PH, Campeau NG (2002) Posterior reversible encephalopathy syndrome: prognostic utility of quantitative diffusion-weighted MR images. AJNR Am J Neuroradiol 23:1038–1048

Dale RC, De Sousa C, Chong WK, Cox TC, Harding B, Neville BG (2000) Acute disseminated encephalomyelitis, multiphasic disseminated encephalomyelitis and multiple sclerosis in children. Brain 123:2407–2422

Dale RC, Brilot F, Banwell B (2009) Pediatric central nervous system inflammatory demyelination: acute disseminated encephalomyelitis, clinically isolated syndromes, neuromyelitis optica, and multiple sclerosis. Curr Opin Neurol 22:233–240

Daxecker F, Felber S (1993) Magnetic resonance imaging features of congenital anophtalmia. Ophtalmologica 206: 139–142

Di Carlo P, Cabibi D, Casuccio A, Mazzola A, Romano A, Titone L et al (2008) Features in tubercular meningoencephalitis diagnosis: 18 childhood cases. Am J Infect Dis 4:187–192

Donmez FY, Aslan H, Coskun M (2009) Evaluation of possible prognostic factors of fulminant acute disseminated encephalomyelitis (ADEM) on magnetic resonance imaging with fluid-attenuated inversion recovery (FLAIR) and diffusion-weighted imaging. Acta Radiol 50(3):334–339

Doris D et al (2003) Proton MR spectroscopy in the diagnostic evaluation of suspected mitochondrial disease. AJNR Am J Neuroradiol 22:33–41

Druhan SM, Shiels WE, Kang DR, Elton SW, Koranyi K (2006) Successful sonographically guided drainage of epidural abscess. AJR Am J Roentgenol 187:512–514

Duchowny M (2009) Et al Clinical, functional, and neurophysiologic assessment of dysplastic cortical networks: implications for cortical functioning and surgical management. Epilepsia 50:19–27

Enberg RN, Kaplan RJ (1974) Spinal epidural abscess in children:early diagnosis and inmediate surgical drainage is essential to forestall paralysis. Clin Pediatr 13:247–253

Farinha NJ, Razali KA, Holzel H, Morgan G, Novelli VM (2000) Tuberculosis of the central nervous system in children: a 20-year survey. J Infect 41:61–68

Filippi M (2008) Multiple sclerosis, Part I: Background and conventional MRI. Preface. Neuroimaging Clin N Am 18:XV–XVI

Fischer EG, Greene CS, Winston KR (1981) Spinal epidural abscess in children. Neurosurgery 9:257–260

Fok W, Sun L, Wong N, Lau P, Cheung H (2007) Spontaneous spinal epidural haematoma in a 15-month-old boy presenting with a wry neck: a case report. J Orthop Surg (Hong Kong) 15:373–375

Goto Y, hoarai S, Matsuoka T et al (1992) Mitochondrial myopathy, encephalopathy, lactic acidosis, and stroke-like episodes (MELAS): a correlative study of the clinical features and mitochondrial DNA mutation. Neurology 42:545–550

Gotway MB, Araoz PA, Macedo TA, Stanson AW, Higgins ChB, Ring EJ et al (2005) Imaging findings in Takayasu´s arteritis. AJR Am J Roentgenol 184:1945–1950

Gundlach KK, Guthoff RF, Hingst VH, Schittkowski MP, Bier UC (2005) Expansion of the socket and orbit for congenital clinical anophthalmia. Plat Reconstr Surg 116:1214–1222

Hailong F, Guangfu H, Haibin T, Hong P, Yong C, Weidong L, Dongdong Z (2008) Endoscopic third ventriculostomy in the management of communicating hydrocephalus: a preliminary study. J Neurosurg 109:923–930

Hoffmann M, Corr P, Robbs J (2000) Cerebrovascular findings in Takayasu disease. J Neuroimaging 10:84–90

Honkaniemi J, Dastidar P, Kähärä V, Haapasalo H (2001) Delayed MR imaging changes in acute disseminated encephalomyelitis. AJNR Am J Neuroradiol 22:1117–1124

Hopper K, Sherman JL, Boal DK, Eggli KD (1992) CT and MR imaging of the pediatric orbit. Radiographics 12:485–503

Huynh W, Cordato DJ, Kehdi E, Masters LT, Dedousis C (2008) Post-vaccination encephalomyelitis: literature review and illustrative case. J Clin Neurosci 15:1315–1322

Inglese M, Salvi F, Iannucci G, Mancardi GL, Mascalchi M, Filippi M (2002) Magnetization transfer and diffusion tensor MR imaging of acute disseminated encephalomyelitis. AJNR Am J Neuroradiol 23:267–272

Jacobsen FS, Sullivan B (1994) Spinal epidural abscess in children. Orthopedics 17:1131–1134

Jones BP, Ganesan V, Saunders DE, Chong WK (2010) Imaging in childhood arterial ischaemic stroke. Neuroradiology 52:577–589

Kaltreider SA (2000) The ideal ocular prosthesis: analysis of prosthetic volume. Ophthal Plast Reconstr 16:388–392

Kaltreider SA, Jacobs JL, Hughes MO (1999) Predicting the ideal implant size before enucleation. Ophthal Plast Reconstr 15:37–43

Katrak SM, Shembalkar PK, Bijwe SR, Bhandarkar LD (2000) The clinical, radiological and pathological profile of tuberculous meningitis in patients with and without human inmunodeficiency virus infection. J Neurol Sci 181:118–126

Kiminobu Y et al (2001) Diffusion-weighted MR imaging in a case of mitochondrial myopathy, encephalopathy, lactic acidosis, and strokelike episodes. AJNR Am J Neuroradiol 22:269–272

Klimo P, Goumnerova LC (2006) Endoscopic third ventriculocisternotomy for brainstem tumors. J Neurosurg 105:271–274

Kwon S, Koo J, Lee S (2001) Clinical spectrum of reversible posterior leukoencephalopathy syndrome. Pediatr Neurol 24: 361–364

Lamy C, Oppenheim C, Méder JF, Mas JL (2004) Neuroimaging in posterior reversible encephalopathy syndrome. J Neuroimaging 14:89–96

Lee VH, Wijdicks EF, Manno EM, Rabinstein AA (2008) Clinical spectrum of reversible posterior leukoencephalopathy syndrome. Arch Neurol 65:205–210

Lipina R, Reguli S, Dolezilová V, Kucíková M, Podesvová H (2008) Endoscopic third ventriculostomy for obstructive hydrocephalus in children younger than 6 months of age: is it a first-choice method? Childs Nerv Syst 24:1021–1027

Martínez-León MI (2002) Microftalmía quística bilateral: ojo quístico clínico. Radiología 44(1):41–42

Matsunaga N, Hayashi K, Sakamoto I, Matsuoka Y, Ogawa Y, Honjo K et al (1998) Takayasu arteritis: MR manifestations and diagnosis of acuete and chronic phase. J Magn Reson Imaging 8:406–414

Miller DH, Grossman RI, Reingold SC, McFarland HF (1998) The role of magnetic resonance techniques in understanding and managing multiple sclerosis. Brain 121:3–24

Mukherjee P, McKinstry RC (2001) Reversible posterior leukoencephalopathy syndrome: evaluation with diffusion-tensor MR imaging. Radiology 219:756–765

Nastri MV, Baptista LP, Baroni RH, Blasbalg R, de Avila LF, Leite CC et al (2004) Gadolinium-enhanced three-dimensional MR angiography of Takayasu arteritis. Radiographics 24: 773–786

O Brien DF, Seghedoni A, Collins DR, Hayhurst C, Mallucci CL (2006) Is there an indication for ETV in young infants in aetiologies other than isolated aqueduct stenosis? Childs Nerv Syst 22:1565–1572

Oberhansli C, Charles-Messance D, Munier F, Spahn B (2003) Management of microphthalmos and anophthalmos: prosthetic experience. Klin Monatsbl Augenheilkd 220:134–137

Offenbacher H, Fazekas F, Schmidt R, Kleinert R, Payer F, Kleinert G et al (1991) MRI in tuberculous meningoencephalitis: report or four cases and review of the neuroimaging literature. J Neurol 238:340–344

Ozates M, Kemaloglu S, Gurkan F, Ozkan U, Hosoglu S, Simsek MM (2000) CT of the brain in tuberculous meningitis. A review of 289 patients. Acta Radiol 41:13–17

Palmini A, Najm I, Avanzini G et al (2004) Terminology and classification of the cortical dysplasias. Neurology 62:S2–S8

Phelan JA et al (2008) Pediatric neurodegenerative white matter processes: leukodystrophies and beyond. Pediatr Radiol 38:729–749

Poser CM, Paty DW, Scheinberg L, McDonald WI, Davis FA, Ebers GC et al (1983) New diagnostic criteria for multiple sclerosis: guidelines for research protocols. Ann Neurol 13:227–331

Provenzale JM, Petrella JR, Cruz LC Jr, Wong JC, Engelter S, Barboriak DP (2001) Quantitative assessment of diffusion abnormalities in posterior reversible encephalopathy syndrome. AJNR Am J Neuroradiol 22:1455–1461

Rajan J, Kannan K, Kesavadas C, Thomas B (2009) Focal Cortical Dysplasia (FCD) lesion analysis with complex diffusion approach. Comput Med Imaging Graph 33:553–558

Ranasuriya DG, Feld RJ, Nairn SJ (2008) A case of acute disseminated encephalomyelitis in a 12-year-old boy. Pediatr Emerg Care 24(10):697–699

Rastorgi S, Lee Ch, Salamon N (2008) Neuroimaging in pediatric epilepsy: a multimodality approach. Radiographics 28:1079–1095

Ringleb PA, Strittmatter EI, Loewer M, Hartmann M, Fiebach JB, Weber R et al (2005) Cerebrovascular manifestations of Takayasu arteritis in Europe. Rheumatology (Oxford) 44:1012–1015

Río J, Rovira A, Tintoré M, Huerga E, Nos C, Tellez N et al (2008) Relationship between MRI lesion activity and response to IFN-beta in relapsing-remitting multiple sclerosis patients. Mult Scler 14:479–484

Ros-Lopez B, Jaramillo-Dallimonti AM, de Miguel-Puello LS, Rodríguez-Barceló S, Domínguez Páez M, Ibáñez-Botella G et al (2009) Ventricular haemorrhage in preterm neonates and posthemorrhagic hydrocephalus. Proposal of a management protocol based on early ventriculo-peritoneal shunt. Neurocirugía 20:15–24

Rossi A (2008) Imaging of acute disseminated encephalomyelitis. Neuroimaging Clin N Am 18:149–161

Rovira A, Swanton J, Tintoré M, Huerga E, Barkhof F, Filippi M et al (2009) A single, early magnetic resonance imaging study in the diagnosis of multiple sclerosis. Arch Neurol 66:587–592

Rubin G, Michowiz SD, Ashkenasi A, Tadmor R, Rappaport ZH (1993) Spinal epidural abscess in the pediatric age group: case report and review of the literature. Pediatr Infect Dis J 12:1007–1011

Ryutarou U, Kushihashi T, Tanaka E, Baba M, Usi N, Fujisawa H et al (2006) Diffusion-weighted MR imaging of early-stage

Creutzfeldt-Jakob disease: typical and atypical manifestations. Radiographics 26:S191–S194

Saenz RC (2005) The disappearing basal ganglia sign. Radiology 234:242–243

Scaglia F et al (2005) Predominant cerebellar volume loss as a neuroradiologic feature of pediatric respiratory chain defects. AJNR Am J Neuroradiol 26:1675–1680

Schlaug G, Diewert B, Benfield A, Edelman RR, Warach S (1997) Time course of the apparent diffusion coefficient (ACD) abnormality in human stroke. Neurology 49:113–119

Schmidt WA, Nerenheim A, Seipelt E, Poehls C, Gromnica-Ihle E (2002) Diagnosis of early Takayasu arteritis with sonography. Rheumatology 41:496–502

Schoeman J, Hewlett R, Donald P (1988) MR of childhood tuberculous meningitis. Neuroradiology 30:473–477

Schroff MM, Soares-Fernandez JP, Whyte H, Raybaud C (2010) MR imaging for diagnostic evaluation of encephalopathy in the newborn. Radiographics 30:763–780

Seyfert S, Klapps P, Meísel C, Fisclier T, Junghan U (1990) Multiple sclerosis and other iminunologic diseases. Acta Neurol Scand 81:37–42

Sikaroodi H, Motamedi M, Kahnooji H, Gholamrezanezhad A, Yousefi N (2007) Stroke as the first manifestation of Takayasu Arteritis. Acta Neurol Belg 107:18–21

Stingh I, Haris M, Husain M, Husain N, Rastogi M, Gupta RK (2008) Role of endoscopic third ventriculostomy in patients with communicating hydrocephalus: an evaluation by MR ventriculography. Neurosurg Rev 31:319–325

Stivaros SM, Sinclair D, Bromiley PA, Kim J, Thorne J, Jackson A (2009) Endoscopic third ventriculostomy: predicting outcome with phase-contrast MR imaging. Radiology 252:825–832

Stott VL, Hurrell MA, Anderson TJ (2005) Reversible posterior leukoencephalopathy syndrome: a misnomer reviewed. Intern Med J 35:83–90

Sue CM et al (1998) Neuroradiological features of six kindreds with MELAS tRNA^{Leu} A3243G point mutation: implications for pathogenesis. J Neurol Neurosurg Psychiatry 65:233–240

Tassil L, Colombo N, Garbelli R et al (2002) Focal cortical dysplasia: neuropathological subtypes, EEG, neuroimaging and surgical outcome. Brain 125:1719–1732

Taylor DC, Falconer MA, Bruton CJ, Corsellis JA (1971) Focal dysplasia of the cerebral cortex in epilepsy. J Neurol Neurosurg Psychiatry 34:369–387

Tenembaum S, Chitnis T, Ness J, Hahn JS (2007) Acute disseminated encephalomyelitis. Neurology 17(68):S23–S36

Traboulsee AL, Li DK (2006) The role of MRI in the diagnosis of multiple sclerosis. Adv Neurol 98:125–146

Tur C, Téllez N, Rovira A, Tintoré M, Río J, Nos C et al (2008) Acute disseminated encephalomyelitis: study of factors involved in a possible development towards multiple. Neurologia 23(9):546–554

Walter RS, King JC, Manley J, Rigamonti D (1991) Spinal epidural abscess in infancy: successful percutaneous drainage in a nine-month-old and review of the literature. Pediatr Infect Dis J 10:860–864

Yamada I, Numano F, Suzuki S (1993) Takayasu arteritis: evaluation with MR imaging. Radiology 188:89–94

Zivadinov R, Cox JL (2007) Neuroimaging in multiple sclerosis. Int Rev Neurobiol 79:449–474

Thorax

Contents

M.I. Martínez-León et al., *Learning Pediatric Imaging*, Learning Imaging,
DOI: 10.1007/978-3-642-16892-5_4, © Springer-Verlag Berlin Heidelberg 2011

Case 4.1
Parapneumonic Pleural Effusion
■
Pablo Valdés Solís

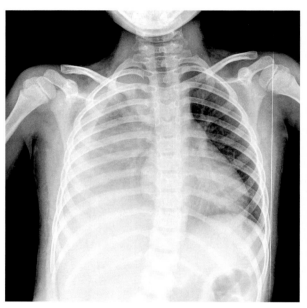

Fig. 4.1

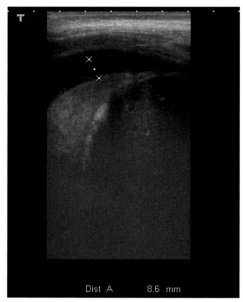

Fig. 4.2

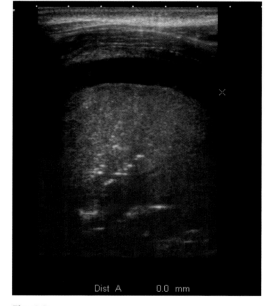

Fig. 4.3

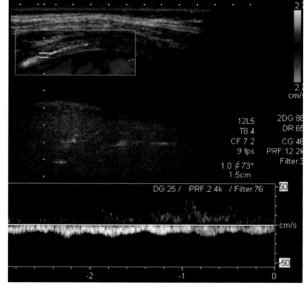

Fig. 4.4

A 5-year-old girl presents with a 4-day history of fever. Routinely recommended immunizations were complete. Blood work showed 24,500 leukocytes with 89% neutrophils. A plain chest radiograph was performed and antibiotic treatment was initiated. Thoracic ultrasound was ordered due to poor clinical evolution.

Parapneumonic pleural effusion and empyema are seen as a complication of approximately 40% of bacterial pneumonias in children that require hospital admission. The presence of effusion worsens the clinical prognosis of lower respiratory tract infections. Currently, a greater number of cases of empyema have been documented, which may be related to pneumococcal vaccination. However, it has not been determined whether there is a greater incidence of pneumonia or whether a greater percentage of them present complications such as theses.

Parapneumonic pleural effusion evolves through exudative, fibropurulent (infected and loculated), and proliferative (fibroblast proliferation) stages. Although plain chest radiography is the study of choice for pneumonias, thoracic ultrasound is a useful complement that aids in evaluating pulmonary parenchyma and pleural effusion. Certain characteristics are assessed in order to determine whether the effusion is simple or complex. Complex effusions show mobile internal echos, fibrinous bands, septations, and honeycomb patterns. On ultrasound, both transudate and exudate may appear anechoic, yet features compatible with complex effusions always indicate exudative fluid. When a moderate amount of fluid is identified, a diagnostic and therapeutic thoracentesis should be performed. Indications for invasive treatment (thoracostomy tube + fibrinolytics, or surgery) include loculated effusions that occupy 50% or more of the hemithorax and have positive cellular cultures.

AP chest radiograph reveals a right lower lobe consolidation and associated pleural effusion with mediastinal displacement to the left (Fig. 4.1). Thoracic ultrasound shows pleural effusion with thin fibrous bands (Fig. 4.2). On follow-up ultrasound performed 5 days later, the effusion has organized and shows fibrous septations that loculate the fluid (Fig. 4.3). Additionally, adjacent pulmonary consolidation with sonographic air bronchogram can be seen. Doppler shows an increase in pleural flow due to inflammatory changes (Fig. 4.4).

Figure 4.1
Figure 4.2
Figure 4.3
Figure 4.4

Case 4.2
Primary Pulmonary Tuberculosis
◼
Cristina Serrano García

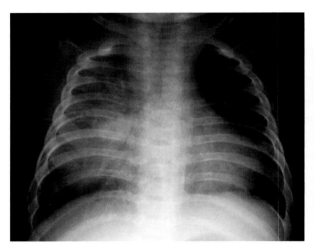

Fig. 4.5

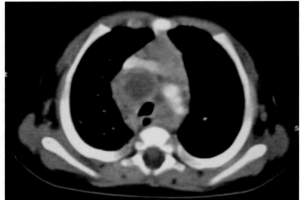

Fig. 4.6

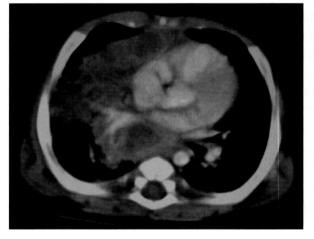

Fig. 4.7

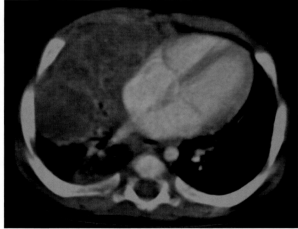

Fig. 4.8

A 5-month-old girl presents with progressive breathing difficulty and high fever. Complementary tests demonstrate leukocitosis, PPD test with 10 mm at 48 h, and PCR positive to Mycobacterium Tuberculosis.

Comments

Primary pulmonary tuberculosis (TB) is the most common form in childhood, and has the highest prevalence in children less than 5 years of age. It manifests as four main entities:

- Lymphadenopathy: Mediastinal or hilar lymphadenopathy with central necrosis is the most frequent radiologic finding in children. They are typically unilateral and right sided (hilum and right paratracheal region). Computed tomography (CT) shows nodes with low-attenuation center secondary to caseous necrosis and peripheral rim enhancement, and frequently suggests active disease. They usually calcify 6 months or more after the initial infection.
- Parenchymal disease: It manifests as dense, homogeneous parenchymal consolidation with predominance in the lower and middle lobes. Lobar or segmental atelectasis is frequently seen in children under 2 years of age. The parenchymal focus resolves without sequelae at chest radiographs. A radiologic scar persists in 15% of cases (Ghon focus). Tuberculomas are seen in 9% of the cases.
- Miliary disease: It refers to widespread dissemination of TB by hematogenous spread. It manifests within 6 months of initial exposure. High-resolution CT is more sensitive than plain films. The typical radiographic findings are diffuse small 2–3 mm nodules with lower lobe predominance and random distribution. They usually resolve within 2–6 months with treatment. In children under 5 years is recommended a cranial CT because there is a high prevalence of CNS dissemination in miliary disease.
- Pleural effusions: It is a very uncommon finding in children, more frequent in adolescents, usually unilateral. Ultrasound demonstrates a complex septated effusion.

Chest radiographs play a major role in the screening and diagnosis in children with TB. They may be normal or show nonspecific findings in patients with active disease. CT scans can detect the extent of disease and can reveal lymphadenopathy, calcifications, bronchogenic nodules, and complications better than chest conventional radiography.

Imaging Findings

Conventional chest radiograph shows a large parenchymal consolidation in right middle and lower lobes (Fig. 4.5). Contrast-enhanced CT demonstrates mediastinal lymphadenopathy in right paratracheal region (Fig. 4.6) and subcarinal (Fig. 4.7), with low-attenuation center secondary to necrosis and peripheral rim enhancement. Extensive parenchymal consolidation in the middle and lower lobes with hypoattenuated areas due to necrosis and mass effect with mild mediastinal shift (Fig. 4.8).

Figure 4.5
Figure 4.6
Figure 4.7
Figure 4.8

Case 4.3
Viral Infections
■
María Isabel Padín Martín

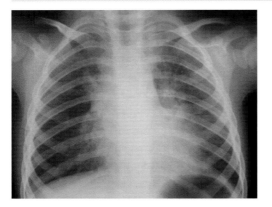

Fig. 4.9

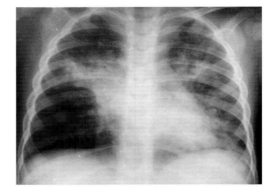

Fig. 4.10

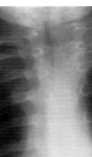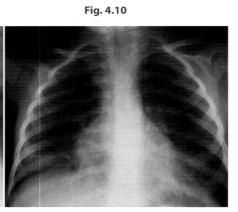

Fig. 4.11

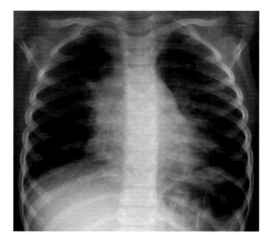

Fig. 4.12

Case 1: Measles,
Case 2: Measles with bacterial coinfection,
Case 3: Upper respiratory tract infection by respiratory syncytial virus (RSV),
Case 4: RSV pneumonia.

Comments

Viruses are the most common cause of respiratory tract infections in childhood. In immunocompetent infants and small children, the most frequently implicated viral pathogens include RSV, influenza, parainfluenza, and adenovirus. The severity of clinical presentation depends on the virulence of the infectious agent and the immunocompetence of the host. Diagnosis is based on cellular culture and serologic analysis results, and bacterial coinfection is considered the most common complication. Long-term pulmonary sequelae may result from the inflammatory effects of viral infection with associated bacterial coinfection on the airways.

The main clinical manifestations of respiratory tract infections are tracheobronchitis, bronchiolitis, and pneumonia.

Radiologic findings of viral pneumonia do not tend to indicate a specific pathogen. Plain chest radiographs show disseminated, patchy consolidations that may display varying degrees of confluence. On occasion, they may present an ill-defined nodular pattern. Bronchial wall thickening and peribronchial shadows are a common characteristic of viral pneumonias. Air entrapment may occur in infections that compromise small caliber airways. Adenopathies are usually rare findings, although they are commonly seen in measles and mononucleosis. On CT images, septal thickening, nodules with associated halo sign, and centrilobular nodules may also be seen.

Imaging Findings

Measles is an infection caused by a myxovirus that may produce pneumonia in 3–4% of cases, along with other systemic and cutaneous manifestations. Radiologically, measles pneumonia displays a reticular pattern with peribronchovascular thickening, patchy consolidations, and associated adenopathies (Fig. 4.9). Bacterial coinfection is with measles pneumonia (Fig. 4.10). RSV is responsible for approximately 15% of mild upper respiratory tract infections and around 45% of lower respiratory tract infections. This virus causes stridorous laryngitis and presents radiologically with the steeple or pencil sign. Furthermore, it is an important cause of bronchiolitis and pneumonia. Plain chest radiographs show peribronchial thickening, pulmonary hyperinflation, lobar collapse and, occasionally, consolidations (Figs. 4.11 and 4.12).

Figure 4.9
Figure 4.10
Figure 4.11
Figure 4.12

Case 4.4
Pulmonary Aspergillosis
■
Gustavo Albi Rodríguez

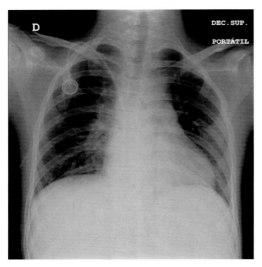

Fig. 4.13

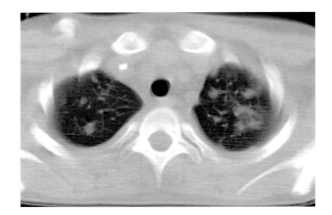

Fig. 4.14

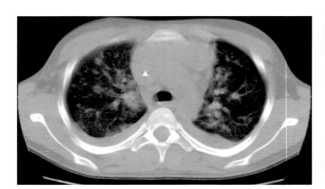

Fig. 4.15

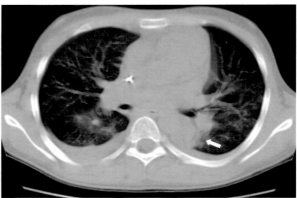

Fig. 4.16

A 15-year-old boy diagnosed with acute myeloblastic leukemia and treated with bone marrow transplantation presents with diarrhea and abdominal pain, as well as graft rejection and pancytopenia. Upon examination, cough and respiratory distress are observed without associated fever.

Comments

The main risk factor for pulmonary fungal infection is neutropenia, which frequently occurs with oncologic patients, especially those diagnosed with leukemia and receiving bone marrow transplants.

The most commonly implicated pulmonary fungal pathogens in these patients are species of *Aspergillus*.

Two separate types of invasive pulmonary aspergillosis have been described, one that affects the respiratory tract and the other that involves the blood vessels. Angioinvasive aspergillosis occurs almost exclusively in immunosuppressed patients with severe neutropenia and it generally develops early on in the post-bone marrow transplant period. Invasion and occlusion of small and medium caliber airways by fungal hyphae cause peripleural necrotic nodules and hemorrhagic pulmonary infarcts.

On the other hand, pulmonary aspergillosis is histologically characterized by the presence of *Aspergillus* beyond the basement membrane of the tracheobronchial tree. Patients with neutropenia and AIDS are most frequently affected. Definitive diagnosis is achieved by histological and/or microbiological studies of pulmonary tissue obtained by open, transbronchial, or percutaneous biopsy.

Imaging Findings

Chest radiography shows nonspecific findings, including consolidations, perihilar infiltrates, and pleural effusion. Aspergillosis should be considered in patients with clinical suspicion and presence of large peripleural consolidations and multiple nodules on radiologic studies. Frequently, chest radiographs are normal (Fig. 4.13) and additional imaging is indicated. CT reveals ill-defined nodules with associated halo sign consistent with hemorrhagic infarcts surrounding necrosed pulmonary parenchyma (Figs. 4.14 and 4.15). Other findings on CT include parenchymal consolidations (arrow) and pleural effusion (Fig. 4.16). At approximately 2–3 weeks after treatment, which coincided with resolution of the patient's neutropenia, the nodules presented cavitation ("air crescent" sign), a finding that is uncommon in children.

Figure 4.13
Figure 4.14
Figure 4.15
Figure 4.16

Case 4.5
Cystic Fibrosis
■
María Isabel Padín Martín

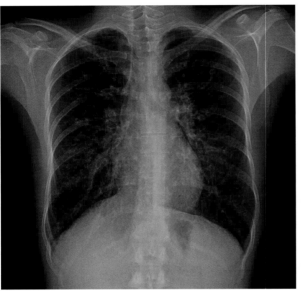

Fig. 4.17

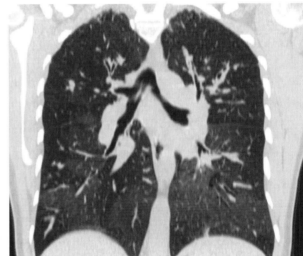

Fig. 4.18

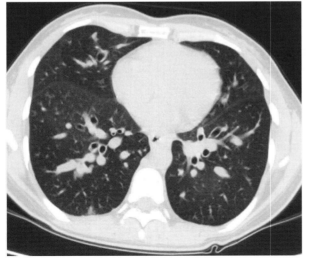

Fig. 4.19

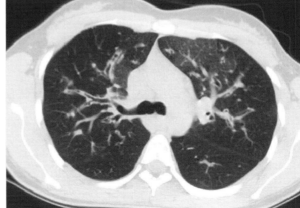

Fig. 4.20

A 12-year-old girl with known diagnosis of cystic fibrosis (CF) presents with respiratory tract infection.

CF or mucoviscidosis is an autosomal recessive disorder caused by a mutation of the trans-membrane conductance regulator gene (CFTR) found in chromosome 7, known as ΔF508. The defective CFTR protein serves as a chlorine ion channel, affecting the chemical composition of mucous secretions and altering pancreatic function.

CF usually presents with abnormal electrolyte levels in sweat, poliposis, sinusitis, varying degrees of pulmonary compromise, exocrine pancreatic insufficiency and infertility in males. Nevertheless, it may affect practically any organ of the body.

Respiratory tract infections continue to be the main cause of morbidity and mortality in patients with CF. During the first decade of life, *Staphylococccus aureus* and *Haemophilus influenzae* are the most frequently implicated pathogens. Later on, *Pseudomona aeruginosa* and *Burkholderia* sp. are more common.

Radiologic manifestations of CF include:

1. Thickening of bronchial walls and dilatation of bronchi (bronchiectasis, bronchiolectasis) due to thick mucus plugs and chronic infection
2. Gloved finger opacities consistent with mucus plugging
3. Cystic lesions consistent with bronchiectasis, abscesses and pulmonary bulla
4. Intermittent atelectasis and focal consolidations
5. Increase in hilar size with adenopathies and dilatation of pulmonary arteries
6. Pulmonary hyperinflation due to obstruction of small caliber airways (mosaic pattern)

The most commo cations of CF are pneumothorax caused by cystic rupture and hemoptysis due to bronchial artery hypertrophy.

CT imaging allows for a more detailed visualization of pulmonary abnormalities. On the other hand, its usefulness in acute exacerbations is limited.

Although several classification systems have been proposed, the Bhalla system is most widely used due to the excellent correlation seen between CT scoring and functional analysis results.

Chest radiography shows air entrapment, bronchial dilatation, and nodules adjacent to secretion-filled bronchi (Fig. 4.17). Coronal CT image shows a mosaic pattern (Fig. 4.18). Axial CT images reveal evidence of mucus impaction and bronchial dilatation (tramlines) (Figs. 4.19 and 4.20).

Figure 4.17
Figure 4.18
Figure 4.19
Figure 4.20

Case 4.6
Cystic Pleuropulmonary Blastoma
■

Héctor Cortina Orts and Laura Pelegrí Martínez

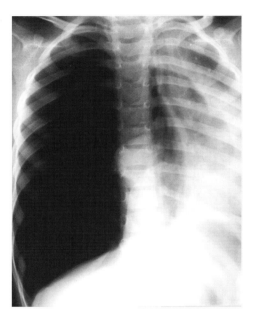

Fig. 4.21

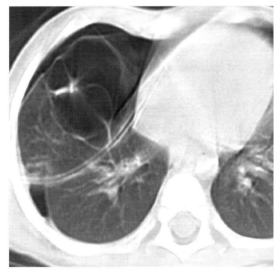

Fig. 4.22

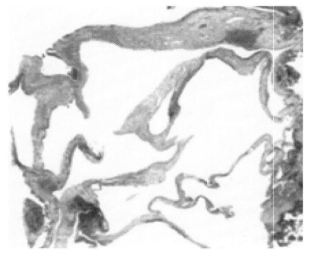

Fig. 4.23

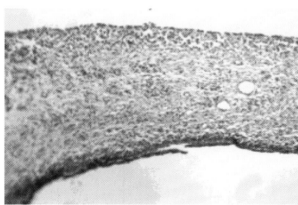

Fig. 4.24

An 18-month-old boy presents with respiratory distress. Chest radiography reveals signs of pneumothorax.

Pleuropulmonary blastoma is a dysontogenetic tumor that arises from embryonic precursors, as do neuroblastomas, Wilm's tumors, and nephroblastomas. The age of onset is approximately 5–6 years. Its origin is found to be the pulmonary blastoma and the primitive esplacnopleural and somatopleural mesoderm. This explains its variable location (pleural, pulmonary, or mixed) as well as its ability to differentiate into various mesenchymal lines (rhabdomyosarcoma, chondrosarcoma, or angiosarcoma). These characteristics and the histological absence of epithelial elements distinguish it from pulmonary blastoma, a tumor that generally occurs during adulthood.

Pleuropulmonary blastoma has been classified in three categories based on age of presentation and degree of aggressiveness. The type I, entirely cystic variant, occurs in children under 1 year. In 10% of cases, it presents with spontaneous pneumothorax. However, advances in prenatal screening hope to reduce the incidence of these unexpected complications. The type II, mixed cystic and solid form of the tumor usually presents in children 2–3 years of age. Finally, the type III, entirely solid variant is generally very large in size and appears in slightly older children.

Type I pleuropulmonary blastomas show up on imaging studies as lesions with an overlapping appearance with cystic adenomatous malformation. Nevertheless, this finding has only been observed in prenatal screening analyses. However, even if it appears later than cystic adenomatoid malformation (i.e., second trimester of the intrauterine period), it is impossible to differentiate by current imaging modalities (i.e., US), so a surgical management is usually required. Type I lesions are usually low-grade malignancies in comparison to multilocular cystic nephromas, cystic nephroblastomas, and thyroglossal cyst papillary carcinomas. This finding raises the question about the connection between these malformations and their malignant transformation.

Plain chest radiography shows signs of pneumothorax (Fig. 4.21). CT image performed after evacuation shows residual pneumothorax and a multi-septated cyst suggestive of cystic adenomatous malformation (Fig. 4.22). Pathological findings were of a cystic membrane composed of ciliated epithelium and filled with multiple undifferentiated small cells (Figs. 4.23 and 4.24). Final diagnosis of pleuropulmonary blastoma was made.

Figure 4.21
Figure 4.22
Figure 4.23
Figure 4.24

Case 4.7

Endobronchial Tumor: Mucoepidermoid Carcinoma

Pilar García-Peña and Ana Coma Muñoz

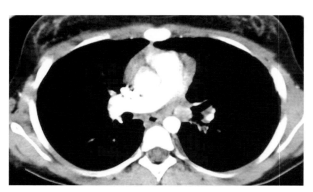

Fig. 4.25

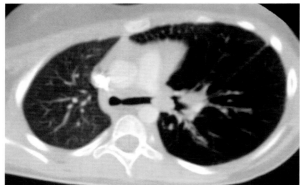

Fig. 4.26

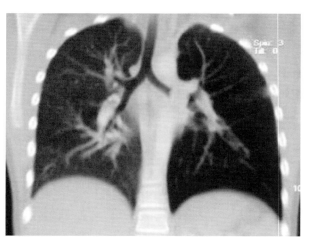

Fig. 4.27

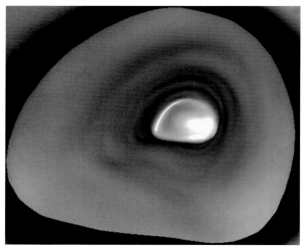

Fig. 4.28

A 10-year-old girl presented repeated episodes of cough and lung collapse. Hemoptysis was present in the last episode. The physical examination showed no stridor or wheezing, and she had no fever. However, during the last episode, breath sounds were clearly decreased in the left hemithorax.

Comments

Endobronchial tumors are rare in the pediatric population. The most common are squamous papilloma, bronchial carcinoid, mucoepidermoid carcinoma, and leiomyoma. Adenoid cystic carcinoma and hamartoma are less frequent. Endobronchial lesions generally arise in a main-stem bronchus or in the proximal portion of the lobar bronchi. Clinical symptoms and radiologic findings are related to bronchial obstruction. In addition to airway foreign bodies, these tumors should be considered in the differential diagnosis of persistent or recurrent symptoms and chest radiography abnormalities.

Mucoepidermoid carcinoma represents about 10% of primary pulmonary malignant neoplasms occurring in children. Patients typically present with cough, fever, expectoration, wheezing, hemoptysis, and chest pain. Hemoptysis occurs in at least 50% of patients, reflecting the highly vascular nature of these neoplasms. Persistent lung collapse, as in aspirated foreign body, leads to bronchoscopy, which often establishes the diagnosis. About 25% of patients are asymptomatic, so that mucoepidermoid carcinomas are found incidentally.

Chest radiography is the initial investigation of choice in most cases. Although most mucoepidermoid carcinomas are primarily endobronchial lesions, they may extend into the adjacent parenchyma ("iceberg" lesion). Bronchoscopy shows an intraluminal component, whereas computed tomography (CT) and magnetic resonance (MR) imaging provide better anatomic delineation of both the intraluminal and extraluminal components. Moreover, CT postprocessing techniques, such as multiplanar reformatting, volume rendering, and virtual bronchoscopy, assist in surgical planning by providing a better representation of the three-dimensional anatomy.

Imaging Findings

Axial contrast-enhanced CT demonstrates an enhancing endobronchial lesion arising from the left main-stem bronchus. There is no lymphadenopathy or extramural extension (Fig. 4.25). Axial oblique CT reconstruction through the left main-stem bronchus axis shows the endobronchial lesion located 1 cm from the carina, and secondary obstructive emphysema in the left lung (Fig. 4.26). Reconstructed coronal CT image provides a good depiction of the tumor and the obstructive emphysema (Fig. 4.27). Virtual bronchoscopy demonstrates obstruction of the left main-stem bronchus (Fig. 4.28).

Figure 4.25
Figure 4.26
Figure 4.27
Figure 4.28

Case 4.8
Pulmonary Artery Sling

Carlos Santiago Restrepo and Susana Calle Restrepo

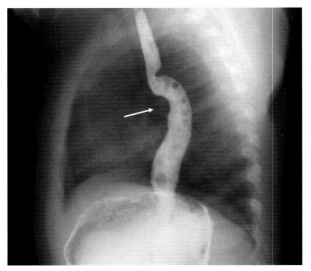

Fig. 4.29

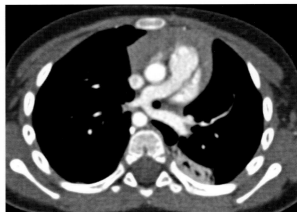

Fig. 4.30

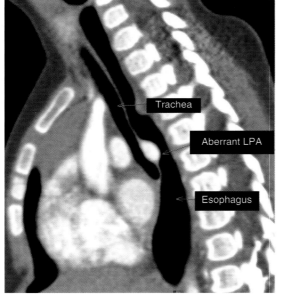

Fig. 4.31

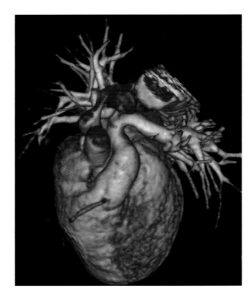

Fig. 4.32

An infant presents with recurrent respiratory stridor.

Pulmonary artery sling or aberrant origin of the left pulmonary artery is characterized by an abnormal origin of the left pulmonary artery from the right pulmonary artery. Axial contrast-enhanced CT of the chest at the level of the pulmonary hila reveals an abnormal origin of the left pulmonary artery from the right pulmonary artery running laterally to distal trachea. The aberrant left pulmonary artery typically passes above the right mainstem bronchus and courses between the trachea and the esophagus to the left pulmonary hilum, explaining the abnormal finding in the esophagogram. Chest X-ray film may show hyperlucency of the right lung and deviation of the trachea to the left, with narrowing of the distal tracheal air column. A barium esophagogram is often diagnostic, showing an anterior indentation of the esophagus, a finding that is only seen in this type of vascular ring.

Associated anomalies of the tracheobronchial tree are seen in 50% of affected patients. The most common malformation being hypoplasia of the distal trachea or right main-stem bronchus usually associated with complete cartilaginous rings ("napkin ring cartilage"), tracheomalacia, and tracheal bronchus. Cardiovascular anomalies are also common (>50%), including persistent left superior vena cava that drains into the coronary sinus, atrial and ventricular septal defects, patent ductus arteriosus, aortic arch anomalies, and tetralogy of Fallot. The majority of these patients present with respiratory symptoms during the first year of life and despite significant improvement with early surgical correction, mortality remains high.

Lateral projection esophagogram with oral contrast demonstrates a vascular structure that indents the anterior aspect of the medial–proximal portion of the esophagus (arrow) (Fig. 4.29). Contrast-enhanced cardiac gated axial CT demonstrates the abnormal origin of the left pulmonary artery from the right, encircling a narrowed distal trachea (Fig. 4.30). Sagittal reconstruction shows the abnormal position of the left pulmonary artery between the trachea and the air-distended esophagus (Fig. 4.31). Volume-rendered 3D reconstruction illustrates the abnormal branching pattern of the pulmonary trunk (Fig. 4.32).

Figure 4.29
Figure 4.30
Figure 4.31
Figure 4.32

Case 4.9

Partial Anomalous Pulmonary Venous Return (PAPVR)

Carlos Santiago Restrepo and Susana Calle Restrepo

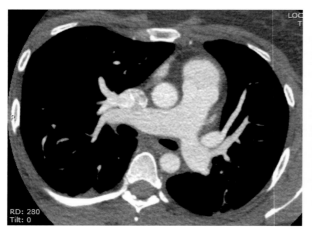

Fig. 4.33

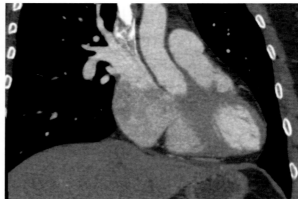

Fig. 4.34

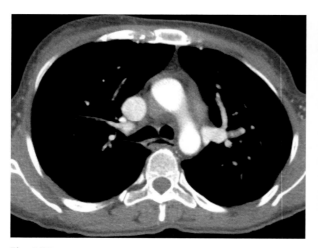

Fig. 4.35

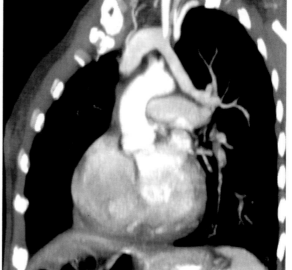

Fig. 4.36

Case 4.9a: A 16-year-old female presents with fatigue.

Case 4.9b: A 17-year-old female presents with arrythmia.

Partial anomalous venous return is characterized by abnormal drainage of one, two, or three pulmonary veins into the systemic circulation, as opposed to total anomalous pulmonary venous return (TAPVR) in which all four pulmonary veins drain into the systemic venous system.

Partial anomalous pulmonary venous return (PAPVR) is an uncommon condition with a prevalence of <1% and the right lung is more commonly affected. Anomalous right lung veins can drain into the systemic circulation via the SVC, azygos vein, right atrium, coronary sinus, or IVC. Association with an atrial septal defect is common. Clinical presentation is similar to that of an intracardiac shunt with manifestations including fatigue, chest pain, dyspnea, and heart murmurs. Right upper lobe PAPVR is commonly associated with sinus venosus ASD. Anomalous veins in the left side are more commonly seen in the upper lobe and are associated with ostium secundum ASD. Left upper lobe PAPVR is usually asymptomatic, and therefore an incidental finding. A PAPVR in the right lung, draining into veins below the diaphragm (IVC, hepatic veins, or other veins), is typically associated with hypoplastic right lung and is known as hypogenetic lung syndrome, venolobar syndrome, or scimitar syndrome because of the appearance of the anomalous vein on chest X-rays.

The presence of an anomalous venous connection can also be suspected when the anomalous vein is canalized by a central venous catheter revealing an abnormal position.

Case 4.9a: Axial contrast-enhanced CT image (Fig. 4.33) and coronal reconstruction (Fig. 4.34) reveal an anomalous connection of the right upper lobe pulmonary veins to the superior vena cava consistent with PAPVR.

Figure 4.33

Figure 4.34

Case 4.9b: Axial contrast-enhanced CT image (Fig. 4.35) and oblique planar MIP reconstruction (Fig. 4.36) demonstrate anomalous venous return from the left upper lobe to a vertical vein that drains into the left innominate artery consistent with left upper lobe PAPVR.

Figure 4.35

Figure 4.36

Case 4.10
Coarctation of the Aorta
■
Carlos Marín

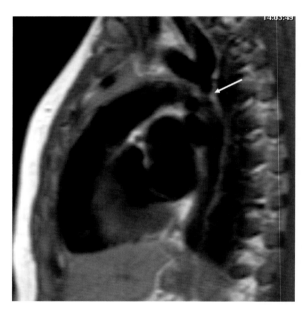

Fig. 4.37

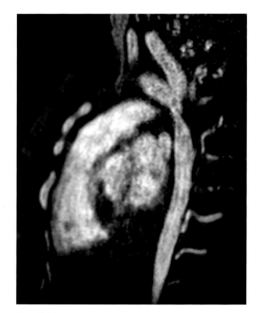

Fig. 4.38

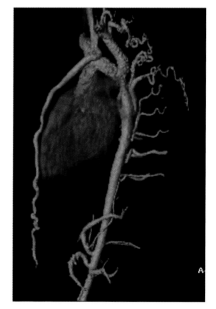

Fig. 4.39

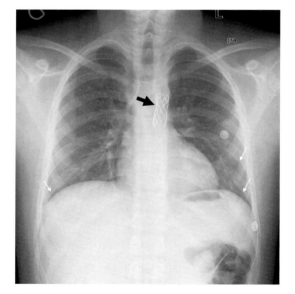

Fig. 4.40

A 12-year-old male presents with hypertension and asymmetric pulses. Transthoracic ultrasound was limited due to poor acoustic window.

Coarctation of the aorta (CoAo) is a congenital obstruction of the aorta, almost invariably located at the insertion of the ductus arteriosus. It represents the eighth most common cardiac malformation and 4% of children with congenital heart disease present some degree of CoAo. It has been divided into four subtypes: uncomplicated coarctation of older children, neonatal coarctation (with or without ventricular septal defect), CoAo with valvular or complex heart disease, and atypical coarctation of the aorta (thoracic or abdominal CoAo, mainly associated with Williams syndrome and other diseases). Different treatment approaches are applied according to the specific variant. This section will focus on uncomplicated coarctation in older children.

Since most patients are asymptomatic, CoAo is usually diagnosed when patients presenting asymmetric pulses or rib notching on chest radiograph undergo further work-up in search of heart murmurs and arterial hypertension.

In neonatal coarctation, cardiac US is usually sufficient to establish diagnosis. On the other hand, in older children, poor acoustic windows and large patient size preclude adequate visualization of the aortic isthmus and descending aorta. Chest radiography in young children is usually normal. Indentation in the aortic arch or rib notching can be seen in older patients, generally children over the age of 12. CT and MR are effective studies for accurate visualization of the thoracic aorta. Lack of ionizing radiation is a major advantage of MR over CT, especially in this age group since frequent posttreatment follow-up imaging is often needed. MR images provide morphologic information of the ascending aorta, transverse arch, isthmus, and descending aorta diameters, as well as the presence of collateral blood vessels. Functional MR imaging adds invaluable data on pressure gradient, hemodynamic significance of collateral circulation and heart function.

Conventional black-blood spin echo imaging usually suffices for CoAo diagnosis (arrow) (Fig. 4.37). However, contrast-enhanced MR angiography better depicts the diameter of the aortic segments and collateral vessels (Fig. 4.38). Rendered images show increased circulation through the internal thoracic arteries, intercostal arteries, and cervical plexus (Fig. 4.39). Chest radiography, taken after endovascular repair, displays the location of the endovascular stent (black arrow) and rib notching of the lower ribs (white arrows) (Fig. 4.40).

Figure 4.37
Figure 4.38
Figure 4.39
Figure 4.40

Further Reading

Books

Donelly L et al (2005) Diagnostic imaging. Pediatrics, vol 2. Amirsys, Salt Lake City, UT, pp 90–92

Hansell Armstrong Lynch Mc Adams. Torax diagnóstico radiológico. 4º ed 2007, Ed. Marban SL

Keane JF, Lock JE, Flyer DC (2006) Nadas pediatric cardiology, 2nd ed. W.B. Saunders, Philadelphia, ISBN: 978-1416023906

Lee J, Sagel SS, Stanley RJ, Heiken JP (eds) (2003) Computed body tomography with MRI correlation, 4th edn. Lippincott Williams & Wilkins, Philadelphia, PA

Lucaya J, Strife JL (2002) Pediatric chest imaging. Chest imaging in infants and children. Springer, Berlin

Lucaya J, Strife JL (2007) Pediatric chest imaging. Springer, Berlin

McHugh K (2008) Chest tumours other than Lymphoma. In: Lucaya J, Strife JL (eds) Pediatric chest imaging, 2nd edn. Springer-Verlag, Berlin, Heidelberg, pp 263–2287

Restrepo CS, Bardo DME (2010a) Cardiac imaging, RadCases Series. Thieme Medical Publishers, New York

Restrepo CS, Bardo DME (2010b) Cardiac imaging: RadCases series. Thieme Medical Publishers, New York

Salcedo Posadas A, García Novo MD (1997) Fibrosis Quística. Ed Roche, 1º edición

Web Link

http://www.uptodate.com/home/index.html
http://www.searchingradiology.com/
http://chestjournal.chestpubs.org/
http://www.uptodate.com/home/index.html
www.thorax.bmj.com
http://www.uptodate.com/home/index.html
http://www.emedicine.medscape.com/article/405994-overview

Berger S (2010) Pulmonary artery sling. Emedicine: WebMD. Last updated March 25, 2010, http://emedicine.medscape.com/article/898075-overview

Gupta M (2010) Partial anomalous pulmonary venous connection. Emedicine: WebMD. Last updated: May 24, 2010, http://emedicine.medscape.com/article/897686-overview

http://www.emedicine.medscape.com/article/150369-diagnosis. Accessed December 5, 2009

Articles

Abbruzzese PA, Aidala E (2007) Aortic coarctation: an overview. J Cardiovasc Med Hagerstown 8:123–128

Ampofo K, Byington C (2007) Management of parapneumonic empyema. Pediatr Infect Dis J 26:445–446

Andronikou S, Kader E (2001) Bronchial mucoepidermoid tumour in a child presenting with organomegaly due to secondary amyloidosis: case report and review of the literature. Pediatr Radiol 31:348–350

Andronikou S, Joseph E, Lucas S, Brachmeyer S, Du Toit G, Zar H et al (2004) CT scanning for the detection of tuberculous mediastinal and hilar lymphadenopathy in children. Pediatr Radiol 34:232–236

Berko NS (2009) Partial anomalous pulmonary venous return: more common from the left or right lung? Anat Sci Int 84(4):327

Berndon WE (2000) Rings, slings and other things: vascular compression of the infant trachea updated from the mid-century to the millennium – the legacy of Robert E. Gross, MD and Edward B.D. Neuhauser MD. Radiology 216:624–632

Berndon WE, Baker DH, Wung J et al (1984) Complete cartilage-ring tracheal stenosis associated with anomalous left pulmonary artery: The ring-sling complex. Radiology 152:57–64

Bhalla M, Turcios N, Aponte V, Jenkins M, Leitman BS, McCaulley DI et al (1991) Cystic fibrosis: scoring system with thin-section CT. Radiology 179:783–788

Brodoefel H, Vogel M, Hebart H, Einsele H, Vonthein R, Claussen C et al (2006) Long-term CT follow-up in 40 non-HIV immunocompromised patients with invasive pulmonary aspergillosis: kinetics of CT morphology and correlation with clinical findings and outcome. AJR Am J Roentgenol 187:404–413

Brody AS (2004) Scoring systems for CT in cystis fibrosis: who cares? Radiology 231:296–298

Burrill J, Williams CJ, Bain G, Conder G, Hine AL, Misra RR (2007) Tuberculosis: a radiologic review. Radiographics 27:1255–1273

Cademartiri F, Luccichenti G, Palumbo AA, Maffei E, Pisi G, Zompatori M et al (2008) Predictive value of chest CT in patients with cystic fibrosis: a single-center 10-year experience. AJR Am J Roentgenol 190:1475–1480

Cameron R, Davies HR (2004) Intra-pleural fibrinolytic therapy versus conservative management in the treatment of parapneumonic effusions and empyema. Cochrane Database Syst Rev 2:CD002312

Cohen MD (1992b) vol 3. Mosby Year Book, pp 20–38

Collins J, Müller NL, Leung AN, McGuinness G, Mergo PJ, Flint JD et al (1998) Epstein-Barr-virus associated lymphoproliferative disease of the lung: CT and histologic findings. Radiology 208:749–759

Cowley CG, Orsmond GS, Feola P, McQuillan L, Shaddy RE (2005) Long-term, randomized comparison of balloon angioplasty and surgery for native coarctation of the aorta in childhood. Circulation 111:3453–3456

Curtis JM, Lacey D, Smyth R, Carty H (1998) Endobronchial tumours in childhood. Eur J Radiol 29:11–20

de Jong PA, Ottink MD, Robben SG, Lequin MH, Hop WC, Hendriks JJ et al (2004) Pulmonary disease assessment in cystic fibrosis: comparison of CT socring systems and value of bronchial and arterial dimension measurements. Radiology 231:434–439

Deiros Bronte L, Baquero-Artigao F, García-Miguel MJ, Hernández González N, Peña García P, del Castillo Martín F (2006) Parapneumonic pleural effusion: an 11-year review. Pediatr Barc 64:40–45

Demos TC, Posniak HV, Pierce KL, Olson MC, Muscato M (2004) Venous anomalies of the thorax. AJR Am J Roentgenol 182:1139–1150

Donnelly L (1999) Maximizing the usefulness of imaging in children with community-acquired pneumonia. AJR Am J Roentgenol 172:505–512

DS LK, Levett JM, Replogle RL (1985) Partial anomalous pulmonary venous return: a ten year experience. Tex Heart Inst J 12(3):239–243

Fauroux B, Aynie V, Larroquet M et al (2005) Carcinoid and mucoepidermoid bronchial tumours in children. Eur J Pediatr 164:748–752

Festa P, Ait-Ali L, Cerillo AG, De Marchi D, Murzi B (2006) Magnetic resonance imaging is the diagnostic tool of choice in the preoperative evaluation of patients with partial anomalous pulmonary venous return. Int J Cardiovasc Imaging 22(5):685–693

Flume PA (2003) FCCP: pneumothorax in cystic fibrosis. Chest 123:217–221

Franquet T, Muller NL, Gimenez A, Guembe P, de La TJ, Bague S (2001) Spectrum of pulmonary aspergillosis: histologic, clinical, and radiologic findings. Radiographics 21:825–837

Franquet T, Gimenez A, Hidalgo A (2004) Imaging of opportunistic fungal infections in immunocompromised patient. Eur J Radiol 51:130–138

Gikonyo BM, Jue KL, Edwards JE (1989) Pulmonary vascular sling: Report of seven cases and review of the literature. Pediatr Cardiol 10:81–89

Greenberg SB (1991) Viral pneumoia. Infect Dis Clin North Am 5:603–621

Greene R (2005) The radiological spectrum of pulmonary aspergillosis. Med Mycol 43(Suppl 1):S147–S154

Gurney JW, Habbe TG, Hicking J (1997) Distribution of disease in cystis fibrosis: correlation with pulmonary function. Chest 112:357–362

Hachem R, Sumoza D, Hanna H, Girgawy E, Munsell M, Raad I (2006) Clinical and radiologic predictors of invasive pulmonary aspergillosis in cancer patients: should the European Organization for Research and Treatment of Cancer/Mycosis Study Group (EORTC/MSG) criteria be revised? Cancer 106:1581–1586

Hamm H, Light RW (1997) The pleura: the outer space of pulmonary medicine. Eur Respir J 10:2–3

Han BK, Son JA, Yoon HK, Lee SI (1998) Epidemic adenoviral lower respiratroy tract infection in pediatric patients:- radiographic and clinical characteristics. AJR Am J Roentgenol 170:1077–1080

Hardie W, Bokulic R, Garcia VF, Reising SF, Christie CD (1996) Pneumococcal pleural empyemas in children. Clin Infect Dis 22:1057–1063

Harisinghani MG, McLoud TC, Shepard JA, Ko JP, Shroff MM, Mueller PR (2000) Tuberculosis from head to toe. Radiographics 20:449–470

Hisatomi K, Eishi K, Hashizume K, Miura T, Taniguchi S, Hashimoto W (2010) Partial anomalous pulmonary venous return. Asian Cardiovasc Thorac Ann 18(2):203–204

Hollingsworth CL, Yoshizumi TT, Frush DP, Chan FP, Toncheva G, Nguyen G et al (2007) Pediatric cardiac-gated CT angiography: assessment of radiation dose. AJR Am J Roentgenol 189:12–18

Hom JJ, Ordovas K, Reddy GP (2008) Velocity-encoded cine MR imaging in aortic coarctation: functional assessment of hemodynamic events. Radiographics 28:407–416

Hornung TS, Benson LN, McLaughlin PR (2002) Interventions for aortic coartation. Cardiol Rev 10:139–148

Indolfi P, Casale F, Bisogno G, Ninfo V, Cecchetto G, Bagnulo S et al (2000) Pleuropulmonary blastoma management in prognosis of 11 cases. Cancer 89:1396–1401

Jeong YJ, Lee KS (2008) Pulmonary tuberculosis: up-to-date imaging and management. AJR Am J Roentgenol 191:834–844

Karnak I, Akçören Z, Senocak ME (2000) Endobronchial leiomyoma in children. Eur J Pediatr Surg 10:136–139

Katz SL, Das P, Ngan BY et al (2005) Remote intrapulmonary spread of recurrent respiratory papillomatosis with malignant transformation. Pediatr Pulmonol 39:185–188

Kim WS, Moon WK, Kim IO, Lee HJ, Im JG, Yeon KM et al (1997) Pulmonary tuberculosis in children: evaluation with CT. AJR Am J Roentgenol 168:1005–1009

Kim HY, Song KS, Goo JM, Lee JS, Lee KS, Lim TH (2001) Thoracic sequelae and complications of tuberculosis. Radiographics 21:839–858

Kim EA, Lee KS, Primack SL, Yoon HK, byun HS, Kim TS et al (2002) Viral pneumonias in adults: radiologic and pathologic findings. Radiographics 22:s137–s149

Kim WS, Choi JI, Cheon JE, Kim IO, Yeon KM, Lee HJ (2006) Pulmonary tuberculosis in infants: radiographic and CT findings. AJR Am J Roentgenol 187:1024–1033

Kobayashi D, Cook AL, Williams DA (2010) Anomalous origin of left pulmonary artery from the aorta with partial anomalous pulmonary venous return. Pediatr Cardiol 31(4):560–561

Kocaoglu M, Bulakbasi N, Soylu K et al (2006) Thin-section axial multidetector computed tomography and multiplanar reformatted imaging of children with suspected foreign-body aspiration: Is virtual bronchoscopy overemphasized? Acta Radiol 47:746–751

Konen E, Merchant N, Provost Y, McLaughlin PR, Crossin J, Paul NS (2004) Coarctation of the aorta before and after correction: the role of cardiovascular MRI. AJR Am J Roentgenol 182:1333–1339

Kula S, Sanli C, Oner AY, Oltuntürk R (2010) Partial anomalous pulmonary venous return associated with coarctation of the aorta. Anadolu Kardiyol Derg 10(1):1–2

Langston C (2003) New concepts in the pathology of congenital lung malformations. Semin Pediatr Surg 12:17–37

Lapierre C, Siles A, Bigras JL (2010) Partial anomalous pulmonary venous return to the azygos vein: an unusual case. Pediatr Cardiol 31(5):749–750, Epub 2010 Feb 27

Lee EY (2007) MDCT and 3D evaluation of type 2 hypoplastic pulmonary artery sling associated with right lung agenesis, hypoplastic aortic arch, and long segment tracheal stenosis. J Thorac Imaging 22(4):346–350

Lee KH, Yoon CS, Choe KO, Kim MJ, Lee HM, Yoon HK, Kim B (2001) Use of imaging for assessing anatomical relationships of tracheobronchial anomalies associated with left pulmonary artery sling. Pediatr Radiol 31(4):269–278

Lee YR, Choi YW, Lee KJ, Jeon SC, Park CK, Heo JN (2005) CT halo sign: the spectrum of pulmonary diseases. Br J Radiol 78:862–865

Leung AN, Müller NL, Pineda PR, FitzGerald JM (1992) Primary tuberculosis in childhood: radiographic manifestations. Radiology 182:87–91

Lin CJ, Chen PY, Huang FL, Lee T, Chi CS, Lin CY (2006) Radiographic, clinical, and prognostic features of complicated and uncomplicated community-acquired lobar pneumonia in children. J Microbiol Immunol Infect 39:489–495

Linnae B, Robinson P, Ranganathan S, Stick S, Murray C (2008) Role of high-resolution computed tomography in the detection of early cystic fibrosis lung disease. Paediatr Respir Rev 9:168–175

MacSweeney F, Papagianopouos K, Goldstraw P, Sheppard MN, Corrin B, Nicholson AG (2003) An assessment of the expanded classification of congenital cystic adenomatoid malformations and their relationship to malignant transformation. Am J Surg Pathol 27:1139–1146

Manivel JC, Priest JR, Watterson BA, Steiner M, Woods WG, Wick MR et al (1988) Pulmonary blastoma: the so-called pulmonary blastoma of childhood. Cancer 62:1516–1526

Marais BJ, Gie RP, Schaaf HS, Starke JR, Hesseling AC, Donald PR et al (2004) A proposed radiological classification of childhood intra-thoracic tuberculosis. Pediatr Radiol 34:886–894

Margolin FR, Gandy TK (1979) Pneumonia of atypical measles. Radiology 131:653–655

Maziak DE, Todd TR, Keshavjee SH et al (1996) Adenoid cystic carcinoma of the airway: thirty-two-year experience. J Thorac Cardiovasc Surg 112:1522–1531

McIntosh K (2002) Community-acquired pneumonia in children. N Engl J Med 346:429–437

Miniati DN, Chintagumpala M, Langston C, Dishop MK, Olutoye OO, Nuchetern JG et al (2006) Prenatal presentation and outcome of children with pleuropulmonary blastoma. J Pediatr Surg 41:66–71

Mitnick J, Becker MH, Rothberg M, Genieser NB (1980) Nodular residua of atipycal measles pneumonia. AJR Am J Roentgenol 134:257–260

Muller FM, Trusen A, Weig M (2002) Clinical manifestations and diagnosis of invasive aspergillosis in immunocompromised children. Eur J Pediatr 161:563–574

Naffaa LN, Donelly LF (2005) Imaging findings in pleuropulmonary blastoma. Pediatr Radiol 35:387–391

Newman B, Cho Y (2010) Left pulmonary artery sling–anatomy and imaging. Semin Ultrasound CT MR 31(2):158–170

Newman B, Meza MP, Towbin RB, Del Nido P (1996) Left pulmonary artery sling: diagnosis and delineation of associated tracheobronchial anomalies with MR. Pediatr Radiol 26:661–668

Nielsen JC, Powell AJ, Gauvreau K, Marcus EN, Prakash A, Geva T (2005) Magnetic resonance imaging predictors of coarctation severity. Circulation 111:622–628

Ogra PL (2004) Respiratory syncytial virus: the virus, the disease and the immune response. Paediatr Respir Rev 5(Suppl A):s119–s126

Olson MA, Becker GJ (1986) The scimitar syndrome: CT findings in partial anomalous pulmonary venous return. Radiology 159:25–26

Orazi C, Inserra A, Schingo PM, De Sio L, Cutrera R, Boldrini R et al (2007) Pleuropulmonary blastoma, a distinctive neoplasm of childhood: report of three cases. Pediatr Radiol 37:337–344

Ortigado Matamala A, García García A, Galicia Poblet G, Jiménez Bustos JM, De Juan Sánchez C (2010) Asymptomatic pulmonary artery sling: noninvasive diagnosis. Pediatr Barc 72(3):205–209

Papagianopoulos PA, Shepard M (2001) Pleuropulmonary blastoma: is prophylactic resection of congenital cyst effective? Ann Thorac Surg 72:604–605

Parrón M, Torres I, Pardo M (2008) The halo sign in computed tomography images: differential diagnosis and correlation with pathology findings. Arch Bronconeumol 44:386–392

Priest JR, McDermott MB, Bhatia S, Watterson J, Manivel JC, Dehner LP (1997) pleuropulmonary blastoma: a clinico-pathological study of 50 cases. Cancer 80:147–161

Primack SL, Hartman TE, Lee KS, Muller NL (1994) Pulmonary nodules and the CT halo sign. Radiology 190:513–515

Quimbao BP, Gatchalian SR, Halonen P, Lucero M, Sombrero L, Paladin Fj et al (1998) Coinfection is common in measles-associated pneumonia. Pediatr Infect Dis J 17:89–93

Ramnath RR, Heller RM, Ben-Ami T et al (1998) Implications of early sonographic evaluation of parapneumonic effusions in children with pneumonia. Pediatrics 101:68–71

Ratjen F, Döping G (2003) Cystic fibrosis. Lancet 361:681–689

Riesenkampff EM, Schmitt B, Schnackenburg B, Huebler M, Alexi-Meskishvili V, Hetzer R, Berger F, Kuehne T (2009) Partial anomalous pulmonary venous drainage in young pediatric patients: the role of magnetic resonance imaging. Pediatr Cardiol 30(4):458–464

Rosenthal E (2005) Coarctation of the aorta from fetus to adult: curable condition or life long disease process? Heart 91:1495–1502

Salcedo Posadas A, Neira Rodríguez MA, Sequeiros González A, Girón Moreno R (1996) Transition between childhood and adulthood in cystic fibrosis. An Esp Pediatr 45:455–458

Shah RM, Sexauer W, Ostrum BJ, Fiel SB, Friedman AC (1997) High-resolution CT in the acute exacerbation of cystic fibrosis: evaluation of acute findings, reversibility of those findings, and clinical correlation. AJR Am J Roentgenol 169:375–380

Shih MC, Tholpady A, Kramer CM, Sydnor MK, Hagspiel KD (2006) Surgical and endovascular repair of aortic coarctation: normal findings and appearance of complications on CT angiography and MR angiography. AJR Am J Roentgenol 187:W302–W312

Soldatski IL, Onufrieva EK, Steklov AM, Schepin NV (2005) Tracheal, bronchial, and pulmonary papillomatosis in children. Laryngoscope 115:1848–1854

Tanaka N, Matsumoto T, Miura G, Emoto T, Matsunaga N (2002) HRCT findings of chest complications in patients with leukemia. Eur Radiol 12:1512–1522

Tateishi A, Kawada M (2009) Partial form of a pulmonary artery sling. Ann Thorac Surg 87(3):965

Thomas KE, Owens CM, Veys PA, Novelli V, Costoli V (2003) The radiological spectrum of invasive aspergillosis in children: a 10-year review. Pediatr Radiol 33:453–460

Van Dyck P, Vanhoenacker FM, Van den Brande P, De Schepper AM (2003) Imaging of pulmonary tuberculosis. Eur Radiol 13:1771–1785

von Schulthess GK, Higashino SM, Higgins SS, Didier D, Fisher MR, Higgins CB (1986) Coarctation of the aorta: MR imaging. Radiology 158:469–474

Welsh JH, Maxson T, Jaksic T et al (1998) Tracheobronchial mucoepidermoid carcinoma in childhood and adolescence: case report and review of the literature. Int J Pediatr Otorhinolaryngol 45:265–273

Wennergren G, Kristjánsson S (2001) Relationship between respiratory syncytial virus bronchiolitis and future obstructive airway diseases. Eur Respir J 18:1044–1058

Wright JR (2000) Pleuropulmonary blastoma. A case report documenting transition from type I (cystic) to type III (solid). Cancer 88:2853–2858

Yedururi S, Guillerman RP, Chung T et al (2008) Multimodality imaging of tracheobronchial disorders in children. Radiographics 28:e29

Zhong YM, Jaffe RB, Zhu M, Gao W, Sun AM, Wang Q (2010) CT assessment of tracheobronchial anomaly in left pulmonary artery sling. Pediatr Radiol, May 19

Contents

M.I. Martínez-León et al., *Learning Pediatric Imaging*, Learning Imaging,
DOI: 10.1007/978-3-642-16892-5_5, © Springer-Verlag Berlin Heidelberg 2011

Case 5.1

Intussusception

■

Pascual García-Herrera Taillefer and Cristina Bravo Bravo

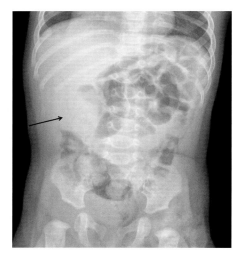

Fig. 5.1

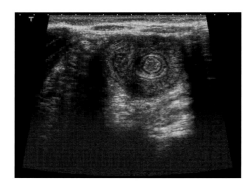

Fig. 5.2

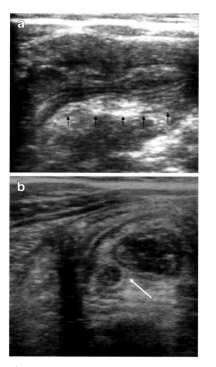

Fig. 5.3

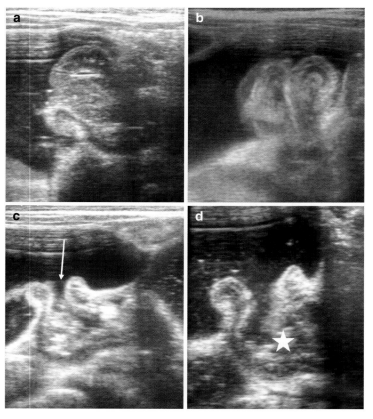

Fig. 5.4

An 18-month-old boy presents with abdominal pain, incessant crying, and lower extremity flexion.

Comments

Intussuception is one of the most frequent causes of acute abdomen in childhood. This occurs when a portion of the intestine (intussusceptum) invaginates into a distal section of bowel (intussuscipiens). The usual age of presentation is between 6 months and 2 years and it is generally idiopathic in nature. The ileocecal region is the most common location. Ultrasound has replaced radiography and barium enema as a non-radiation alternative that serves both as a diagnostic tool (sensibility 98–100%, specificity 88–100%) and as a guide in reduction procedures.

The classic clinical presentation includes colic-type abdominal pain with a palpable mass and bloody stool. Since this triad is present in less than 50% of patients, imaging studies are essential in establishing diagnosis. Abdominal radiography is used in cases of low-suspicion or in order to detect associated complications (perforation or intestinal obstruction). Appearance on ultrasound depends on the location and plane used to evaluate the bowel.

Hydrostatic reduction consists of applying pressure directly to the invaginated intestine without exceeding 120 mmHg (150 cm on saline solution barometry) in order to protect against possible perforation. Ultrasound-guided hydrostatic reduction using saline enema is often effective. Absolute contraindications include: dehydration, shock, and evidence of perforation. If after a 10-min attempt, reduction of the invaginated bowel is not attained, the procedure should be suspended. Furthermore, if the intussuscipiens has been displaced into the base of the cecum, reduction should be reattempted after a few hours, when edema has subsided. Although resolution is obtained in up to 95% of cases, the condition may recur.

Imaging Findings

Radiography of the abdomen shows changes in the normal distribution of bowel gas with an appearance resembling a soft-tissue mass, usually in the right upper quadrant (arrow) (Fig. 5.1). Meniscus sign may or may not be present. Ultrasound reveals a complex mass with a concentric ring pattern (Fig. 5.2) and an echogenic center with a hypoechoic halo. These findings correspond to invaginated mesointestine with associated lymphadenopathies (white arrow). A sandwich-like appearance is revealed on the longitudinal plane view (black arrows) (Fig. 5.3a, b). Real-time ultrasound guides hydrostatic reduction and shows reopening of the ileocecal valve (white arrow) and filling of the terminal ileum (asterisk) (Fig. 5.4a–d).

Figure 5.1
Figure 5.2
Figure 5.3
Figure 5.4a–d

Case 5.2

Hypertrophic Pyloric Stenosis

■

Pascual García-Herrera Taillefer and Cristina Bravo Bravo

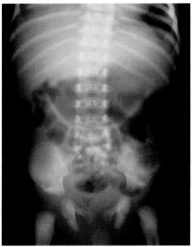

Fig. 5.5

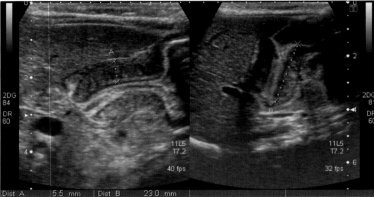

Fig. 5.6

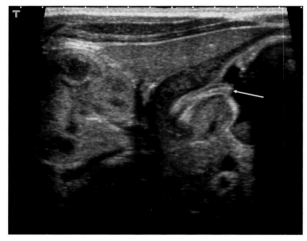

Fig. 5.7

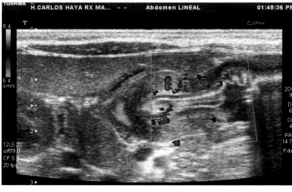

Fig. 5.8

A 3-week-old boy presents with progressively worsening vomiting after feeding and associated weight loss.

Hypertrophic pyloric stenosis (HPS) represents the most common surgically treated cause of vomiting in infants and is more frequent in males and in patients with genetic susceptibility. This condition generally presents during the first weeks of life caused by an idiopathic lack of antro-pyloric muscle relaxation, which leads to progressive hyperplasia and hypertrophy and ultimately, obstructed gastric emptying.

Clinically, previously healthy infants present with non-bilious vomiting that turns projectile. Associated irritability, due to hunger and related electrolyte disturbances, dehydration, and malnutrition, can also be seen. Physical examination may reveal a palpable pyloric "olive" or, in advanced cases, visualization of gastric contraction through the abdominal wall.

Radiography of the abdomen shows gastric distension (Fig. 5.5). On occasion, evidence of distal gas may be absent. Currently, diagnosis of HPS is established by ultrasound, which provides useful information without the use of ionizing radiation or contrast agents. Direct signs include: thickening (>11 mm) and elongation (>15 mm) of the pyloric canal, as well as hypoechoic thickening of the musculature (>3–4 mm) (Fig. 5.6). The gastric mucosa presents hypertrophy and prolapses toward the antrum (arrow); this is known as the "nipple sign" (Fig. 5.7). Color Doppler shows increased vascularization of both the muscular and mucosal layers (Fig. 5.8). Real-time imaging may reveal indirect signs such as gastric distension, defective opening of the distal stomach as peristaltic waves approach, and associated gastroesophageal reflux.

Barium studies are reserved for nonconclusive cases or for when other causes of upper digestive tract obstruction are being evaluated (gastric or duodenal membranes). Classic findings of these studies include: an elongated pyloric canal with a double linear image that appears train track-like, extrinsic bulging of the musculature on the antrum ("shoulder sign"), and vigorous peristalsis.

Figure 5.5
Figure 5.6
Figure 5.7
Figure 5.8

Case 5.3
Mesenteric Lymphadenopathy in Children
Pablo Valdés Solís

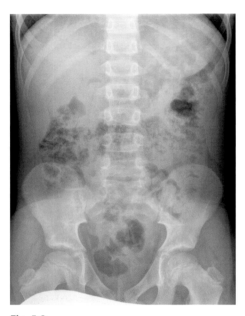

Fig. 5.9

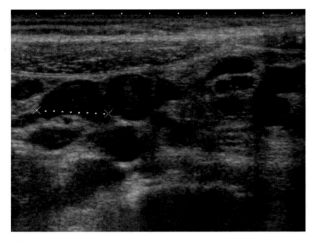

Fig. 5.10

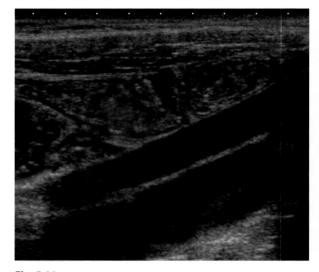

Fig. 5.11

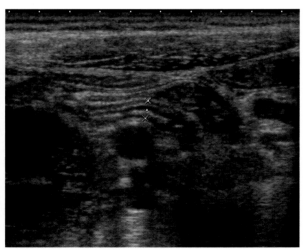

Fig. 5.12

A 5-year-old boy presents with a 24-h history of right lower quadrant pain and low fever. Blood work reveals moderate leukocytosis.

Inflammation of mesenteric lymph nodes is a common cause of abdominal pain in children. Although usually caused by viral infection, it may also develop secondary to pathogens such as *Yersinia enterocolitica*, *Campylobacter jejuni*, and different species of Salmonella. It has also been documented in children with streptococcal pharyngitis or with ileocolitis. Clinical presentation is often nonspecific. Classic symptoms include abdominal pain, fever, nausea, and occasionally diarrhea.

Mesenteric lymphadenopathy is considered a self-limiting condition and its main difficulty is differentiating it from cases of acute appendicitis. Imaging studies are essential for establishing the correct diagnosis. Both ultrasound and CT reveal enlarged mesenteric lymph nodes. Since it represents a diagnosis of exclusion, a normal-appearing appendix must be demonstrated.

The presence of enlarged lymph nodes is a common finding in children. No definite node size criteria have been established to diagnose mesenteric lymphadenopathy. However, values of >8 mm on the minor axis and >20 mm on the mayor axis are generally considered pathological. Apart from size, other characteristics such as number, morphology (rounded), and associated clinical presentation (pain during ultrasound probing) may aid in the final diagnosis.

Radiograph of the abdomen shows the large bowel with fecal matter and nonspecific gas distribution, except for a relative absence of luminal air in the right lower quadrant (Fig. 5.9). Linear ultrasound reveals enlarged mesenteric lymph nodes (Fig. 5.10). This finding is more evident at the right lower quadrant, although it may also be seen in other mesenteric regions. The intestinal bowel shows normal thickness and no significant abnormalities (Fig. 5.11). The appendix is clearly seen with a caliber of less than 4 mm and normal echogenicity (Fig. 5.12). Findings of a normal appendix and non-inflamed bowel established the diagnosis of mesenteric lymphadenopathy.

Figure 5.9
Figure 5.10
Figure 5.11
Figure 5.12

Case 5.4
Acute Appendicitis
Pablo Valdés Solís

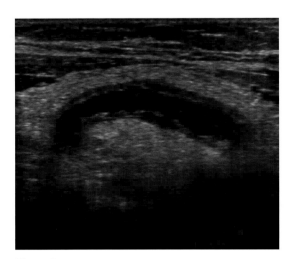

Fig. 5.13

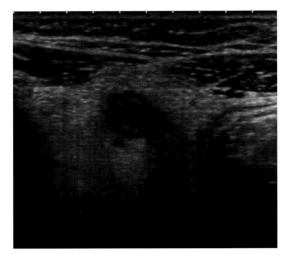

Fig. 5.14

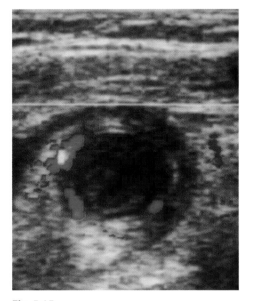

Fig. 5.15

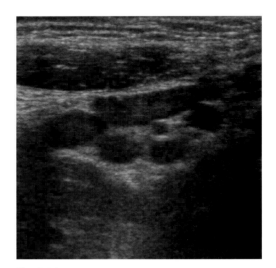

Fig. 5.16

A 12-year-old boy presents with a 36-h history of right lower quadrant pain and fever. Blood work revealed leukocytosis and a differential shift to the left.

Pathogenesis of acute appendicitis is poorly understood. An obstructive cause is considered the most likely theory. Blockage of the appendicular lumen secondary to appendicoliths, fecal matter, lymphoid hyperplasia, and tumors lead to distension of the appendix. A distended appendix is susceptible to infection and mucosal damage. Inflammatory changes lead to increased vascularization, mucosal ulceration, and ultimately perforation. Cases related to systemic, usually viral, infections have also been documented.

Typical clinical presentation consisting of right lower quadrant pain, vomiting, and fever is not always present in children, especially younger patients. In atypical cases, imaging studies are essential in determining an accurate diagnosis. Evidence suggesting the most effective imaging study is scarce. CT is generally considered to be superior to ultrasound in evaluating for possible appendicitis. Nevertheless, given the great disadvantage that ionizing radiation represents to this age group, ultrasound is usually the initial study of choice. CT would then be reserved for nonconclusive cases.

Dynamic ultrasound shows an inflamed, noncompressible appendix with increased caliber (>6 mm), rounded morphology, and peristaltic wave absence. Increased vascular flow seen by Doppler aids in the final diagnosis. Ultrasound also allows for the identification of appendicoliths, even those that are not calcified. In more advanced cases, there is notable lack of definition between the layers of the appendix wall. CT findings include distension, wall thickening (which may present contrast enhancement), and periappendicular inflammatory changes.

B-mode ultrasound of the right lower quadrant shows a noncompressible, fixed, tubular structure, which can be visualized completely (Fig. 5.13). Its wall is thickened and the mucosa is irregular. The mesoappendix shows increased echogenicity secondary to inflammatory changes. The distal end is ill-defined (real-time image not obtained), a finding that suggests perforation. Transverse planes allow for accurate measurements of the caliber of the appendix, in addition to showing its rounded morphology and noncompressible nature (Fig. 5.14). Doppler (Fig. 5.15) displays wall vascularization and adjacent reactive lymphadenopathies can be seen (Fig. 5.16).

Figure 5.13
Figure 5.14
Figure 5.15
Figure 5.16

Case 5.5
Inflammatory Bowel Disease
■
Juio Rambla Vilar and Cinta Sangüesa Nebot

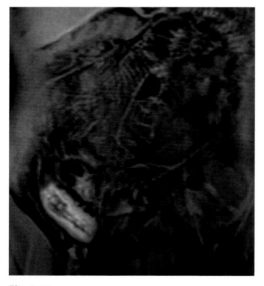

Fig. 5.17

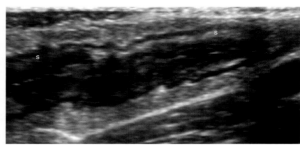

Fig. 5.18

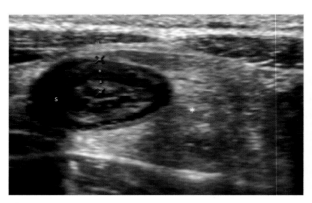

Fig. 5.19

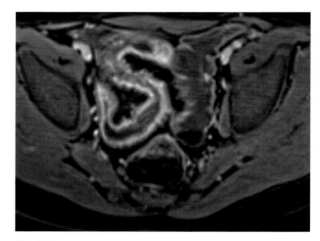

Fig. 5.20

A 12-year-old boy presents with abdominal pain during last 2 months and weight loss of 4 kg.

Inflammatory bowel diseases (IBDs) are complex genetic disorders that include Crohn's disease (CD) and ulcerative colitis (UC). In children, CD is more frequent than UC.

CD is characterized by chronic segmental inflammation that may progressively extend through all layers of the intestinal wall and involve extraintestinal structures. It has recurrent episodes of exacerbation and remission. CD may involve any part of the gastrointestinal tract, but distal ileum and colon are the most frequently affected parts.

Children with CD most often present with several symptoms including abdominal pain, diarrhea, perianal lesions, growth retardation, and weight loss. Because these symptoms are common in children, the diagnosis is often delayed by several months.

The goal of imaging studies in the evaluation of CD is an early diagnosis, complete demonstration of the extent of the disease, detection of its extramural complications, periodic revaluation, and identification of recurrence.

Absence of ionizing radiation and the ability to evaluate both gut wall and extramural extension make sonography a valuable imaging technique. The abnormal segment appears stiff and thickened, with lumen narrowing. At the onset, stratification is preserved and the submucosa thickened and seen as a hyperechoic band. It can be interrupted by deep ulcers. Transmural inflammation extends to all layers and to the surrounding mesentery. Stratification may disappear in severe CD. Doppler US is an excellent method of assessing disease activity.

MRI shows the extension, the activity, and the CD complications especially fistulas, abscesses, and phlegmons. The bowel wall enhancement by gadolinium indicates active disease, a factor of great importance as it could alter disease management.

Ultrasound: Transversal and longitudinal views of the terminal ileum show wall thickening with preserved stratification. Submucosa appears as a hyperechoic band (s) (Figs. 5.17 and 5.18). Surrounding mesenteric fat is thickened due to transmural inflammation (*) (Figs. 5.19 and 5.20). MRI: Axial and coronal FAST contrast-enhanced images. The distal ileum shows marked contrast enhancement in the wall. MRI demonstrates the extension and the activity of the disease perfectly.

Figure 5.17
Figure 5.18
Figure 5.19
Figure 5.20

Case 5.6
Pancreatic Trauma
◼
Inés Solís Muñiz

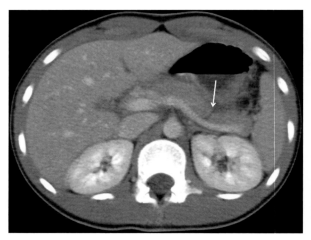

Fig. 5.21

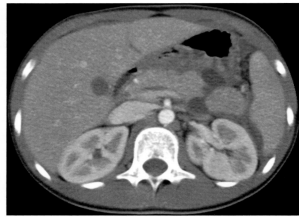

Fig. 5.22

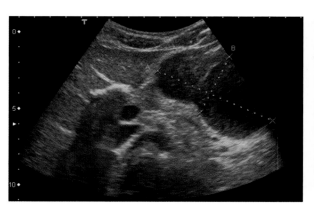

Fig. 5.23

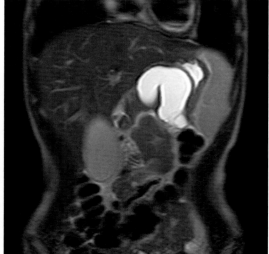

Fig. 5.24

A 14-year-old boy presents with abdominal trauma due to a biking accident. The patient complains of epigastric pain associated to vomiting and shows elevation of serum amylase levels.

Approximately 3–12% of cases of blunt abdominal trauma in the pediatric population present pancreatic involvement, which leads to a mortality rate of 8–10%. The most frequent causes include motor vehicle collisions, bicycle handlebar injuries, and child abuse.

Given the nonspecific clinical manifestations of pancreatic trauma, a thorough clinical history should be obtained. Low-velocity biking accidents with handlebar trauma to the abdomen are a common cause. The neck and body of the pancreas are frequently affected due to a compressive effect against the spinal column. Children are especially susceptible because of their low amount of intra-abdominal adipose tissue.

Absence of abdominal visceral abnormalities and findings of peripancreatic fluid (in the pararenal region and/or lesser sac) suggest possible pancreatic trauma.

Although imaging studies constitute an essential diagnostic tool, findings may be minimal during the first 24 h. Ultrasound is used as the initial imaging technique in evaluating abdominal trauma. The presence of free fluid, clinical suspicion, and suggestive paraclinical test results warrant contrast-enhanced CT imaging. When damage of the main pancreatic duct (Wirsung) is suspected, MR cholangiopancreatography (MRCP) and endoscopic retrograde cholangiopancreatography (ERCP) are indicated, as it is a surgically treated condition. The most frequent complications include the development of pancreatitis, pseudocysts, hemorrhage, fistulas, and sepsis. Pseudocysts are pathological unwalled collections of varying internal content depending on associated hemorrhage or infection.

Contrast-enhanced CT taken 12 h after trauma shows a hypodense linear lesion of the body of the pancreas, consistent with laceration (arrow). A small amount of fluid can be seen in the lesser sac (Fig. 5.21). Contrast-enhanced CT taken 10 days after trauma shows the development of cystic collections on both sides of the pancreas, consistent with pseudocysts (Fig. 5.22). Follow-up ultrasound imaging was performed displaying a progressive enlargement of the cyst (Fig. 5.23). Standard abdominal MRI sequences and MRCP ruled out pancreatic duct lesions (Fig. 5.24).

Figure 5.21
Figure 5.22
Figure 5.23
Figure 5.24

Case 5.7
Focal Nodular Hyperplasia
◼

María Vidal Denis and María I. Martínez León

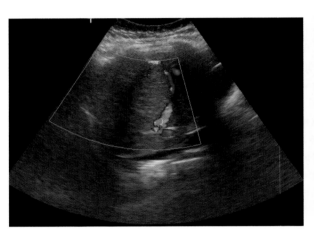

Fig. 5.25

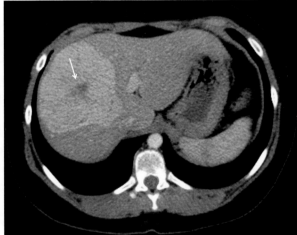

Fig. 5.26

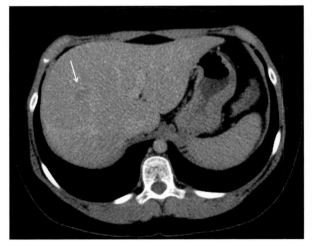

Fig. 5.27

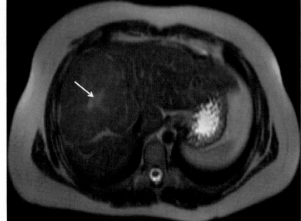

Fig. 5.28

A 13-year-old boy presents with nonspecific abdominal discomfort. Examination reveals excess weight and there are no paraclinical result abnormalities.

Focal nodular hyperplasia (FNH) is not considered a true neoplasm but rather a hyperplastic response of the hepatic parenchyma to a congenital vascular abnormality. This condition results in the formation of a hepatic nodule composed, histologically, by hepatocytes and Kupffer cells (abnormal but not neoplastic), as well as abundant malformed biliary ducts. Additionally, these nodules present a star-like central scar within which evidence of thickened arteries run from its center to the periphery.

Up to 8% of cases present in children under the age of 15 years and it constitutes approximately 2–7.5% of hepatic tumors in childhood, although it is typically seen in women of reproductive age.

FNH tends to have a stable clinical evolution and no cases of malignant transformation have been reported.

Close clinical follow-up is the preferred management in asymptomatic cases (up to 90% of patients) and surgery is reserved for symptomatic patients (usually cholestasis due to compressive effect on the biliary tract) or when diagnosis is uncertain. Differential diagnoses include benign hepatic tumors such as hemangiomas, adenomas, and hamartomas, as well as malignant neoplasms like fibrolamellar carcinoma.

Ultrasound reveals an isoechoic lesion of the hepatic parenchyma with evidence of peripheral and central vessels seen on the Doppler study (Fig. 5.25).

CT imaging without contrast (not shown) shows a well-delineated mass of isodense signal in relation to the surrounding parenchyma, with a pseudocapsule that corresponds to compressed liver tissue. With contrast administration, the lesion presents intense, homogeneous enhancement in the arterial phase (Fig. 5.26), with the exception of the central scar, which shows characteristically delayed uptake (arrow) (Fig. 5.27).

On MR imaging, the FNH appears isointense to adjacent parenchyma and the central scar is hyperintense on T2-weighted sequences (arrow) (Fig. 5.28), which corresponds with the presence of vascular channels and biliary ducts.

Figure 5.25
Figure 5.26
Figure 5.27
Figure 5.28

Case 5.8
Ascariasis
■
Silvia Villa Santamaría and Susana Calle Restrepo

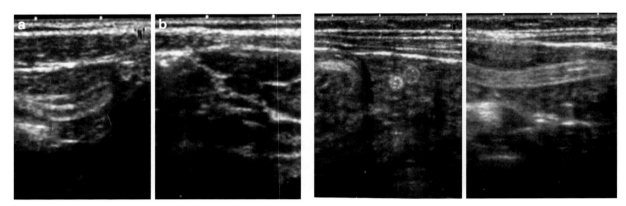

Fig. 5.29

Fig. 5.30

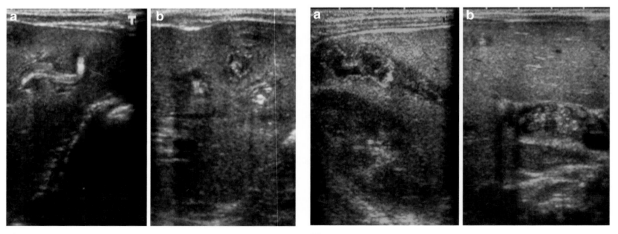

Fig. 5.31

Fig. 5.32

A 2-year-old male patient with grade III malnutrition and failure to thrive presents with several months of abdominal pain, vomiting, increase in abdominal diameter, and during the last 8 days, a fever of 38.5°C and marked pallor.

Comments

Ascaris lumbricoides is a parasite found in soil and human feces and is the nematode most commonly found in the gastrointestinal tract of humans. This parasitic worm is transmitted by an oral–fecal route, with an increased prevalence in developing nations, tropical climates, and regions with poor hygiene. Furthermore, children are at a greater risk of developing this infection.

Ascariasis occurs when the parasite's eggs are ingested, then travel to the duodenum and, by gastric enzyme activity, release larva that then penetrate the intestinal mucosa and reach portal circulation, which delivers the worm to the liver where it may remain up to 96 h. Later, the infection may travel to the heart and lungs by means of pulmonary circulation, where the larva may penetrate the alveoli and bronchi, then reach the pharynx where they may be ingested and reach the duodenum in their adult state where they can remain for months in the intestinal lumen. The infection may produce symptoms such as abdominal pain, changes in bowel habits including bowel obstruction, severe inflammatory processes, and migration to the biliary tract that may cause jaundice, cholangitis, stone formation, and hepatic abscesses.

Treatment of this condition is done with antiparasitic drugs that aid in the elimination of the nematode, and in certain cases, depending on the clinical presentation, surgical management is required.

Imaging Findings

Ultrasound image shows a hypoechoic tubular structure with echogenic, moving walls within an intestinal loop, which corresponds to *Ascaris lumbricoides* (Fig. 5.29a). Associated right lower quadrant lymphadenopathies are seen (Fig. 5.29b). Transverse and longitudinal ultrasound views of the parasite can be seen (Fig. 5.30). Hepatobiliary ultrasound reveals the parasite ascending through the intrahepatic biliary tract (Fig. 5.31a). Transverse views show hepatic abscesses with Ascaris worms within (Fig. 5.31b). A hepatic abscess caused by ascariasis (Fig. 5.32a) and parasites within the gall bladder are also shown (Fig. 5.32b).

Figure 5.29a, b
Figure 5.30
Figure 5.31a, b
Figure 5.32a, b

Case 5.9

Congenital Imperforate Hymen with Hydrocolpos

Pascual García-Herrera Taillefer and Cristina Bravo Bravo

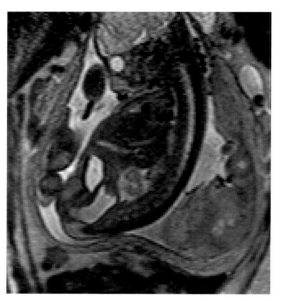

Fig. 5.33

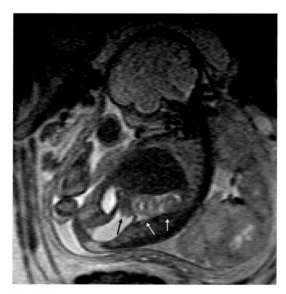

Fig. 5.34

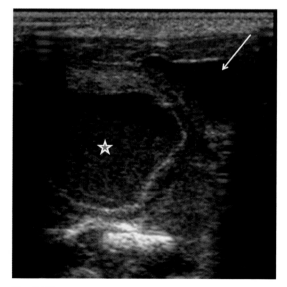

Fig. 5.35

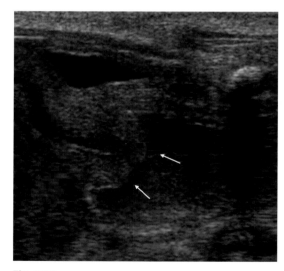

Fig. 5.36

Pregnant woman, whom after an abnormal ultrasound exam at 36 week of gestation that revealed a pelvic cystic lesion, absence of the left kidney, and a single umbilical artery is referred for a fetal MRI.

Comments

The vagina is canalized during the fifth month of fetal age and its embryonic origin is the Müllerian duct and urogenital sinus. The hymen is a remnant of the urogenital sinus that should ultimately develop a lumen. When this perforation fails to occur, secretions build up inside the vagina (hydrocolpos) and, in more advanced cases, affect the uterus as well (hydrometrocolpos). Complex manifestations include urinary tract and cloacal involvement.

Congenital utero-vaginal obstructions present in the third trimester of pregnancy as pelvic cystic lesions. Suggestive prenatal findings can be confirmed at birth by thorough physical examination of the newborn and postnatal ultrasound used to evaluate the urinary tract.

Imaging Findings

Sagittal, T2-weighted fetal MR image shows a cystic mass at the posterior aspect of the bladder, with a normal uterus and the cervix making a mark at its most cranial portion (arrow) (Figs. 5.33 and 5.34). The main differential diagnoses include type III teratoma (it shows more heterogeneity, septations, and solid components) and anterior myelomeningocele (dysraphism is invariably present). Crossed renal ectopia may also be observed (double arrow).

Postnatal axial ultrasound of the pelvis minor reveals a thin-walled, finely echogenic, cystic lesion (asterisk) at the posterior aspect of the bladder (arrow) occupying the vaginal canal and prolapsing toward the vulva (Fig. 5.35). With the sagittal plane view, a normal neonatal uterus (arrows) is seen at the cranial end of the lesion (Fig. 5.36)

Figure 5.33
Figure 5.34
Figure 5.35
Figure 5.36

Case 5.10
Intrauterine Spermatic Cord Torsion

◼

Francisco Pérez Nadal

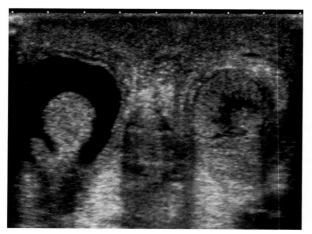

Fig. 5.37

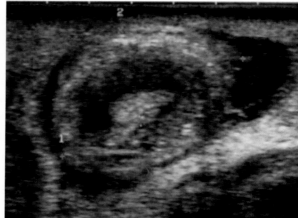

Fig. 5.38

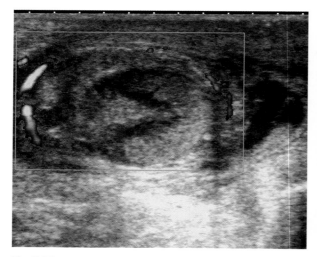

Fig. 5.39

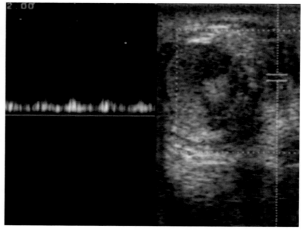

Fig. 5.40

A 39-week full-term neonate, born by eutocic delivery, and weighing 3,375 g presents with a painless, non-inflamed enlargement of the left hemiscrotum.

Testicular torsion can be extravaginal (intrauterine-neonatal) or intravaginal (seen in older children), as well as complete or incomplete.

Extravaginal testicular torsions are idiopathic and occur before the vaginal tunic contains the scrotal structures. This disturbance causes hemorrhagic necrosis, calcifications, and atrophy that affect the testicle, epididymis, and vaginal tunic, ultimately leading to anorchism. They represent approximately 5–12% of testicular torsions in infancy.

Generally, extravaginal torsions are prenatal and unilateral. However, they may occasionally occur bilaterally and synchronously, the asynchronous presentation being uncommon. At birth the testicle is nonviable, presenting a hardened increase in size without evidence of inflammation. Acute forms of torsion, developing after birth, are a clinical emergency and require immediate intervention in order to save the functionality of the testicle. Differential diagnoses include hernias, orchiepididymitis, testicular appendix torsion, trauma, hydrocele, meconial peritonitis, and scrotal tumors, among others. Doppler serves as an essential tool in establishing diagnosis. Findings consistent with changes in echogenicity, hematoma, hydrocele, hyperechoic rings, albugineal tunic calcifications, and decreased Doppler flow suggest testicular torsion. On the other hand, other conditions present more frequently with increased vascularization, peristasis, and fluid collections. Although their incidence is low in children under the age of 1 month, the presence of neoplasms must be ruled out. During the initial stage of testicular torsion, the testes may be viable, with normal echogenicity but no visible blood flow. Chronic forms may show collateral vessel formation. In incomplete torsions, venous flow may be interrupted while arterial flow remains, although with high resistance and inverted diastole.

In the acute phase, treatment is surgical correction with testicular fixation to the scrotum. On the other hand, surgery while in the chronic period is currently controversial.

Heterogeneous testicle surrounded by a hyperechoic ring and mild hydrocele with debris (Fig. 5.37). Hyperechoic mediastinum testis is shown (Fig. 5.38) with an increase in size, no visible testicular blood flow, and presence of collateral arteries (Fig. 5.39) and veins (Fig. 5.40) in the scrotal walls.

Figure 5.37
Figure 5.38
Figure 5.39
Figure 5.40

Further Reading

Books

Botero D, Restrepo M (2003a) Parasitosis humanas, 4th edn. Corporación para Investigaciones Biológicas, Medellin, Colombia

Fiocchi C (2007a) "Una visión integrada de la fisiopatología de la enfermedad inflamatoria intestinal". In: Casullo MA, Gomollón F, Hinojosa J, Obrador A (eds) enfermedad inflamatoria intestinal, 3rd edn. Ed Arán, Madrid, pp 117–129

Haaga J, Lanzieri C, Gilkeson R. TC y MR (2001) Diagnóstico por imagen del cuerpo humano. Madrid, Elsevier España, 4 ed, p 1271

Siegel MJ (1991) Pediatric sonography. Raven, Capítulo, p 11

Siegel MJ (2002a) Pediatric sonography. Lippincott Williams & Wilkins, Philadelphia, PA

Siegel MJ, Babyn PS, Lee EY (2008a) Pediatric body CT. Lippincott Williams & Wilkins, Philadelphia, PA, pp 449–452

Sivit CJ, Siegel MJ (2004a) Invaginación intestinal. In: Siegel MJ (ed) Ecografía Pediátrica, 2nd edn., pp 355–358

Sivit CJ, Siegel MJ (2004b) Estenosis hipertrófica de píloro. In: Siegel MJ (ed) Ecografía Pediátrica, 2nd edn., pp 340–344

Swischuk LE (1986a) Emergency radiology of the acutely ill or injured child, 2nd edn. Williams & Wilkins, Baltimore, MD

Swischuk LE (2005) Malformaciones del útero y la vagina. En: Swischuk, ed. Radiología en el niño y en el recién nacido, pp 681–685

Sivit CJ, Siegel MJ (2004c) Invaginación intestinal. In: Siegel MJ (ed) Ecografía Pediátrica, 2nd edn., pp 355–358

Sivit CJ, Siegel MJ (2004d) Estenosis hipertrófica de píloro. In: Siegel MJ (ed) Ecografía Pediátrica, 2nd edn., pp 340–344

Siegel MJ (2002b) Pediatric sonography. Lippincott Williams & Wilkins, Philadelphia, PA

Swischuk LE (1986b) Emergency radiology of the acutely ill or injured child, 2nd edn. Williams & Wilkins, Baltimore, MD

Fiocchi C (2007b) "Una visión integrada de la fisiopatología de la enfermedad inflamatoria intestinal". In: Casullo MA, Gomollón F, Hinojosa J, Obrador A (eds) Enfermedad inflamatoria intestinal, 3rd edn. Ed Arán, Madrid, pp 117–129

Siegel MJ, Babyn PS, Lee EY (2008b) Pediatric body CT. Lippincott Williams & Wilkins, Philadelphia, PA, pp 449–452

Haaga J, Lanzieri C, Gilkeson R. TC y MR (2001) Diagnóstico por imagen del cuerpo humano. Madrid, Elsevier España, 4 ed, p 1271

Botero D, Restrepo M (2003b) Parasitosis humanas, 4th edn. Corporación para Investigaciones Biológicas, Medellin, Colombia

Swischuk LE (2005) Malformaciones del útero y la vagina. En: Swischuk, ed. Radiología en el niño y en el recién nacido, pp 681–685

Siegel MJ (1991) Pediatric sonography. Raven, Capítulo, p 11

Web Link

www.emedicine.medscape.com/article/930708-overview
www.emedicine.medscape.com/article/929829-overview
http://emedicine.medscape.com/article/411043-overview
http://emedicine.medscape.com/article/773895-overview
http://www.uptodate.com

http://emedicine.medscape.com/article/821995-overview
http://journals.lww.com/jpgn/Fulltext/2001/04000/Focal_Nodular_Hyperplasia_in_Children.17.aspx
http://www.medigraphic.com/pdfs/circir/cc-2003/cc034i.pdf
Montiel-Jarquín A, Carrillo-Ríos C, Flores-Flores J (2010) Ascaridiasis vesicular asociada a hepatitis aguda. Manejo conservador. Cir Ciruj 2003;71:314–318
www.emedicine.medscape.com/article/954252-overview
http://emedicine.medscape.com/article/438817-overview
www.medigraphic.com/espanol/e-htms/e-circir/e-cc2004/e-cc04-1/em-cc041h.htm

Articles

Adaleti I, Ozer H, Kurugoglu S, Emir H, Madazli R (2007) Congenital imperforate hymen with hydrocolpos diagnosed using prenatal MRI. AJR Am J Roentgenol 189:W23–W25

Alexopoulou E, Roma E, Loggitsi D, Economopoulos N, Papakonstantinou O, Panagiotou I et al. (2009) Magnetic resonance imaging of the small bowel in children with idiopathic inflammatory bowel disease: evaluation of disease activity. Pediatr Radiol. Published on line: 19 May 2009

Alison M, Kheniche A, Azoulay R (2007) Ultrasonography of Crohn disease in children. Pediatr Radiol 37:1071–1082

Applegate K, Maglinte D (2008) Imaging of the bowel in children: new imaging tecniques. Pediatr Radiol 38(Suppl 2): S272–S274

Arcement CM, Meza MP, Arumanla S, Towbin RB (2001) MRCP in the evaluation of pancreaticobiliary disease in children. Pediatr Radiol 31:92–97

Aso C, Enríquez G, Fité M, Torán N, Piró C, Piqueras J, Lucaya J (2005) Gray-scale and color doppler sonography of scrotal disorders in children: an update. Radiographics 25:1197–1214

Babyn PS, Kellenberger CJ, Dick PT et al (2006) US or CT for diagnosis of appendicitis in children and adults? A meta-analysis. Radiology 241:83–94

Baldisserotto M (2009) Scrotal emergencias. Pediatr Radiol 39:516–521

Barret Connor E (1982) Parasitic pulmonary disease. Am Rev Respir Dis 126:558–563

Bay YZ, Qu RB, Wang GD, cols y (2006) Ultrasoud-guided hydrostatic reduction of intussusceptions by saline enema: a review of 5.218 cases in 17 years. Am J Surg 192(3):273–275

Bhargava P, Dighe M (2009) Prenatal US diagnosis of congenital imperforate hymen. Pediatr Radiol 39:1014

Bogen DL, Gehris RP, Bellinger MF (2000) Special feature: picture of the month. Denouement and discussion: imperforate hymen with hydrocolpos. Arch Pediatr Adolesc Med 154(9):959–960

Bosboom D, Braam AW, Blickman JG, Wijnen RM (2006) The role of imaging studies in pancreatic injury due to blunt abdominal trauma in children. Eur J Radiol 59:3–7

Bremmer A, Griffiths M, Argent J (2006) Sonographic evaluation of inflammatory bowel disease: a prospective, blinded, comparative study. Pediatr Radiol 36:947–953

Brown SM, Casillas VJ, Montalvo BM, Albores-Saavedra J (1990) Intrauterine spermatic cord torsion in the newborn: sonographic and pathologic correlation children. Radiology 177:755–757

Buetow PC, Pantongrag-Brown L, Buck JL, Ros PR, Goodman ZD (1996) Focal nodular hyperplasia of the liver: radiologic-patologic correlation. Radiographics 16:369–388

Callahan MJ, Rodriguez DP, Taylor GA (2002) CT of appendicitis in children. Radiology 224:325–332

Carrasco Torres R, Castañón García-Alix M, San Vicente Vela B, Montaner Brunat A, Morales Fochs L (2001) Focal nodular hyperplasia of the liver. An Esp Pediatr 55:569–572

Catalano O, Forcione D, Czermak B, Sahani D, Liu C, Muller P (2009) Biliary infections: spectrum of imaging management. Radiographics 29:2059–2080

Chicano Marín FJ, Torroba Carón A, Aranda García MJ, Ruiz Jiménez JI, Jiménez Abadía MA (2000) Focal nodular hyperplasia. A report of a new case. An Esp Pediatr 52:279–280

Choi CS, Freeny PC (1998) Triphasic helical CT of hepatic focal nodular hyperplasia: incidence of atypical findings. AJR Am J Roentgenol 170:391–395

Crystal P, Hertzanu Y, Farber B, cols y (2002) Sonographi-cally guided hydrostatic reduction of intussusception in children. J Clin Ultrasound 30(6):343–348

Cuervo JL, Grillo A, Vecchiarelli C, Osio C, Prudent L (2007) Perinatal testicdular torsión: a unique strategy. J Pediatr Surg 42(4):699–703

Daneman A, Navarro O (2003) Intussusception. Part 1: a review of diagnostic aproaches. Pediatr Radiol 33(2):79–85

de Silva NR, Guyatt HL (1997) Budny dA: morbidity and mortality due to ascaris-induced intestinal obstruction. Trans R Soc Trop Med Hyg 91:31–36

Del Pozo G, Albillos JC, Tejedor D, Calero R, Rasero M, De la Calle U, Lopez-Pacheco U (1999) Intussusception in children: current concepts in diagnosis and enema reduction. Radiographics 19:299–319

Doria AS (2009) Optimizing the role of imaging in appendicitis. Pediatr Radiol 39(Suppl 2):S144–S148

Evans TN, Poland ML, Boving RL (2001) Vaginal malformations. Am J Obstet Gynecol 15:910–920

Gaca AM, Jaffe T, Delaney S, Yoshizumi T, Toncheva G, Nguyen G et al (2008) Radiation doses from small-bowel follow-through and abdomine/pelvis MDCT in pediatric Crohn disease. Pediatr Radiol 38:285–291

Garcia P, Barbara M, Cook EF, Mandl KD (2004) Selective imaging strategies for the diagnosis of appendicitis in children. Pediatrics 113:24–28

Garel L, Dubois J, Grignon A, Filiatrault D, Van Vliet G (2001) US of the pediatric female pelvis: a clinical perspective. Radiographics 21:1393–1407

Gimondo P, Mirk P, Messina G, Pizzi C (1996) Abdominal lymphadenopathy in benign diseases: sonographic detection and clinical significance. J Ultrasound Med 15:353–359

Gross JA, Vaughan MM, Johnston BD, Jurkovich G (2002) Handlebar injury causing pancreatic contusion in a pediatric patient. AJR Am J Roentgenol 179:222

Grove DI (2010) Helmintic diseases in the abdomen: an epidemiologic and radiologic overview. Radiographics 30:253–267

Grübner R, Pistor G, Abou-Touk B, Alcen G (1986) Significance of ultrasound for the diagnosis of hypertrophic pyloric stenosis. Pediatr Surg Int 1:130–134

Gupta A, Stuhlfaut JW, Fleming KW, Lucey BS, Soto JA (2004) Blunt trauma of the pancreas and biliary tract: a multimodality imaging approach to diagnosis. Radiographics 24:1381–1395

Hayden CK Jr, Swischuk LE, Lobe TE, Schwartz MZ, Boulden T (1984) Ultrasound: the definive imagin modality in pyloric stenosis. Radiographics 4:517–530

Hernandez JA, Swischuk LE, Angel CA, Chung D, Chandler R, Lee S (2005) Imaging of acute appendicitis: US as the primary imaging modality. Pediatr Radiol 35:392–395

Hernanz-Schulman M (2003) Infantile hipertrophic pyloric stenosis. Radiology 227:319–331

Hernanz-Schulman M (2009) Pyloric stenosis: role of imagin. Pediatr Radiol 39(Suppl 2):S134–S139

Herranz-Schulman M, Zhu Y, Stein SM, Heller RM, Bethel LA (2003) Hypertrophic pyloric stenosis in infants: US evaluation of vascularity of the pyloric canal. Radiology 229:389–393

Hiorns MP (2008) Imaging of inflammatory bowel disease. How? Pediatr Radiol 38 (Suppl 3):S512–S517

Holscher HC, Heij HA (2009) Imaging of acute appendicitis in children: EU versus U.S. or US versus CT? A European perspective. Pediatr Radiol 39:497–499

Hörmann M, Balassy C, Philipp MO, Pumberger W (2004) Imaging of the scrotum in children. Eur Radiol 14:974–983

Hugot JP, Bellaiche M (2007) Inflammatory bowel diseases: the paediatric gastroenterologist´s perspective. Pediatr Radiol 37:1065–1070

Hussain SM, Terkivatan T, Zondervan PE, Lanjouw E, de Rave S, Ijzermans Jn et al (2004) Focal nodular hyperplasia: findings at state-of-the-art MR imagings, US, CT and pathologic analysis. Radiographics 24:3–17

Karakas SP, Guelfguat M, Leonidas JC, Springer S, Singh SP (2000) Acute appendicitis in children: comparison of clinical diagnosis with ultrasound and CT imaging. Pediatr Radiol 30:94–98

Karmazyn B, Werner EA, Rejaie B, Applegate KE (2005) Mesenteric lymph nodes in children: what is normal? Pediatr Radiol 35:774–777

Kenney PJ, Spirt BA, Leeson MD (1984) Genitourinary anomalies: radiologic-anatomic correlations. Radiographics 4 (num 2):233–260

Klim SC, Ferry GD (2004) Inflammatory bowel diseases in paediatric and adolescent patients: clinical, therapeutic and psychosocial considerations. Gastroenterology 126:1550–1560

Koumanidou C, Manoli E, Anagnostara A, Polyviou P, Vakaki M (2004) Sonographic features of intestinal and biliary ascariasis in childhood: case report and review of the literature. Ann Trop Paediat 24(4):329–335

Lucey BC, Stuhlfaut JW, Soto JA (2005) Mesenteric lymph nodes seen at imaging: causes and significance. Radiographics 25:351–365

Martin DR, Danrad R, Hussain SM (2005) MR imaging of the liver. Radiol Clin North Am 43:861–886

Martinez S, Restrepo S, Carillo J, Betancurt S, Franquet T, Varon C, Ojeda P, Gimenez A (2005) Thoracic manifestations of tropical parasitic infections: a pictorial review. Radiographics 25:135–155

Mc Cort J (1958) Ascaris ileus in children. Radiology 70:528–531

Mortelé KJ, Praet M, Van Vlierberghe H, Kunnen M, Ros PR (2000) CT and MR imaging findings in focal nodular hyperplasia of the liver: radiologic-pathologic correlation. AJR Am J Roentgenol 175:687–692

Nijs E, Callahan MJ, Taylor GA (2005) Disorders of the pediatric pancreas: imaging features. Pediatr Radiol 35:358–373

Nussbaum Blask AR, Sanders RC, Gearhart MD (1991) Obstructed uterovaginal anomalies: demonstration with sonography. Part I. Neonates and infants. Radiology 179:79–83

Panteli C (2009) New insights into the pathogenesis of infantile pyloric stenosis. Pediatr Surg Int 25:1043–1052

Poortman P, Oostvogel HJM, Bosma E et al (2009) Improving diagnosis of acute appendicitis: results of a diagnostic pathway with standard use of ultrasonography followed by selective use of CT. J Am Coll Surg 208:434–441

Puylaert JB (2003) Ultrasonography of the acute abdomen: gastrointestinal conditions. Radiol Clin North Am 41:1227–1242, vii

Pylant A, Hinshaw JW, Leonard RB, Zelman S (2006) Intestinal ascariasis: CT findings and diagnosis. S Med J 99(3):317–318

Quillin SP, Siegel MJ (1993) Color Doppler US of children with acute lower abdominal pain. Radiographics 13:1281–1293

Rao PM, Rhea JT, Novelline RA (1997) CT diagnosis of mesenteric adenitis. Radiology 202:145–149

Rathaus V, Zissin R, Werner M (2001) Minimal pelvic fluid in blunt abdominal trauma in children: the significance of this sonographic finding. J Pediatr Surg 36:1387–1389

Rathaus V, Shapiro M, Grunebaum M, Zissin R (2005) Enlarged mesenteric lymph nodes in asymptomatic children: the value of the finding in various imaging modalities. Br J Radiol 78:30–33

Rekhi S, Anderson SW, Rhea JT, Soto JA (2010) Imaging of blunt pancreatic trauma. Emerg Radiol 17:13–19

Riebel TW, Nasir R, Weber K (1993a) US-guided hydrostatic reduction of intussusception in children. Radiology 188(2):513–516

Riebel TW, Nasir R, Weber K (1993b) US-guided hydrostatic reduction of intussusception in children. Radiology 188:513–516

Ripolles T, Martinez MJ, Paredes JM (2009) Crohn disease: correlation of findings at contrast-enhanced US with severity at endoscopy. Radiology 253:241–248

Rohrschneider WK, Mittnacht H, Drage K, Tröger J (1998) Pyloric muscle in asymptomatic infants: sonographic evaluation and discrimination from idiopathic hypertrophic pyloric stenosis. Pediatr Radiol 28:429–434

Ruppert-Kohlmayr AJ, Uggowitzer MM, Kugler C, Zebedin D, Schaffler Gruppert GS (2001) Focal nodular hyperplasia and hepatocellular adenoma of the liver: differentiation with multiphasic helical CT. AJR Am J Roentgenol 176:1493–1498

Sargent MA, Babyn P, Alton DJ (1994) Plain abdominal radiography in suspected intusussusception: a reassessment. Pediatr Radiol 24:17–20

Sargent SK, Foote SL, Mooney DP, Shorter NA (2000) The posterior approach to pyloric sonography. Pediatr Radiol 30:256–257

Schaffer RM, Taylor C, Haller JO, Friedman AP, Shih YH (1983) Nonobstructive hydrocolpos: sonographic appearance and differential diagnosis. Radiology 149:273–278

Shen Z, She Y, Ding W, Wang L (1989) Changes in pyloric tumor of infantile hypretrophic pyloric stenosis before and after pyloromyotomy. Pediatr Surg Int 4:322–325

Shrivastav A, Pal J (2008) Medical image: Ascaris lumbricoides. N Z Med J 121(1285):126–129

Simanovsky N, Hiller N (2007) Importance of sonographic detection of enlarged abdominal lymph nodes in children. J Ultrasound Med 26:581–584

Sivit CJ (2004) Imaging the child with right lower quadrant pain and suspected appendicitis: current concepts. Pediatr Radiol 34:447–453

Sivit CJ, Eichelberger MR (1995) CT diagnosis of pancreatic injury in children: significance of fluid separating the splenic vein and the pancreas. AJR Am J Roentgenol 165:921–924

Sivit CJ, Eichelberger MR, Taylor GA et al (1992) Blunt pancreatic trauma in children: CT diagnosis. AJR Am J Roentgenol 158:1097–1100

Sivit CJ, Newman KD, Chandra RS (1993) Visualization of enlarged mesenteric lymph nodes at US examination. Clinical significance. Pediatr Radiol 23:471–475

Somech R, Brazowski E, Kesller A, Weiss B, Getin E, Lerner A et al (2001) Focal nodular hyperplasia in children. J Pediatr Gastroenterol Nutr 32:480–483

Srinivasan AS, Darge K (2009) Neonatal scrotal abscess: a differential diagnostic challenge for the acute scrotum. Pediatr Radiol 39:91

Stocker JT, Ishak KG (1981) Focal nodular hyperplasia of the liver: a study of 21 pediatric cases. Cancer 48:336–345

Stoker J, van Adrienne R, Boermeester MA, Ubbink DT, Bipat S, Zwinderman AH (2008) Acute appendicitis: meta-analysis of diagnostic performance of CT and graded compression US related to prevalence of disease. Radiology 249:97–106

Sung T, Riedlinger WF, Diamond DA, Chow JS (2006) Solid extratesticular masses in children: radiographic and pathologic correlation. AJR Am J Roentgenol 186:483–490

Swischuk LE, Stanberry SD (1991) Ultrasonographic detection of free peritoneal fluid in uncomplicated intussusception. Pediatr Radiol 21:350–351

Swischuk LE, Hayden CK, Stansberry SD (1989) Sonographic pitfalls in imagin of antropyloric region in infants. Radiographics 9:437–447

Toma P, Granata C, Magnano G, Barabino A (2007) CT and MRI of paedietric Crohn disease. Pediatr Radiol 37:1083–1092

Tran ATB, Arensman RM, Falterman KW (2007) Diagnosis and management of hydrohematometrocolpos syndromes. Am J Dis Child 141:632–634

Traubici J, Daneman A, Navarro O, Mohanta A, García C (2003) Original report. Testicular torsion in neonates and infants: sonographic features in 30 patients. AJR Am J Roentgenol 180:1143–1145

van der Sluijs JW, den Hollander JC, Lequin MH, Nijman RM, Robben SG (2004) Prenatal testicular torsion: diagnosis and natural course. An ultrasonographic study. Eur Radiol 14:250–255

Vayner N, Coret A, Polliack G, Weiss B, Hertz M (2003) Mesenteric lymphadenopathy in children examined by US for chronic and/or recurrent abdominal pain. Pediatr Radiol 33:864–867

Venkatesh SK, Chin Wan JM (2008) CT of blunt pancreatic trauma – a pictorial essay. Eur J Radiol 67:311–320

Villamizar E, Mendez M, Bonilla E, Varon H, de Onatra S (1996) Ascaris lumbricoides infestation as a cause of intestinal obstruction in children: experience with 87 cases. J Pediatr Surg 31:201–205

Watanabe M, Ishii E, Hirowatari Y et al (1997) Evaluation of abdominal lymphadenopathy in children by ultrasonography. Pediatr Radiol 27:860–864

Woo SK, Kim JS, Suh SJ, Paik TW, Choi SO (1992) Childhood intussusception: US-guided hydrostatic reduction. Radiology 182:77–80

Woodward PJ, Sohaey R, Kennedy A, Koeller KK (2005) A comprehensive review of fetal tumors with pathologic correlations. Radiographics 25:215–242

Zelrin JM, DiPietro MA, Grignon A, Shea D (1990) Testicular infarction in the newborn: ultrasound findings. Pediatr Radiol 20:329–330

Contents

M.I. Martínez-León et al., *Learning Pediatric Imaging*, Learning Imaging,
DOI: 10.1007/978-3-642-16892-5_6, © Springer-Verlag Berlin Heidelberg 2011

Case 6.1
Neuroblastoma
■

Julio Rambla Vilar and María Dolores Muro Velilla

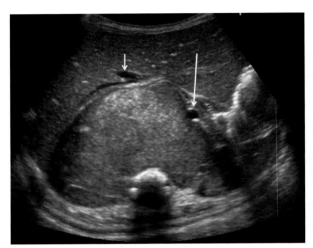

Fig. 6.1

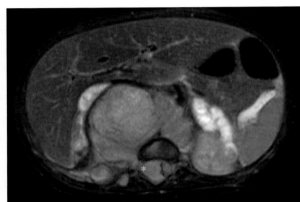

Fig. 6.2

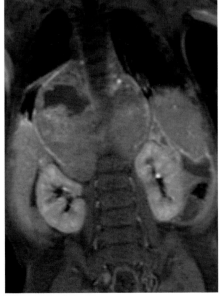

Fig. 6.3

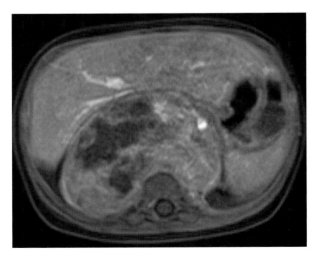

Fig. 6.4

A 3-month-old boy with 10-days liquid diarrhea and fever.

Neuroblastoma (NB) is the most common solid, extracranial tumor in infants and children. NB are of neural crest origin, and most cases arise in the adrenal medulla. Less often, NB may arise in other extra-adrenal sites along the sympathetic chain.

The median age at diagnosis is 22 months, and NB may occur in newborns. The clinical presentation depends on the site of the primary lesion or location of its metastatic spread. The vast majority of NB secrete catecholamine. Vasoactive intestinal peptide (VIP) may be secreted by the tumor and may result in watery diarrhea, hypokalemia, and acidosis. Stage, age at diagnosis, histology, and genetics (MYCN oncogene) are the most significant and clinically relevant prognostic factors.

Local extension usually consists of perivascular extensions with peculiar arterial encasement, infiltration of adjacent soft tissues and organs, and infiltration of foramina and epidural space of the spinal canal when the primary arises from paraspinal sympathetic ganglia.

A new International NB Risk Group Staging System (INRGSS) was recently designed to stratify patients at the time of diagnosis before any treatment. In the INRGSS, extent of locoregional disease is determined by the absence (stage L1) or presence (stage L2) of image-defined risk factors (IDRF). Stage M will be used for widely disseminated disease. Stage MS describes metastatic NB limited to skin, liver, and bone marrow without cortical bone involvement in children aged 0–18 months.

The presence or absence of each individual IDRF should be evaluated by CT or MRI. Distant metastases must be assessed by iodine-123-metaiodobenzylguanidine (MIBG) scintigraphy. Bone marrow involvement must also be assessed by both marrow aspirates and after the age of 6 months, by bone marrow biopsies.

Axial US view through the upper abdomen reveals a big, well-defined, retroperitoneal central mass. The lesion displaces anteriorly the inferior vena cava (IVC) and the aorta (short and long arrows) (Fig. 6.1). Axial T2FS-W shows neural foraminal invasion (*), with marked thecal sac displacement. Both adrenal glands seem to be bigger than normally with cystic lesions (Fig. 6.2). Coronal T1-W IV contrast shows heterogenous enhancement of the large posterior mediastinal and retroperitoneal mass. The right paraspinal musculature is also invaded (Fig. 6.3). T1Gd-W shows intratumoral necrosis (Fig. 6.4).

Figure 6.1
Figure 6.2
Figure 6.3
Figure 6.4

Case 6.2
Hepatoblastoma
■
Sara Picó Aliaga and Cinta Sangüesa Nebot

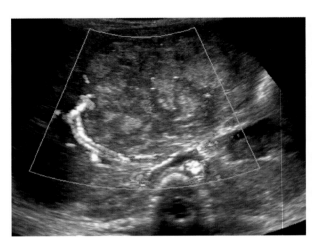

Fig. 6.5

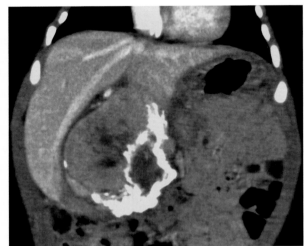

Fig. 6.6

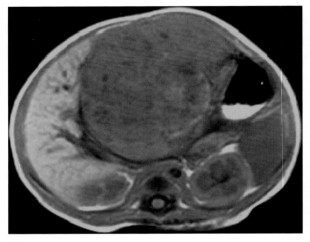

Fig. 6.7

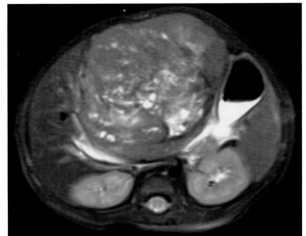

Fig. 6.8

A 5-month-old male with an abdominal mass.

Hepatoblastoma is the most common malignant tumor of the liver in children. Boys are affected about twice as frequently as girls, and the most cases occurring prior to age 5.

Usually is presented as an abdominal mass or abdominal distension. In the majority (90%) of patients, a highly elevated alpha-feto protein is present in the serum, and it is used in both diagnosis and as a marker to monitor treatment effectiveness.

The right lobe is involved three times more commonly than the left, with bilobar involvement seen in 20–30%, and multicentric involvement in 15%.

Metastases at diagnoses occur in 10–20% of patients, with the lung being the predominant site. Although pulmonary metastases are usually accompanied by an increase in AFP, recurrence of pulmonary metastases has been reported to occur without such an increase.

In imaging studies, it usually appears as a focal or multifocal solid tumor, with calcifications in 40–50% of patients. This calcification closely correlates to histologically detected osteoid matrix; however, it is a nonspecific finding and is not particularly helpful in differential diagnosis. Frequently, the initial diagnosis is made by ultrasound in conjunction with color Doppler; it can assign the tumor to the liver and define its relationship to the vascular structures. However, the exact limits of the tumor and, even more important, the amount and anatomical location of the remaining normal liver tissue necessitate the use of MRI and/or CT scan. A single-phase spiral CT is obtained prior to and following intravenous administration of an iodinated contrast material; this technique allows optimal visualization of the tumor during the late arterial/early portal phases. It is recommended at diagnosis to include chest CT to determine if pulmonary metastases are present.

The most important objective of imaging is to define resectability of the tumor. The PRETEXT, based on the Couinaud's system of segmentation of the liver, designed by SIOPEL group, describes tumor extent before any theraphy and is used for staging and risk stratification of liver tumors.

Color US: It has mixed pattern, predominantly increased echoes compared to normal liver (Fig. 6.5). Coronal contrast-enhanced CT scans reveal a hypoattenuated tumor with calcifications in the left lobe abutting the middle hepatic vein (Fig. 6.6). Axial T1-weighted MRI shows a mass with slightly lower intensity than normal liver (Fig. 6.7). Axial T2-weighted MRI, signal intensity is nonhomogeneous as a result of areas of necrosis within it (Fig. 6.8).

Figure 6.5
Figure 6.6
Figure 6.7
Figure 6.8

Case 6.3
Infantile Hemangioendothelioma of the Liver
◼
Susana Calle Restrepo and Jorge Andrés Soto

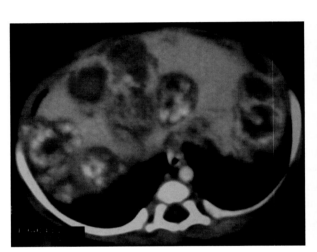

Fig. 6.9

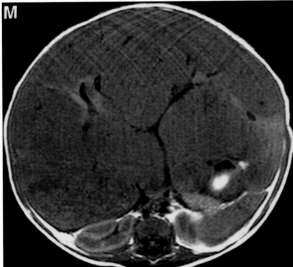

Fig. 6.10

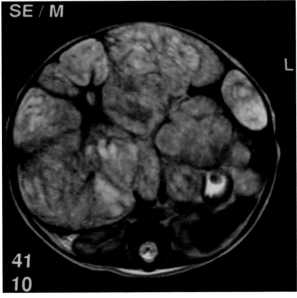

Fig. 6.11

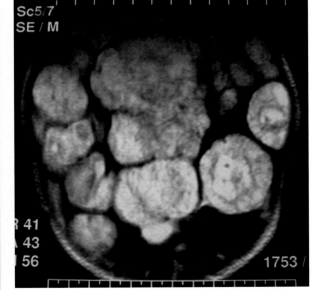

Fig. 6.12

A 12-month-old patient presents with abdominal distension and a palpable abdominal mass.

The infantile hemangioendothelioma is a benign vascular tumor that arises from mesenchymal tissue. This tumor occurs predominantly in the liver and develops more frequently in females. Although considered a benign neoplasm, cases of malignant transformation into sarcomas have been reported. It is the third most common hepatic tumor in childhood, the most common benign vascular tumor in this age group, and the most common symptomatic liver tumor in children under the age of 6 months.

Most patients present symptoms during the first 6 months of life, including abdominal distension and hepatomegaly, and approximately half also have cutaneous hemangiomas. Other findings may include heart failure (due to arteriovenous shunting within the lesion), anemia, thrombocytopenia, jaundice, difficulty breathing, and bowel obstruction. Differential diagnoses include hepatoblastoma and mesenchymal hamartoma.

Histologically, hemangioendotheliomas can be further classified into type I and type II. While type I tumors are composed of multiple vascular channels with immature endothelial linings and fibrous septations containing biliary ducts, type II tumors are more disorganized and hypercellular, and lack biliary ducts.

On ultrasound, the lesion appears as a heterogeneous, predominantly solid mass. On CT studies, the mass presents peripheral enhancement during early phases and later shows central contrast uptake. The tumor is hypointense on T1-weighted and hyperintense on T2-weighted MR images.

Conservative management is usually applied unless life-threatening symptoms warrant surgical resection. The use of steroids and interferon aids in accelerating the natural regression of the lesion, which generally occurs spontaneously after the first year of life.

Axial contrast-enhanced arterial phase CT image depicts marked hepatomegaly and multiple heterogeneous lesions with peripheral contrast uptake (Fig. 6.9). MR shows large masses that are slightly hypointense on T1-weighted images (Fig. 6.10) and hyperintense on axial (Fig. 6.11) and coronal (Fig. 6.12) T2-weighted images.

Figure 6.9
Figure 6.10
Figure 6.11
Figure 6.12

Case 6.4

Endodermal Sinus Tumors (Yolk Sac Tumors)
■

Alejandra Doroteo Lobato and María I. Martínez León

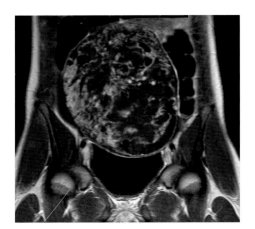

Fig. 6.13

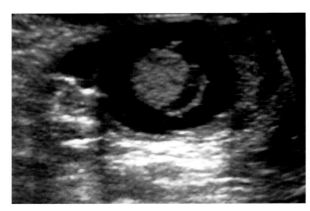

Fig. 6.14

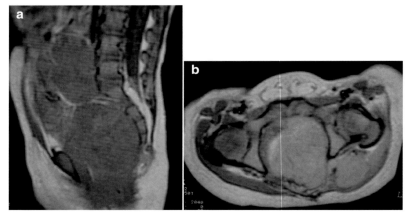

Fig. 6.15

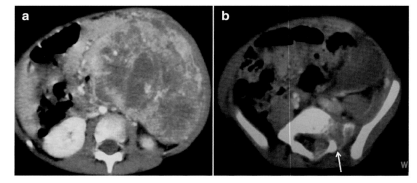

Fig. 6.16

Comments

Endodermal sinus tumors (EST) are a histological subtype of the germ cell tumor (GCT) group of cancer, a heterogeneous variety of neoplasms. GCTs include benign variants (teratoma) as well as malignant tumors (EST, germinoma, choriocarcinoma, embryonal carcinoma). Malignant GCTs are uncommon in children and represent only 3% of all cancerous tumors in the pediatric population. Of the malignant varieties of GCTs, EST is the most frequent. EST, also known as yolk sac tumor (YST), is a malignant neoplasm of non-seminomatous germ cells. They are often gonadal in location, although they may arise anywhere at the midline of the body (extragonadal). These tumors usually present in children under the age of 2 years, and they represent the most common form of testicular cancer in young children. On the other hand, ovarian involvement occurs more frequently in prepubescent females.

Clinical presentation depends on the location and staging of the tumor. Symptoms related to compressive effects of the tumor on adjacent structures can often be seen.

At diagnosis, many patients are classified in advanced stages of the disease (III or IV) with associated organ infiltration and metastases. Usually, testicular tumors are diagnosed in earlier stages (I or II).

Radiologically, ESTs present a heterogeneous appearance with evidence of necrosis, hemorrhage, and cystic degeneration. These findings often make them indistinguishable from other non-seminomatous GCTs and sometimes even difficult to differentiate from other forms of neoplasms (rhabdomyosarcoma, neuroblastoma, lymphoma). A characteristic finding, in up to 90% of cases, is a significant elevation in alpha-fetoprotein levels, which aid in determining the diagnosis, prognosis, and clinical evolution of the tumor.

Imaging Findings

Ovarian EST. Abdominopelvic T1-weighted contrast-enhanced MR image shows a well-delineated, large, solid, heterogeneous mass with cystic areas in its interior arising from the pelvis, specifically from the right adnexa. It ruptured during surgical resection and was classified as a stage III (Fig. 6.13). Testicular EST. Testicular US reveals a complex solid mass with cystic components (Fig. 6.14). Sacrococcygeal EST. Pelvic MR image shows a presacral mass that appears isointense on sagittal T1-weighted images (Fig. 6.15a) and hyperintense on axial T2-weighted MR images (Fig. 6.15b). Retroperitoneal EST. Abdominopelvic axial CT displays a huge retroperitoneal solid mass with areas of necrosis (Fig. 6.16a) producing osseous infiltration of the lamina and pedicle of S1 (arrow) (Fig. 6.16b).

Figure 6.13 Ovárico
Figure 6.14 Testicular
Figure 6.15 Sacrocoxígeo
Figure 6.16 Retroperitoneo

Case 6.5
Adrenocortical Tumors
■
Sonia Romero Chaparro and María I. Martínez León

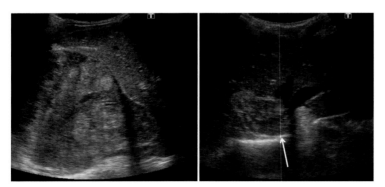

Fig. 6.17

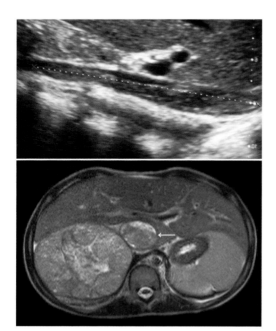

Fig. 6.18

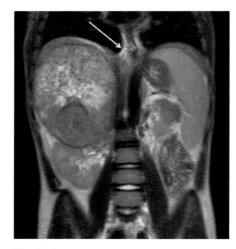

Fig. 6.19

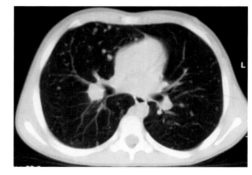

Fig. 6.20

A 11-year-old boy presents with asthenia and anorexia. There are no signs of virilization.

Childhood adrenocortical tumors (ACT) constitute only about 0.2% of all pediatric malignancies. The incidence of ACT is remarkably high in southern Brazil. The clinical presentation in most children includes signs and symptoms of virilization, which may be accompanied by manifestations secondary to hypersecretion of other adrenal cortical hormones. Fewer than 10% of patients with ACT show no endocrine changes at onset and these are often older children and adolescents.

ACT is commonly seen in association with constitutional genetic abnormalities, particularly mutations of the p53 gene.

Given their histological and radiological similarities, differentiating between adenoma and carcinoma may be difficult. The presence of hematogenous metastases and/or vascular infiltration is highly suggestive of malignancy. Other suggestive radiologic findings include a mass with a size greater than 6 cm, heterogeneity of the lesion, and signs of recurrence.

Complete surgical resection is required in order to obtain full ACT remission. The role of chemotherapy or radiotherapy has not yet been established. Nevertheless, treatment with medications such as Mitotane and others has shown promising results.

Among patients who undergo complete tumor resection, favorable prognostic factors include: an age of less than 4 years, small tumor size, signs of virilization as the only manifestation at onset, and adenomatous tumor histology.

The combination of clinical signs of adrenocortical hyperfunction and evidence of an adrenal mass indicates a diagnosis of ACT.

Ultrasound reveals a well-defined, solid, large heterogenous right adrenal mass showing tumor thrombosis of the IVC (arrow) and its relation with the suprahepatic veins in the localized image (Fig. 6.17). Axial and coronal T2-weighted MR image and sagital sonography displays infiltration of the IVC (short arrow in MRI) by the tumor, extending toward the right atrium (long arrow) and caudally to the common iliac (not shown). Displacement of adjacent structures (liver and right kidney) due to secondary mass effect can also be observed (Figs. 6.18 and 6.19). Multiple, bilateral pulmonary nodules consistent with hematogenous metastases can also be seen (Fig. 6.20).

Figure 6.17
Figure 6.18
Figure 6.19
Figure 6.20

Case 6.6

Hodgkin's Lymphoma

Elena Pastor Pons and Antonio Rodríguez Fernández

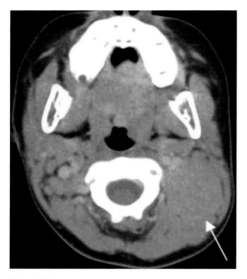

Fig. 6.21

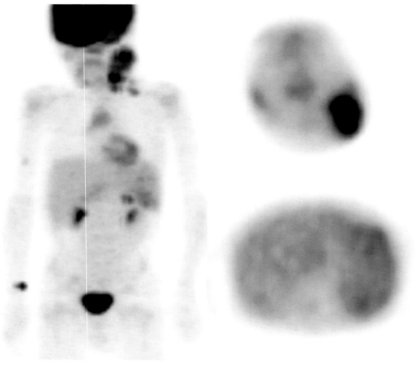

Fig. 6.22

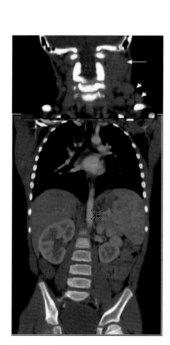

Fig. 6.23

Fig. 6.24

A 7-year-old boy presents with enlarging left-sided cervical lymphadenopathies that did not respond to anti-inflammatory or antibiotic treatment. Lymph node resection revealed grade II nodular sclerosing Hodgkin's lymphoma.

Hodgkin's lymphoma, also known as Hodgkin's disease, may present an exclusively nodal or nodal and splenic origin. The grand majority manifest with cervical or supraclavicular adenopathies. The main objective of imaging techniques in Hodgkin's lymphoma is initial staging. Lymphadenopathies are the most common cause of neck masses in children, and they are generally benign lesions. Ultrasound is essential in establishing superficial lymph node involvement. Lymphomatous nodes are usually solid, round, and show absence or infiltration of the fatty hilum, as well as vascularization abnormalities. The use of whole body CT (optimally, multi-detector CT) or MRI is essential. Positron emission tomography (PET) yields functional images using radionuclide-traced molecules. Recently, x-ray tomography has been incorporated to this study in order to fuse both functional and structural images (PET-CT). The functional image helps to differentiate the tumor from healthy or fibrotic tissue and also helps to characterize lesions that have not responded to treatment. Since 2005, the EuroNet Pediatric Hodgkin's Lymphoma Group has developed a European protocol for children and adolescents suffering from classic Hodgkin's lymphoma (EuroNet-PHL-C1). These guidelines standardize the use of thoracic PET and CT imaging for initial staging. Furthermore, three ways of conducting extension studies have been established: (a) MRI of the neck, thorax (mediastinum), abdomen, and pelvis; (b) CT of the neck, thorax, abdomen, and pelvis with oral and IV contrast, taken from the epipharynx to the pubic symphysis; or (c) a combination of CT and PET techniques, where CT must provide images of equal quality than those of diagnostic CT studies.

Axial MDCT reconstructions of the skull base show a large, rounded lymph node mass with homogeneous enhancement located in the left retrocarotid space (arrow) and in the abdomen (not shown) (Fig. 6.21). Splenomegaly with multiple focal lesions is seen (Fig. 6.22). Coronal reconstruction image shows, in addition to these lesions, multiple latero-cervical, supra and infraclavicular lymphadenopathies (arrows) (Fig. 6.23). Coronal and axial PET images of the neck and spleen reveal a heterogeneous increase in metabolic activity in latero-cervical, supra and infra clavicular regions as well as in the spleen (Fig. 6.24).

Figure 6.21
Figure 6.22
Figure 6.23
Figure 6.24

Case 6.7

Non-Hodgkin Lymphoma

■

Elena Pastor Pons and Antonio Rodríguez Fernández

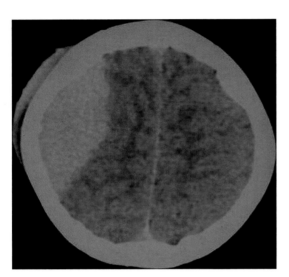

Fig. 6.25

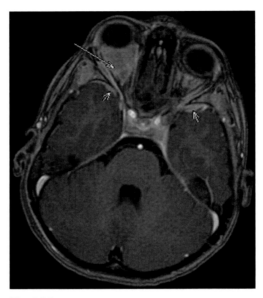

Fig. 6.26

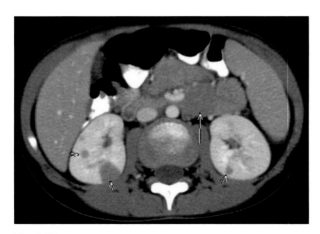

Fig. 6.27

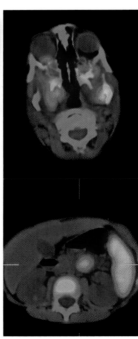
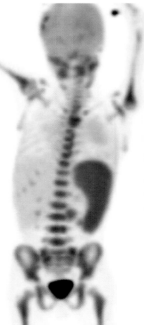

Fig. 6.28

A 6-year-old boy presents with a soft tissue mass located in the right fronto-parietal region associated with proptosis, splenomegaly, and right ocular hyperemia. Both the mass biopsy and bone marrow aspiration showed a Burkitt lymphoma.

Comments

Lymphomas comprise approximately 10–15% of all childhood malignancies and encompass a wide range of pathological subtypes. Any organ or structure may be affected, including the CNS, head, neck, thorax, abdomen, gonads, and bone. Extragonadal involvement is more common in non-Hodgkin lymphoma (NHL). The main objective of imaging is tumor staging. Various protocols have been established for the initial evaluation according to the histological type and associated findings. Ultrasound is essential in assessing superficial lymph node and testicular involvement. It also provides important information on abdominal compromise, although it does not replace CT imaging for this purpose. Multi-detector CT (MDCT) is the main imaging modality utilized to evaluate these patients. If neurological symptoms are present, brain and spine MRI are indicated. Brain MRI should also be performed if blasts are detected in CSF and if there are manifestations of lymphoma in the head and neck. PET yields functional images using radionuclide-traced molecules. Recently, x-ray tomography has been incorporated to this study in order to fuse both functional and structural images (PET-CT). The functional image helps to differentiate the tumor from healthy or fibrotic tissue and also helps to characterize lesions that have not responded to treatment.

Imaging Findings

Brain CT reveals a large fronto-parietal, hyperdense mass with a significant extradural component and a permeative infiltration of the skull (Fig. 6.25). Contrast-enhanced MRI shows multiple, moderately enhancing lesions in the retroconal space of the right orbit with associated proptosis of the ocular globe (arrow) and dural thickening at the anterior aspect of both middle cranial fossae (short arrows) (Fig. 6.26). Body MDCT with contrast reveals hepato-splenomegaly, bilateral hypodense focal lesions with low enhancement (short arrows) and a conglomerate of retroperitoneal lymphadenopathies (arrow) (Fig. 6.27). PET-CT imaging displays increased metabolic activity of the bone marrow with several right fronto-parietal, right orbit, and para-aortic mass foci. In conclusion, these findings were consistent with stage IV Burkitt lymphoma with osseous, neuromeningeal, orbitary, splenic, renal, retroperitoneal, and bone marrow involvement (Fig. 6.28).

Figure 6.25
Figure 6.26
Figure 6.27
Figure 6.28

Case 6.8

Hepatosplenic Candidiasis in Acute Lymphoblastic Leukemia

Luisa Ceres Ruiz

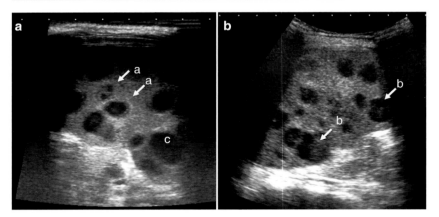

Fig. 6.29

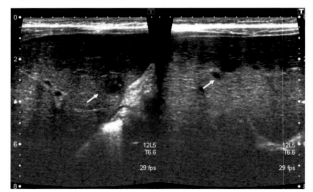

Fig. 6.30

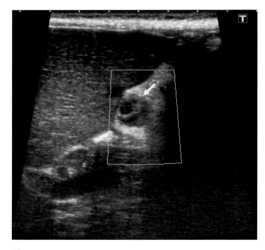

Fig. 6.31

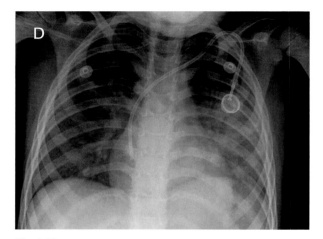

Fig. 6.32

Following two rounds of chemotherapy for acute lymphoblastic leukemia (ALL), a 5-year-old patient presents with recurrent fever, persistent neutropenia, abdominal pain, and hepatosplenic lesions visible on ultrasound.

Comments

Chronic or hepatosplenic candidiasis represents a disseminated form of candidal infection that involves the liver, the spleen, and occasionally, the kidneys. It is generally considered a variant of systemic invasion in immunosuppressed hosts. Prevalence has been shown to rise over the past years, which may be due to an increase in immunosuppressed patients with an elevated risk of developing fungal infections and the use of more intense chemotherapy. Furthermore, now that neutropenic patients show better survival rates, more complications are documented. Finally, diagnostic sensitivity has improved. US, CT, and MR imaging aid in the identification of this condition. In neutropenic patients, dissemination to intra-abdominal organs occurs hematogenously through portal circulation. Fever and bilateral hypochondriac pain may be the only clinical manifestations. However, a blood culture positive for Candida suggests an invasive infectious process. Timely diagnosis and treatment are essential in establishing a favorable prognosis. Diagnostic criteria include the growth of yeast in blood cultures, detection of *Candida* antigen in serum, suggestive findings on imaging studies, and the presence of yeast or pseudohyphae in hepatic tissue.

In the case mentioned above, diagnosis was made by detection of *Candida* in the culture of secretions obtained by bronchial lavage. Coexisting pulmonary symptoms were present in addition to the hepatosplenic lesions. This condition should be suspected in all patients that present persistent fever or fever that reappears after neutropenia has subsided, along with elevated alkaline phosphatase levels. Criteria for remission are based on radiologic findings including eradication of lesions and absence of clinical signs and symptoms of infection.

Imaging Findings

Ultrasound imaging guides the diagnosis by revealing characteristic findings in the liver and spleen. US of the spleen shows: (a) a concentric ring pattern seen in early stages of the condition; (b) target-like lesions; (c) hypoechoic lesions (Fig. 6.29). Ring-like lesions of 1–4 mm in diameter are viewed in the liver on ultrasound (arrow) (Fig. 6.30). A hepatic hilar adenopathy with ring-like lesions in its interior is seen (arrow) (Fig. 6.31). Chest radiograph shows patchy infiltrates at the lung bases, especially on the left side (bronchial lavage was positive for *Candida*) (Fig. 6.32).

Figure 6.29 (**a**) and (**b**)
Figure 6.30
Figure 6.31
Figure 6.32

Case 6.9
Cystic Testicular Teratoma
■

Carolina Torres Alés

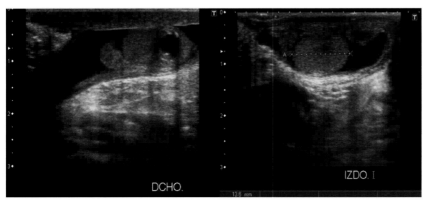

Fig. 6.33

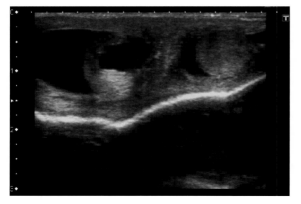

Fig. 6.34

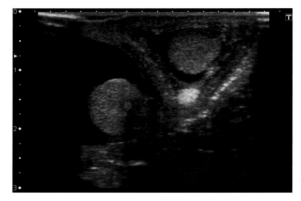

Fig. 6.35

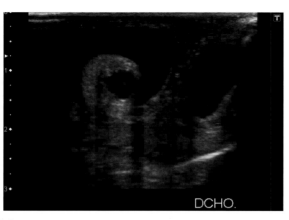

Fig. 6.36

A 15-day-old boy presents with an enlarged scrotum on the right and mild cutaneous erythema.

Teratomas represent the second most frequent type of testicular tumor in patients under the age of 4 years, and testicular tumors in turn comprise 1–2% of solid neoplasms in children (with an increased incidence during the first 3 years of life). The most common form of testicular tumors in the pediatric population are non-seminomatous GCTs (70–90%), with YSTs and teratomas being the most frequent subtypes. Clinical presentation usually consists of a painless testicular mass, and associated risk factors include positive family history, cryptorchidism and intersex syndromes (gonadal dysgenesis, true hermaphroditism, and pseudohermaphroditism).

Teratomas are composed of cells originating from three distinct embryologic germ layers. The mean age at onset is 13 months, and these tumors generally present a benign clinical evolution. They are classified as mature, immature and with malignant components. Teratomas appear as well-defined, solid masses with a cystic component (either simple or complex) and/or with echogenic foci (hemorrhage, cartilage, calcification, fibrosis). They do not present tumor marker elevation. Differential diagnoses include other tumors such as epidermoid cysts (cystic lesion with hyperchoic ring with a typical onionskin appearance) and YSTs (solid, heterogeneous or microcystic lesion with associated elevation of alpha-fetoprotein).

B-mode and color Doppler ultrasound is the diagnostic study of choice due to its ability to determine the location (intra- or extrascrotal), composition (solid or cystic), and vascularization of the tumor (useful for infiltrating tumors). However, US does not differentiate between benign and malignant neoplasms. The use of CT imaging is indicated when there is suspicion of metastases (retroperitoneum, lung, and mediastinum). The first line of treatment is surgical resection by orchidectomy or enucleation. (Teratomas may present malignant transformation in adulthood).

Longitudinal view B-mode ultrasound shows moderate hydrocele and an enlargement of the right testicle in comparison to the left with a single, intratesticular cystic mass located in its inferior pole (Fig. 6.33). The transverse view (Figs. 6.34 and 6.35) reveals well-defined margins with a reinforced posterior echo and echogenic borders (peripheral solid component). The cystic portion is predominantly anechoic with a few echogenic components (Fig. 6.36).

Figure 6.33
Figure 6.34
Figure 6.35
Figure 6.36

Case 6.10

Ovarian Tumor (Yolk Sac Tumor)

Luisa Ceres Ruiz

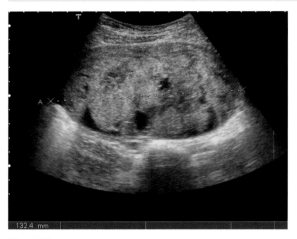

Fig. 6.37

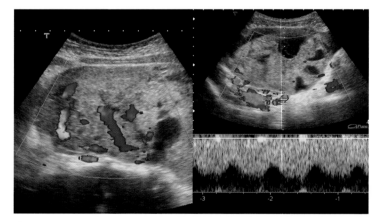

Fig. 6.38

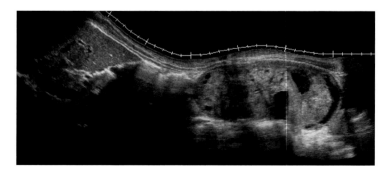

Fig. 6.39

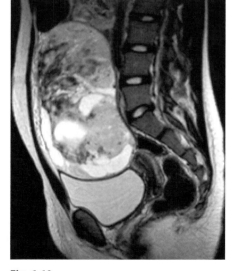

Fig. 6.40

A 13-year-old girl presents with a 10-day history of abdominal pain.

The ovarian/YST arises from the primitive multipotent cell, originating from yolk sac structures and appearing as a hyperproliferation of the yolk sac endoderm (forming alpha-fetoprotein) and with extraembryonic mesoderm. It is considered a rare neoplasm and constitutes approximately 10% of GCTs. They usually appear in young females as large, unilateral, solid/cystic, aggressive masses.

Clinical presentation generally consists of abdominal pain associated with an abdominal or pelvic mass. Approximately 10% of patients present with acute abdomen due to torsion, rupture, or hemorrhaging of the mass. As with any ovarian tumor of malignant characteristics, staging must include dissemination studies, tumor marker levels, and karyotype when a GCT is suspected. Furthermore, dysgerminomas may be associated with gonadal dysgenesis.

A staging system has been developed by the International Federation of Gynecology and Obstetrics:

Stage I: Disease is limited to the ovaries.
Stage II: Disease presents extension to the pelvis.
Stage III: Disease extends to the peritoneal cavity.
Stage IV: Disease presents distant metastases to the liver parenchyma or has spread beyond the peritoneal cavity.

Differential diagnoses include embryonic carcinoma, immature teratoma, intra-abdominal cystic tumors, and other GCTs such as the dysgerminoma. If the mass is small in size, ovarian torsion must be considered. In ovarian torsion, Doppler ultrasound reveals absence of blood flow within the mass, while in ovarian YSTs, a vascularized solid component is seen.

Sagittal view US reveals a well-encapsulated, 13 × 16 × 14 cm solid mass located in the hypogastrium (Fig. 6.37). Duplex US shows significant vascularization and an afferent pedicle originating from the internal iliac artery (right ovarian artery) (Fig. 6.38). Sagittal, extended field-of-view ultrasound displays the extension of the large mass (Fig. 6.39). Sagittal T2-weighted MR image reveals a tumor of mixed components showing high-intensity signal of the solid portion in addition to its cystic areas (Fig. 6.40).

Figure 6.37
Figure 6.38
Figure 6.39
Figure 6.40

Further Reading

Book

Cohen MD (1992a) Imaging of children in cancer. Mosby Year Book, St. Louis

Cohen MD. Imaging of children with cancer. (1992) vol 3. St Louis: Mosby Year Book, pp 20–38

Donnelly LF et al, ed. (2005) Diagnostic imaging: Pediatrics. Salt Lake City, AMIRISYS (Philadelphia: Elsevier)

Hughes WT (1997) Candidiasis. In: Fegin RD (ed) Textbook of pediatric infectious diseases. W.B. Saunders, Philadelphia, pp 1814–1822

Lencioni R, Cioni D, Bartolozzi C (2005) Focal liver lesions: detection, characterization, ablation. Springer-Verlag, Berlin, Heidelberg

Luis Sierrasesúmaga, F. Antillón, E. Bernaola, A. Patiño, M. San Julián (eds.) (2005) Tratado de Oncología Pediátrica. Editorial Pearson Educación, Madrid

Reznek RH, Husband JE Vinnicombe S y (2004) Lymphoma. In: Husband JE, Reznek RH (eds) Imaging in oncology, 2nd edn. Taylor & Francis, London, pp 817–874

Siegel MJ (2004) Ecografía pediátrica, 2nd edn. Marbán, Madrid

Swischuk LE (1997) Imaging of the newborn, infant, and young child, 4th ed. Lippincott Williams & Wilkins, Philadelphia

Web Link

FIGO Staging of Ovarian Cancer. Retrieved March 2, 2000 from the World Wide Web: http://www.figo.org/committees/ovary.asp

http://emedicine.medscape.com/article/1015422-overview

http://www.cancer.gov/cancertopics/types/non-hodgkin

http://www.lymphome.de/Gruppen/GPOH-HD/Protokolle/EuroNet-PHL-C1/Synopsis.pdf

http://www.scielo.br/scielo.php?pid=S0100-879X2000001000013&script=sci_arttext

http://www.uptodate.com/home/index.html

http://www.uptodate.com

Wolf D, Raghuraman U (2009) Hepatic hemangiomas. Emedicine: Web MD. http://emedicine.medscape.com/article/177106-overview. Last updated 8 Dec 2009

www.medigraphic.com/pdfs/patol/pt-2000/pt004d.pdf

www.radiographics.org

Articles

Abramson SJ, Price AP (2008) Imaging of pediatric lymphomas. Radiol Clin North Am 46(2):313–338

Agrons GA, Lonergan GJ, Dickey GE, Perez-Monte JE (1999) Adrenocortical neoplasms in children: radiologic–pathologic correlation. RadioGraphics 19:989–1008

Antilla V, Elonen E, Nordiling (1997) Hepatosplenic candidiasis in patients with acute leukemia: incidence and prognostic implications. Clin Infect Dis 24:375–380

Balu M, Tarrant A, Lenoir M, Ducou Le Pointe H (2008) Ovarian masses imaging before puberty. Arch Pediatr Fr 15(5): 783–785

Barth RA, Teele RL, Colodny A, Retik A, Bauer S (1984) Asimptomatic scrotal masses in children. Radiology 152:65–68

Blade J, Lopez-Guillermo A, Rozman C, Grañena A, Bruguera M, Bordas J et al (1992) Chronic systemic candidiasis in acute leukemia. Ann Hematol 64:240–244

Brammer HM, Buck JL, Hayes WS, Sheth S, Tavassoli FA (1990) Malignant germ cell tumors of the ovary: radiologic–pathologic correlation. RadioGraphics 10:715–724

Brown J, Perilongo G, Shafford E, Keeling J, Pritchard J, Brock P et al (2000) Pretreatment prognostic factors for children with hepatoblastoma-results from the International Society of Paediatric Oncology (SIOP) study SIOPEL 1. Eur J Cancer 36:1418–1425

Celestino Aso MD, Goya Enríquez MD et al (2005) Gray-scale and color Doppler sonography of scrotal disorders in children: an update. RadioGraphics 25:1197–1214

Chang YW, Hong SS, Jeen YM, Kim MK, Suh ES (2009) Bilateral sclerosing stromal tumor of the ovary in a premenarchal girl. Pediatr Radiol 9:731–734

Chen CC, Kong MS, Yang CP, Hung IJ (2003) Hepatic hemangioendothelioma in children: analysis of thirteen cases. Acta Paediatr Taiwan 44(1):8–13

Choyke PL, Hayes WS, Sesterhenn IA (1993) Primary extragonadal germ cell tumors of the retroperitoneum: differentiation of primary and secondary tumors. RadioGraphics 13: 1365–1375

Cohn SL, Pearson AD, London WB, Monclair T, Ambros PF, Brodeur GM et al (2008) The International Neuroblastoma Risk Group (INRG) classification system: an INRG Task Force report. J Clin Oncol 27:289–297

Czauderna P, Otte JB, Roebuck DJ, von Schweinitz D, Plaschkes J (2006) Surgical treatment of hepatoblastoma in children. Pediatr Radiol 36:187–191

David R, Lamki N, Fan S, Singleton EB, Eftekhari F, Shirkhoda A et al (1989) The many faces of neuroblastoma. RadioGraphics 9:859–882

Davidoff AM, Hebra A, Bunin Nancy, Shochat SJ, Schnaufer L, Pennsylvania P (1996) Endodermal sinus tumor in children. J Pediatr Surg 31:1075–1079

Dickson PV, Davidoff AM (2006) Malignant neoplasms of the head and neck. Semin Pediatr Surg 15:92–98

Dogra VS, Gottlieb RH, Oka M, Rubens DJ (2003) Sonography of the scrotum. Radiology 227:18–36

Ein SH, Mancer K, Toronto SDA et al (1985) Malignant sacroccoygeal teratoma, endodermal sinus, yolk sac tumor. in infants and children: a 32-year review. J Pediatr Surg 20(5):473–477

Elsayes KM, Mukundan G, Narra VR, Lewis JS Jr, Shirkhoda A, Farooki A et al (2004) Adrenal masses: MR imaging features with pathologic correlation. RadioGraphics 24(suppl 1):S73–S86

Fleece DM, Faerber EN, de Chadarévian JP (1998) Pathological case of the month. Hepatosplenic candidiasis in a patient with leukemia. Arch Pediatr Adolesc Med 152:1033–1034

Fletcher BD, Magill HL (1988) Wheel-within-a-wheel patterns in hepatosplenic infections. Radiology 169:578–579

Fox MA, Vix VA (1980) Endodermal sinus (yolk sac) tumors of the anterior mediastinum. AJR 135:291–294

Frush DP, Curtis CA (1998) Diagnostis imaging for pediatric scrotal disorders. RadioGraphics 18:969–985

Gámez Cenzano C, Cabrera Villegas A, Sopena Monforte R, García Velloso MJ (2002) Positron emision tomography (PET) in oncology (part 1). Rev Esp Med Nucl 21:41–60

Ganguly R, Mukherjee A (2010) Infantile hemangioendothelioma: a case report and discussion. Pathol Res Pract 206(1):53–58

Halefoğlu AM (2007) Magnetic resonance imaging of infantile hemangioendothelioma. Turk J Pediatr 49(1):77–81

Hamm B (1997) Differential diagnosis of scrotal masses by ultrasound. Eur Radiol 7:668–679

Herzog CE, Andrassy RJ, Eftekhari F (2000) Childhood cancers: hepatoblastoma. Oncologist 5:445–453

Hiorns MP, Owens CM (2001) Radiology of neuroblastoma in children. Eur Radiol 11:2071–2081

Isaacs H Jr (2007) Fetal and neonatal hepatic tumors. J Pediatr Surg 42(11):1797–1803

Isasi CR, Lu P, Blaufox MD (2005) A metaanalysis of 18F-2-deoxy-2-fluoro-D-glucose positron emission tomography in the staging and restaging of patients with lymphoma. Cancer 104:1066–1074

Islam S, Yamout SZ, Gosche JR (2008) Management and outcomes of ovarian masses in children and adolescents. Am Surg 74(11):1062–1065

Juweid ME (2006) Utility of positron emission tomography (PET) scanning in managing patients with Hodgkin lymphoma. Hematol Am Soc Hematol Educ Prog 1:259–265

Kontoyoannis DP, Luna MA, Samuels BI, Bodey GP (2000) Hepatosplenic candidiasis: a manifestation of chronic disseminated candidiasis. Infect Dis Clin North Am 14:721–739

Korobkin M, Francis IR, Kloos RT, Dunnick NR (1996) The incidental adrenal mass. Radiol Clin North Am 34:1037–1054

Krishnan A, Shirkhoda A, Tehranzadeh J, Armin AR, Irwin R, Les K (2003) Primary bone lymphoma: radiographic–mr imaging correlation. RadioGraphics 23:1371–1387

Kurtz AB, Tsimikas JV, Tempany CMC, Hamper UM, Arger PH, Bree RL et al (1999) Diagnosis and staging of ovarian cancer: comparative values of Doppler and conventional US, CT, and MR imaging correlated with surgery and histopathologic analysis – Report of the radiology diagnostic oncology group. Radiology 212:19–27

Lau SK, Weiss LM (2009) The Weiss system for evaluating adrenocortical neoplasms: 25 years later. Hum Pathol 40:757–768

Lee WK, Lau EW, Duddalwar VA, VA SAJ, Ho YY (2008) Abdominal manifestations of extranodal lymphoma: spectrum of imaging findings. AJR 191:198–206

Lehner R, Wenzl R, Heinzl H, Husslein P, Sevelda P (1998) Influence of delayed staging laparotomy after laparoscopic removal of ovarian masses later found malignant. Obstet Gynecol 92:967–971

Lev MH, Blickman JG (1993) Extragonadal yolk sac tumor. AJR 160:370–371

Levitin A, Haller KD, Cohen HL, Zinn DL, O'Connor MTC (1996) Endodermal sinus tumor of the ovary: imaging evaluation. AJR 167:791–793

Lin PC, Chang TT, Jang RC, Chiou SS (2003) Hepatosplenic microabscesses in pediatric leukemia: a report of five cases. Kaohsiung J Med Sci 19:368–374

Lonergan GJ, Schwab CM, Suarez ES, Carlson CL (2002) Neuroblastoma, ganglioneuroblastoma, and ganglioneuroma: radiologic–pathologic correlation. RadioGraphics 22:911–934

Luker GD, Siegel MJ (1994) Pediatric testicular tumors: evaluation with gary-scale and color Doppler US. CT diagnosis. Radiology 191:561–654

Malkin D, Li FP, Strong LC, Fraumeni JF Jr, Nelson CE, Kim Dh et al (1990) Germ line p53 mutations in a familial syndrome of breast cancer, sarcomas, and others neoplasms. Science 250:1233–1238

Martí-Climent JM, García Velloso MJ, Serra P, Boán JF, Richter JA (2005) Positron emission tomography with PET/TAC. Rev Esp Med Nucl 24(1):60–79

Medina LS, D'Alessandro M, Buonomo C (1996) Pediatric case of the day. Adrenocortical adenoma. RadioGraphics 16:449–451

Meuwly JY, Lepori D, Theumann N, Schnyder P, Etechami G, Hohlfeld J, Gudinchet F (2005) Multimodality imaging evaluation of the pediatric neck: techniques and spectrum of findings. RadioGraphics 25:931–948

Mlikotic A, McPhaul L, Hansen GC, Sinow RM (2001) Significance of the solid component in predicting malignancy in ovarian cystic teratomas: diagnostic considerations. J Ultrasound Med 20:859–866

Monclair T, Brodeur GM, Ambros PF, Brisse HJ, Cecchetto G, Holmes K et al (2009) The International Neuroblastoma Risk Group (INRG) staging system: an INRG Task Force report. J Clin Oncol 27:298–303

Ng WH, Ching AS, Chan KF, Fung WT (2003) Infantile hepatosplenic haemangioendotheliomas. Singapore Med J 44(9):491–495

Nuchtern JG (2006) Perinatal neuroblastoma. Semin Pediatr Surg 15:10–16

Olivier P, Colarinha P, Fettich J, Fisher S, Frökier J, Giammarile F et al (2003) Guidelines for radioiodinated MIBG scintigraphy in children. Eur J Nucl Med Mol Imaging 30:B45–B50

Papaioannou G, McHugh K (2005) Neuroblastoma in childhood: review and radiological findings. Cancer Imaging 5:116–127

Papakonstantinou O, Bakantaki A, Paspalaki P, Charoulakis N, Gourtsoyiannis N (2001) High-resolution and color-doppler ultrasonography of cervical lymphadenopathy in children. Acta Radiol 42:470–476

Pellerito JS, Troiano RN, Quedens-Case C, Taylor KJ (1995) Common pitfalls of endovaginal color Doppler flow imaging. RadioGraphics 15:37–47

Ribeiro RC, Figueredo B (2004) Childhood adrenocortical tumours. Eur J Cancer 40:1117–1126

Rodriguez-Galindo C, Figueiredo BC, Zambetti GP, Ribeiro RC (2005) Biology, clinical characteristics, and management of adrenocortical tumors in children. Pediatr Blood Cancer 45:265–273

Roebuck DJ, Perilongo G (2006) Hepatoblastoma: an oncological review. Pediatr Radiol 36:183–186

Roebuck DJ, Olsen O, Pariente D (2006) Radiological staging in children with hepatoblastoma. Pediatr Radiol 36:176–182

Roebuck DJ, Aronson D, Clapuyt P, Czauderna P, de Ville de Goyet J, Gauthier F et al (2007) 2005 PRETEXT: a revised staging system for primary malignant liver tumours of childhood developed by the SIOPEL group. Pediatr Radiol 37:123–132

Roh JL, Huh J, Moon HN (2007) Lymphomas of the head and neck in the pediatric population. Int J Pediatr Otorhinolaryngol 71:1471–1477

Roos JE, Pfiffner R, Stallmach T, Stuckmann G, Marincek B, Willi U (2003) Infantile hemangioendothelioma. RadioGraphics 23(6):1649–1655

Rosado-de-Christenson ML, Templeton PA, Moran CA (1992) Mediastinal germ cell tumors: radiologic and pathologic correlation. RadioGraphics 12:1013–1030

Ross JH, Kay R (2004) Prepuberal testis tumors. Rev Urol 6(1):11–18

Roth LM (2005) Variants of yolk sac tumor. Pathol Case Rev 10:186–192

Royal SA, Joseph DB, Galliani CA (1994) Bilateral testicular teratoma. AJR 163:1130

Salem S, White LM, Lai J (1994) Doppler sonography of adnexal masses: the predictive value of the pulsatility index in benign and malignant disease. AJR 163:1147–1150

Sallah S, Semelka R, Kelekis N, Worawattanakul S, Sallah W (1998) Diagnosis and monitoring response to treatment of hepatosplenic candidiasis in patients with acute leukemia using magnetic resonance imaging. Acta Haematol 100:77–81

Sato M, Ishida H, Konno K, Naganuma H, Hamashima Y, Komatsuda T et al (2000) Liver tumors in children and young patients: sonographic and color Doppler findings. Abdom Imaging 25:596–601

Sauvat F, Sarnacki S, Brisse H, Medioni J, Rubie H, Aigrain Y et al (2002) Outcome of suprarenal localized masses diagnosed during the perinatal period. Cancer 94:2474–2480

Schneider DT, Calaminus G, Koch S, Teske C, Schmidt P, Haas RJ, Harms D, Göbel U (2004) Epidemiologic analyisis of 1442 children and adolescents registered in the German germ cell tumor protocols. Pediatr Blood Cancer 42:169–175

Shirkhoda A, López-Berestein G, Holbert J, Luna M (1996) Hepatosplenic fungal infection: CT and pathologic evaluation after treatment with liposomal amphotericin B. Radiology 159:349–353

Siegelman ES, Outwater EK (1999) Tissue characterization in the female pelvis by means of MR imaging. Radiology 212:5–18

Singh S, Chowdhury V, Prakash A, Aggarwal A (2008) Infantile haemangio-endothelioma of liver: a case report. J Indian Med Assoc 106(2):120–122

Stewart DR, Jones PH, Jolleys A (1974) Carcinoma of the adrenal gland in children. J Pediatr Surg 9:59–67

Stringer MD (2000) Liver tumors. Semin Pediatr Surg 9(4):196–208

Suita S, Tajiri T, Takamatsu H, Mizote H, Nagasaki A, Inomata Y et al (2004) Improved survival outcome for hepatoblastoma based on an optimal chemotherapeutic regimen-a report from the study group for pediatric solid malignant tumors in the Kyushu area. J Pediatr Surg 39(2):195–198

Taskinen S, Fagerholm R, Aroiemi J, Rintala R, Taskinen M (2008) Testicular tumors in children and adolescents. J Pediatr Urol 4:134–137

Teruko U, Tanaka YO, Nagata M, Tsunoda H, Anno I, Ishikawa S, Hawai K, Itai Y (2004) Spectrum of germ cell tumors: from head to toe. RadioGraphics 24:387–404

Toma P, Granata C, Rossi A, Garaventa A (2007) Multimodality imaging of Hodgkin disease and non-Hodgkin lymphomas in children. RadioGraphics 27:1335–1354

Uhl M, Altehoefer C, Kontny U, Il'yasov K, Büchert M, Langer M (2002) MRI-diffusion imaging of neuroblastomas: first results and correlation to histology. Eur Radiol 12:2335–2338

van der Meijs BB, Merks JH, de Haan TR, Tabbers MM, van Rijn RR (2009) Neonatal hepatic haemangioendothelioma: treatment options and dilemmas. Pediatr Radiol 39:277–281

Vázquez E, Lucaya J, Castellote A, Piqueras J, Sainz P, Olive T, Sánchez-Toledo J, Ortega JJ (2002) Neuroimaging in pediatric leukemia and lymphoma: differential diagnosis. RadioGraphics 22:1411–1428

Verdeguer A, Fernandez J, Esquembre C, Ferris J, Ruis J, Castel B (1990) Hepatosplenic candidiasis in children with acute leukemia. Cancer 15:874–877

Walsh R, Harrington J, Beneck D, Ozkaynak MF (2004) Congenital infantile hepatic hemangioendothelioma type II treated with orthotopic liver transplantation. J Pediatr Hematol Oncol 26(2):121–123

Westra SJ, Zaninovic AC, Hall TR, Kangarloo H, Boechat MI (1994) Imaging of the adrenal gland in children. RadioGraphics 14:1323–1340

Wong DC, Masel JP (1995) Infantile hepatic haemangioendothelioma. Australas Radiol 39(2):140–144

Woodward PJ, Sohaey R, O'Donogue MJ, Green DE (2002) Tumors and tumorlike lesions of the tesis: radiologic–pathologic correlation. RadioGraphics 22:189–216

Yang JJ, Lin LW, Lin ZH, Xue ES, Gao SD, He YM (2008) Ultrasonographic diagnosis of hepatic fungal infection. Hepatobiliary Pancreat Dis Int 7:169–173

Zenge JP, Fenton L, Lovell MA, Grover TR (2002) Case report: infantile hemangioendothelioma. Curr Opin Pediatr 14(1):99–102

Contents

M.I. Martínez-León et al., *Learning Pediatric Imaging*, Learning Imaging,
DOI: 10.1007/978-3-642-16892-5_7, © Springer-Verlag Berlin Heidelberg 2011

Case 7.1
Wilms' Tumor
■
Luisa Ceres Ruiz

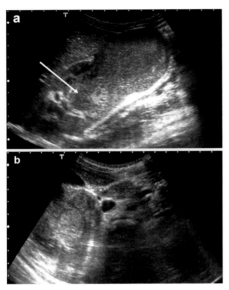

Fig. 7.1

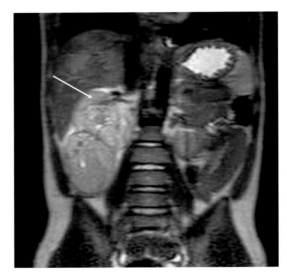

Fig. 7.2

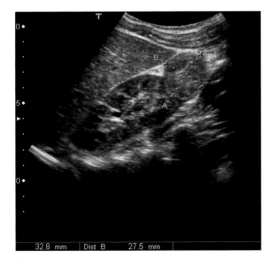

Fig. 7.3

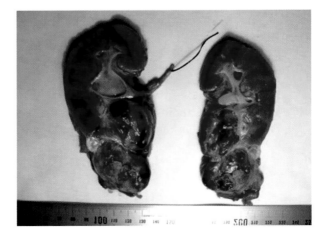

Fig. 7.4

A 7-year-old boy with hematuria and a brother diagnosed with Wilms' tumor.

Wilms' tumor (WT) is the most common intra-abdominal malignancy found in children (0.8 per 100,000 people per year). It originates from the kidney by abnormal proliferation of the metanephric blastema. The histological spectrum of this tumor ranges from elements of the renal blastema to aggressive sarcomatous variants (4–10% of WT). An association has been described between the loss of the WT1 suppressor gene found in chromosome 11 and the development of this tumor, and it may be seen in relation to WAGR syndrome (**W**ilms' tumor, **A**niridia, **G**enitourinary anomalies, and mental **R**etardation). Clinical presentation consists of a flank mass and hematuria, as well as hypertension, fever, and anemia.

Prognosis depends on the histological variant, and the degree of capsular and vascular invasion. If vascular invasion is documented, distant metastases are more frequent. A 90% survival rate can be achieved with surgical management and chemotherapy.

The staging system is as follows: (1) Tumor is limited to the kidney. (2) Tumor extends locally but may be excised. (3) Similar to II but the tumor is unresectable. (4) Lung, liver, brain, or bone metastases are detected. (5) Bilateral renal involvement is present.

Differential diagnoses include neuroblastoma and other renal tumors such as malignant rhabdoid tumor (MRT) and clear cell sarcoma (both are extremely rare). Final diagnosis is made by histological findings. Imaging studies aid in identifying and locating the mass, evaluating the degree of local and vascular extension (may invade the renal vein, the vena cava, and the right atrium), and determining the presence of metastases. Extension assessment must be performed by employing different imaging techniques:

- Retroperitoneal adenopathies (US, CT, MRI)
- Perirenal or capsular involvement (ideally with CT, also with MRI)
- Vascular invasion (Doppler US, contrast-enhanced CT, MRI)
- Contralateral kidney involvement and pulmonary metastases (CT, MRI)
- Hepatic metastases, uncommon (US)
- Bone metastases, exceptional (scintigraphy)

Sagittal and axial US show a solid inferior renal mass that invades the sinus (arrow) (Fig. 7.1a, b). Coronal T2-weighted MR image reveals normal renal parenchyma at the superior pole (arrow) (Fig. 7.2). US displays tumor size reduction post-chemotherapy (Fig. 7.3). A bisection of the anatomical specimen shows a tumor in the inferior pole (Fig. 7.4).

Figure 7.1a, b
Figure 7.2
Figure 7.3
Figure 7.4

Case 7.2

Fetal Rhabdomyomatous Nephroblastoma

Roberto Llorens Salvador and Carolina Ramírez Ribelles

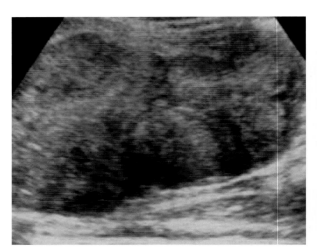

Fig. 7.5

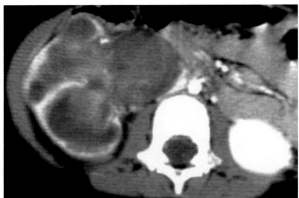

Fig. 7.6

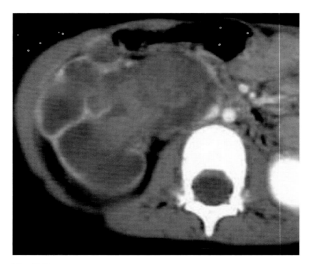

Fig. 7.7

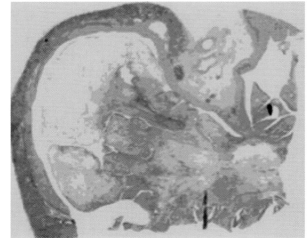

Fig. 7.8

A 3-year-old patient presents with macroscopic hematuria and right palpable abdominal mass.

Renal tumors in children represent approximately 8% of all pediatric malignancies. More than 80% of renal tumors are classic nephroblastomas or WT composed of a combination of blastemal, stromal, and epithelial cell types. Of the histological variants of WT, some present distinct morphologic features and biological behaviors as, for example, the fetal rhabdomyomatous nephroblastoma (FRN), a rare stromal variant that contains at least 30% of fetal striated muscle (rhabdomyoblasts) which is classified as an intermediate-grade malignant tumor by the International Society of Pediatric Oncology (ISPO).

FRN may be radiologically indistinguishable from WT, but it is characterized by appearing at an earlier age than WT (with an increased incidence in children under the age of 2 years). Specific characteristics of this neoplasm include bilateral presentation (seen in one third of cases), large size at diagnosis, tumoral extension to the renal pelvis and ureter, paucity of pulmonary metastases, and poor response to chemotherapy. Clinically, patients present with a palpable mass and abdominal pain. Respiratory distress and fever may also appear.

At the initial evaluation, abdominal ultrasound is necessary to characterize the renal tumor and exclude bilateral involvement. Chest radiography is useful to assess for the presence of pulmonary metastases. Contrast-enhanced body CT and/or abdominal MRI should be performed for tumor staging and a complete abdominal evaluation. Surgical management is elective in these patients.

A large hyperechoic mass is found on ultrasound in the right upper renal pole that expands within the collecting system causing distortion and displacement of the renal parenchyma (Fig. 7.5). Contrast-enhanced CT image shows a large intra-pelvic mass causing secondary hydronephrosis with rim enhancement of the compressed parenchyma (Fig. 7.6). No adenopathies, venous extension, contralateral involvement, or metastases were detected. After a month of preoperative chemotherapy, another CT study was performed showing no significant changes in the right renal tumor (Fig. 7.7). These findings were suggestive of FRN. Final diagnosis is usually determined by open biopsy or nephrectomy. The histological specimen is shown revealing the tumor's extension to the renal collecting system (Fig. 7.8).

Figure 7.5
Figure 7.6
Figure 7.7
Figure 7.8

Case 7.3

Mesoblastic Nephroma

Lourdes Parra Ruiz and María I. Martínez León

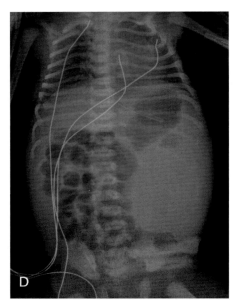

Fig. 7.9

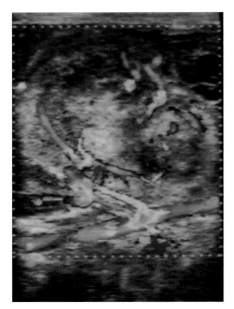

Fig. 7.10

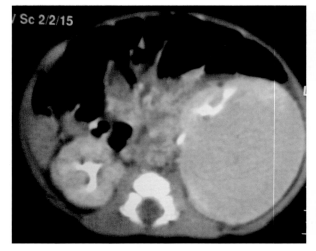

Fig. 7.11

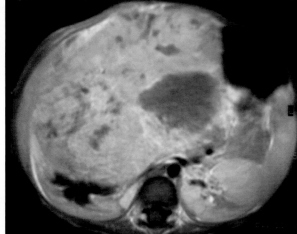

Fig. 7.12

Premature female newborn with palpable solid left intra-abdominal mass.

Mesoblastic nephroma (MN) is a mesenchymal renal tumor of early life. It is an uncommon benign neoplasm that comprises 3% of renal tumors of childhood but as many as 56% in the first 3 months of life and nearly 90% of patients present in the first year. This tumor is the most common solid renal tumor in the neonate. Clinically, the most reliable differential feature is the patient's age. MN is the primary consideration in a neonate and young infant with a palpable renal mass, the differential diagnosis is WT with neonatal presentation. The most common clinical presentation is a palpable abdominal mass.

Many cases are detected at prenatal US. Plain radiography shows a large soft-tissue mass, visible calcification is rare. The sonography appearance or this tumor varies from a homogeneously hypoechoic lesion to a complex, heterogeneous mass with cystic formation and areas of hemorrhage. Hydronephrosis is usually absent. CT and MRI also demonstrate a hypervascular mass, neovascularity, and displacement of adjacent vessels without invasion.

Histologically, MN may show a classical, cellular or mixed pattern. Histologic characteristics are not reliable for predicting the biologic behavior of the tumor. Nephrectomy with wide surgical margin is necessary due to the infiltrative nature of the lesion. Chemotherapy is occasionally used for cellular histology, tumor rupture, or incomplete surgical excision. Local recurrence occurs within 12 months following surgery; therefore, it is currently recommended that patients be closely followed up for 1 year after surgical resection.

X-ray film: large soft-tissue left mass without calcifications, displacing adjacent bowels (Fig. 7.9). Doppler color ultrasound: Hypervascular solid heterogeneous renal mass involving the sinus. Non-nephroblastomatous foci or renal vein invasion (not shown) (Fig. 7.10). CT with contrast: large left homogeneous well-defined renal mass, minimum dilatation of superior callicial groups, light pseudocapsula enhanced, no perirenal extension, no extension through the midline (Fig. 7.11). MR T1 with contrast (other case): huge right solid renal mass with cystic/necrotic degeneration and medium enhancement. There is minimum dilatation of inferior callicial groups. MN is bulking across midline without adjacent infiltration (Fig. 7.12).

Figure 7.9
Figure 7.10
Figure 7.11
Figure 7.12

Case 7.4

Malignant Rhabdoid Tumor of the Kidney
■

María I. Martínez León

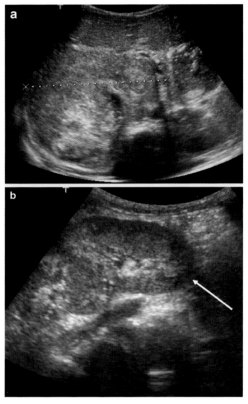

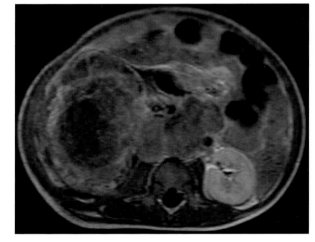

Fig. 7.13

Fig. 7.14

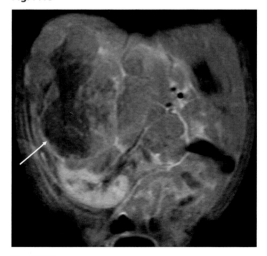

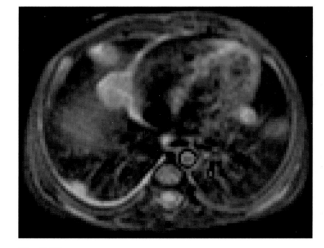

Fig. 7.15

Fig. 7.16

A 1-year-old boy is sent to the emergency room by his pediatrician for presenting an abdominal mass.

Comments

The Malignant Rhabdoid Tumor (MRT) represents approximately 2% of renal malignancies. Also, it has the worst prognosis and is considered the most aggressive neoplasm. MRT was initially described in 1978 as a rhabdomyosarcomatoid variant of the WT because of its occurrence in the kidney and its cells' resemblance to rhabdomyoblasts. The lack of muscular differentiation led to the coining of the term Rhabdoid tumor of the Kidney in 1981, as a separate entity from WT. Now, it is called the MRT of the kidney. MRT occurs exclusively in infancy, with a mean age of 11 months and a survival rate of less than 20%.

Clinical presentation usually consists of a palpable abdominal mass, with other, less frequent symptoms such as hematuria, fever, and hypercalcemia (caused by ectopic production of parathyroid hormone). MRT presents an aggressive behavior with vascular and lymphadenopatic invasion, and early metastases to lung, bone, lymphatics, liver, and brain.

Characteristic imaging findings allow for the differentiation between MRT and other, more frequent tumors at this age, such us WT and MN. These tumors usually show a lobular outline with internal heterogeneity due to hemorrhage and necrosis. Calcifications are seen with a higher prevalence than in WT. A subcapsular fluid collection has been described as a characteristic finding.

Since nearly 15% of MRTs are associated with synchronic or metachronic midline brain neoplasms, CNS CT or MRI is recommended in these cases.

An association with tumoral gene suppression (hSNF5/INI1) has been described, a feature that provides additional genetic and molecular information about the tumor.

Imaging Findings

Axial US reveals an extensive heterogeneous right renal mass. Coronal US shows the relation between the mass and the kidney, with inferior displacement and rotation of the kidney (arrow) (Fig. 7.13a, b). Axial T1-weighted contrast-enhanced MR displays an image similar to the first US, with the MRT displacing the mesenteric vessels (Fig. 7.14). Coronal T1-weighted contrast-enhanced MR image shows the renal origin of the mass, crossing the midline and encasing the renal artery and vein. A peripheral necrotic collection is seen (arrow) (Fig. 7.15). T2-weighted MR image of the lung bases reveals parenchymal lung metastases (Fig. 7.16).

Figure 7.13a, b
Figure 7.14
Figure 7.15
Figure 7.16

Case 7.5

Megacystis-Microcolon-Intestinal Hypoperistalsis Syndrome (Berdon Syndrome)
■
Luisa Ceres Ruiz

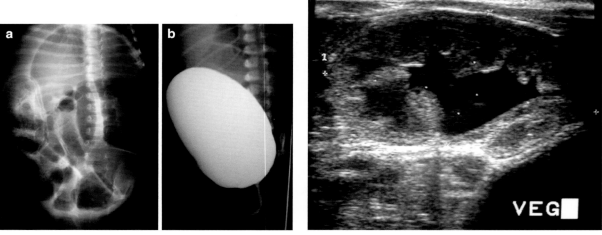

Fig. 7.17

Fig. 7.18

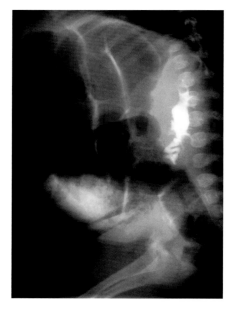

Fig. 7.19

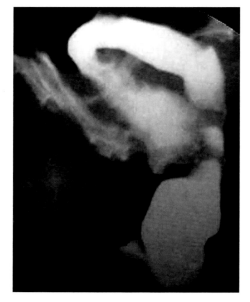

Fig. 7.20

A 1-month-old boy presents to the emergency department with abdominal distension, bilious vomiting, constipation, and incessant crying.

Megacystis-microcolon-intestinal hypoperistalsis syndrome (MMIH) is a rare and serious autosomal recessive entity, described by Berdon in 1976. It occurs more frequently in females with a ratio of 4:1 and is produced by vacuolar degeneration of the intestinal and vesical smooth muscle cells with the presence of ganglionar cells in the myenteric and submucosal plexi (may be increased or decreased in some cases). Recently, the primary myocellular defect has been demonstrated to occur in the synthesis of contractile fibers due to a mutation in the genes coding for the $\alpha 3$ and $\beta 4$ subunits of the nicotinic-acetylcholine neuronal receptor in chromosome 15q24.

Muscular tone is decreased in both the urinary and intestinal tracts. Patients present with abdominal distension, intestinal hypoperistalsis and malrotation, microcolon, dilatation of the proximal ileum, hydronephrosis, and megacystis (due to transmural interstitial fibrosis of the bladder).

Diagnosis should be suspected if findings of constipation, and meconium and urinary retention are documented. Clinical manifestations may develop at birth or shortly after.

During routine pregnancy sonographic exploration, suggestive prenatal findings include megacystis and abdominal distension. Differential diagnoses include prune belly syndrome, posterior urethral valves (PUVs), vaginal atresia, and large ovarian cysts. Distinguishing between them is essential due to the fact that MMIH presents a less favorable outcome. Diagnostic confirmation is determined by histological and immunohistochemical (decreased actin in smooth muscle) data collected from intestinal biopsy or autopsy that demonstrates intestinal and vesical myopathy.

Abdominal radiography is suggestive of MMIH if abdominal distension with small bowel dilatation, and occasionally intestinal perforation is identified (Fig. 7.17a). Voiding cystourethrogram (VCUG) shows significant megacystis, and vesicourethral reflux is uncommon (Fig. 7.17b). Ultrasound reveals megacystis with low-grade (I/IV) hydronephrosis (Fig. 7.18) due to defective urethral drainage. Intravenous urography shows minimal urethral ectasia, which is always less severe than that observed in prune belly syndrome and PUV (Fig. 7.19). Barium enema (Fig. 7.20) displays microcolon with a significant disparity in relation to the caliber of the small bowel. The small intestine presents a greater dilatation of its middle portion than of the distal ileum.

Figure 7.17a, b
Figure 7.18
Figure 7.19
Figure 7.20

Case 7.6
Ossifying Renal Tumor of Infancy
■
Silvia Villa Santamaría and Susana Calle Restrepo

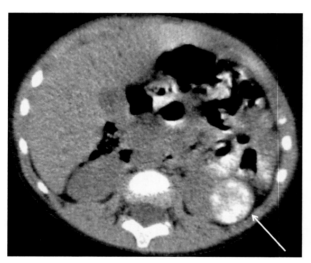

Fig. 7.21

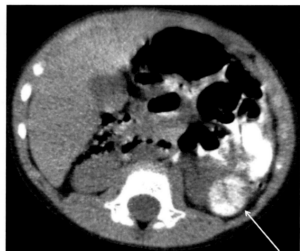

Fig. 7.22

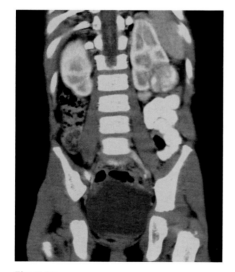

Fig. 7.23

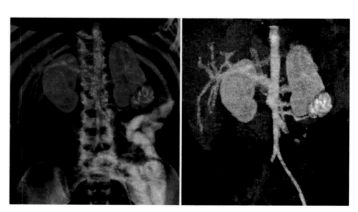

Fig. 7.24

A 5-year-old black female patient presents with hematuria. Upon physical examination, no changes are observed. Further studies, including CT, detect a calcified renal mass.

The ossifying renal tumor of infancy (ORTI) is an extremely rare neoplasm, which was first described in 1980 and has since had few reported cases. The peak of incidence is reached at 14 months of age, and the condition is more frequent in males.

ORTI originates from the urothelium and affects the renal medulla, more specifically the papilla, and may extend itself to the calyceal system. Due to its location, it may mimic staghorn calculi, which can be ruled out because of the patient's age.

Although the etiology of the lesion is poorly understood, some authors believe it is caused by osteogenic changes of the urothelial cells, while others have described the presence of fusiform cells similar to those found in the spectrum of the Wilm's tumor. Nevertheless, to date, no WT transformation has been reported in patients affected by ORTI.

Histologically, this tumor is comprised of hypocellular areas made up of cells with small, rounded or oval nuclei within a pale cytoplasm immersed in a dense bone matrix. Also, the tumor presents an osteoblastic osteoid component without osteoclasts or cartilaginous tissue. Furthermore, few to none mitoses are detected. Macroscopically, ORTI is an irregular calcified mass.

The neoplasm is classified as a benign tumor since at up to 23 years of follow-up neither recurrence nor metastases have been documented. Surgical resection and close clinical monitoring are considered the first line of treatment.

Non-contrast CT shows a solid, calcified heterogeneous mass located at the inferior pole of the left kidney (Figs. 7.21 and 7.22). A contrast-enhanced coronal CT view shows a calcified heterogeneous renal mass that does not exhibit contrast uptake (Fig. 7.23). Coronal 3D reconstructions show the anatomic location of the mass and its relation to neighboring structures (Fig. 7.24).

Figure 7.21
Figure 7.22
Figure 7.23
Figure 7.24

Case 7.7

Xanthogranulomatous Pyelonephritis
■

Alejandra Doroteo Lobato and María I. Martínez León

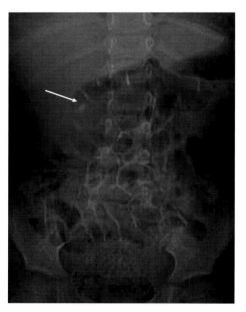

Fig. 7.25

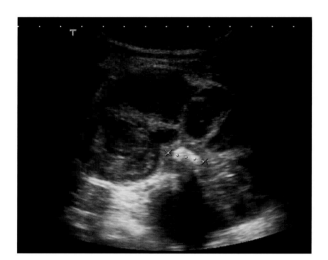

Fig. 7.26

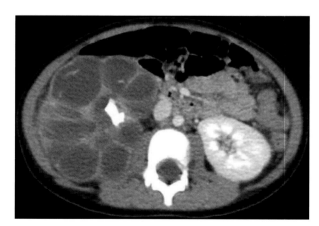

Fig. 7.27

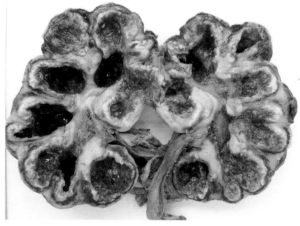

Fig. 7.28

A 4-year-old girl presents with a 4-month history of recurrent urinary tract infections, fever, and clinical deterioration. Upon examination, a right hypochondriac mass is palpated.

Xanthogranulomatous pyelonephritis (XP) is a serious and chronic inflammatory process of the kidney characterized by a destruction of the renal parenchyma with infiltration by lipid-charged macrophages. It is considered a rare entity that usually occurs in adults, predominantly women in the sixth to seventh decade of life. XP is uncommon in children, and only few cases have been reported. Although the pathogenesis is unclear, up to 76% have been documented in relation to obstruction of the pyeloureteral junction, generally by calculi. Also, congenital cases have been reported. The most frequently implicated pathogens include *Escherichia coli* and *Proteus mirabilis*. XP can be divided into two subtypes: diffuse and focal.

XP is usually unilateral and presents initially as a pyonephrosis. Clinical manifestations include fever, flank pain, weight loss, failure to thrive, urinary symptoms, and palpable flank mass. It may be associated with anemia, leukocytosis, increased globular sedimentation rates, and urinary sediment abnormalities.

Neither the clinical presentation nor the imaging findings are specific to this entity. Nevertheless, a combination of both may help in guiding the diagnosis. Manifestations such as urinary infections, lithiasis, and impaired renal excretion in a patient presenting chronic obstruction with infection and a poor response to antibiotic treatment suggest a diagnosis of XP. Unfortunately, the treatment of choice for this condition is nephrectomy and definitive diagnosis is established by histological examination.

Localized abdominal radiograph shows a staghorn calculus superimposed on the right renal silhouette (arrow) (Fig. 7.25). Abdominal ultrasound reveals an enlarged right kidney with a thinning cortex and echogenic elements within dilated calyces. Lithiasis within the renal pelvis is observed (Fig. 7.26). Abdominopelvic contrast-enhanced CT shows right nephromegaly with a thin rim of cortex, delayed enhancement in comparison to the contralateral kidney, and distended calyces occupied by material. Renal pelvis lithiasis is revealed (Fig. 7.27). A bisected macroscopic specimen of the right kidney is shown (Fig. 7.28).

Figure 7.25
Figure 7.26
Figure 7.27
Figure 7.28

Case 7.8

Ureteral Duplications

■

Luisa Ceres Ruiz

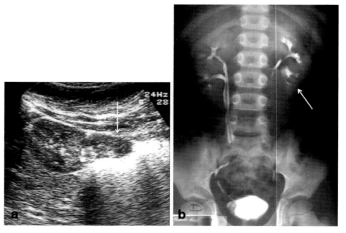

Fig. 7.29

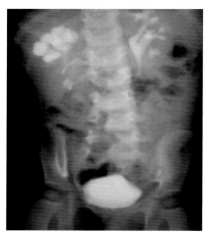

Fig. 7.30

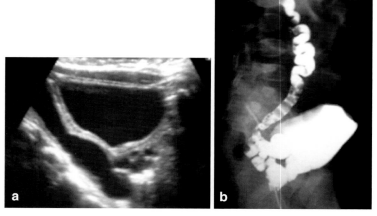

Fig. 7.31

Fig. 7.32

Ureteral duplications consist of the presence of two excretory systems originating from a single kidney. It is termed incomplete duplicity or bifid ureter when both drain into the bladder via a common ureter and complete duplicity occurs when both ureters drain separately. The pathogenesis of this condition is due to the premature division of the ureteral bud originating from the Wolffian duct. The Weigert–Meyer rule states that the ureter collecting from the superior pole of the kidney usually opens inferiorly and medially in relation to that of the lower pole. The superior ureter tends to drain ectopically in the vesical trigone, urethra, or other Wolffian duct structures in males and Müllerian structures in females. Furthermore, it has a higher susceptibility to become obstructed and if distension occurs at its intravesical portion, ureterocele develops.

Anomalies associated with a double collecting systems include:

- Hydronephrosis of the upper renal pole due to stenosis of the ureteral opening
- Ectopic insertion of the superior ureter
- Ectopic ureterocele of the superior system
- Reflux to the inferior system due to valvular incompetence

The treatment of choice is surgical correction, namely, heminephroureterectomy when dysfunctional parenchyma of a renal pole is detected. The endoscopic management of the refluxing ureter is usually curative in low-grade cases.

US imaging in complete duplication reveals an evident differentiation between the renal poles. On the other hand, incomplete duplication may be confused with Bertin column hypertrophy. When the superior system displays dilatation, the bladder must be evaluated for ureterocele. A single intravenous urography (IVU) image taken 20 min post-contrast or MRI may aid in establishing the diagnosis. VCUG is indicated in assessing for reflux when the collecting systems present dilatation. IVU, MRI, and/or vaginogram is useful in evaluating ectopic insertions. Differential diagnoses include cystic adrenal masses, non-acute hemorrhage, cystic neuroblastoma, and segmental multicystic kidney.

US and IVU show incomplete duplication of the right collecting system and complete duplication of the left with inferior pole nephropathy (arrow in both) (Fig. 7.29a, b). IVU shows right duplication with inferior pole reflux nephropathy (Fig. 7.30). US and VCUG display ureteral duplication with an ectopic insertion at the seminal vesicles (Fig. 7.31a, b). Ureteral duplication with a large ureterocele (arrow) is seen causing obstruction and associated dysfunction of the superior renal pole (asterisk) (Fig. 7.32).

Figure 7.29a, b
Figure 7.30
Figure 7.31a, b
Figure 7.32

Comments

Imaging Findings

Case 7.9
Renal Trauma
■
Luisa Ceres Ruiz

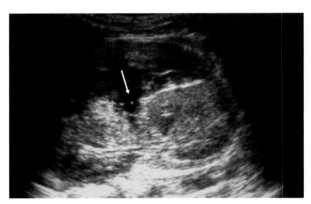

Fig. 7.33

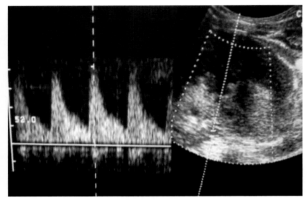

Fig. 7.34

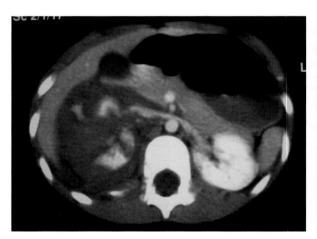

Fig. 7.35

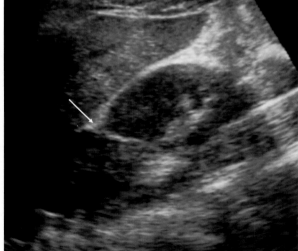

Fig. 7.36

A 5-year-old girl presents with lumbar region contusion and associated malaise due to a fall 4 days prior.

Approximately 80–85% of renal lesions occur secondary to blunt trauma to the abdomen, flank, and/or dorsal region. Compression causes direct organ damage, which in turn produces lacerations, hematomas, contusions, fractures, and thromboses.

Ultrasound is typically used as the initial imaging technique and aids in determining the need for further studies. The preliminary use of US decreases the amount of normal CT studies. The Injury Severity Score, which incorporates clinical and sonographic data, ultimately determines the use of additional diagnostic imaging by CT or MRI.

The manner in which renal lesions occur is generally trauma by compression or deceleration mechanisms, and less frequently in children, penetrating injuries.

Imaging for this clinical entity must evaluate parenchymal lesions, the integrity of the collecting system and vascular pedicle, urine excretion, perirenal extension, and active hemorrhage. Renal trauma can be classified into four grades by severity:

1. Minor renal injury – includes subcapsular hematomas, small lacerations, and segmental infarcts. Conservative treatment is generally employed.
2. Major renal injury – includes lacerations that affect over 50% of the renal parenchyma, involves the collecting system with associated leakage of urine and/or presents with large perirenal hematomas. Surgery is indicated in hemodynamically unstable patients.
3. Catastrophic kidney damage that requires surgical intervention. Findings include fragmentation of the renal parenchyma with large para- or perinephric hematomas, and venous or arterial vascular pedicle lesions.
4. Pyeloureteral junction avulsion.

Sagittal US of the right kidney shows an extensive subcapsular and perirenal hematoma with a severe lesion of the renal parenchyma that involves the sinus (arrow) (Fig. 7.33). Doppler of the renal artery reveals integrity of the vascular pedicle (Fig. 7.34). Contrast-enhanced CT shows multiple renal lesions with a large perirenal hematoma. The patient remained stable after blood transfusion, and conservative management was followed (Fig. 7.35). Follow-up US 4 months later revealed a scar (arrow) located in the middle region of the kidney as the only sequelae of the trauma (Fig. 7.36).

Figure 7.33
Figure 7.34
Figure 7.35
Figure 7.36

Case 7.10
Renal Candidiasis
■
Silvia Villa Santamaría and Susana Calle Restrepo

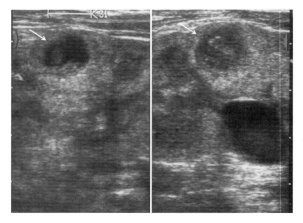

Fig. 7.37

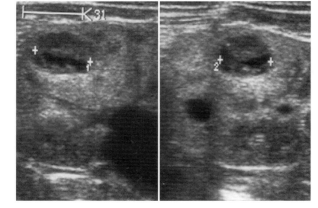

Fig. 7.38

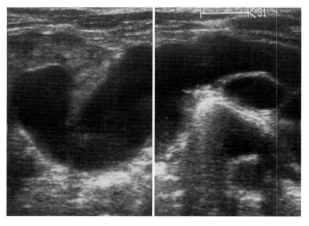

Fig. 7.39

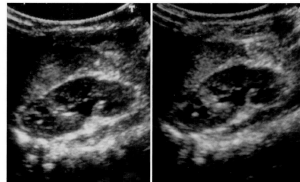

Fig. 7.40

A 45-day-old male patient with a history of PUVs presents with fever and vomiting. Upon physical examination, the patient was irritable and laboratory results showed a urinary infection. Renal ultrasound identified pelvicalyceal dilatation and a renal abscess, culture of which grew *Candida albicans*.

Comments

C. albicans is a fungus that makes up part of the normal human flora and usually does not cause symptoms. Nevertheless, it may manifest as an opportunistic disease in individuals with compromised immune response. Neonates are at greater risk due to their immune immaturity. Other factors such as antibiotic use, prematurity, and indwelling catheters also contribute to the development of candidiasis in newborns.

Infections caused by *C. albicans* have been described in almost all organs including the meninges, eyes, kidneys, and heart, as well as in other less common locations, such as the joints. Renal compromise may occur by hematogenous spread of the pathogen from septic foci elsewhere in the body. Also, an ascending infection originating from a urinary infection, urinary tract instrumentation or urinary obstruction may ultimately colonize the kidneys.

Renal candidiasis may manifest itself as pyelonephritis, papillary necrosis, a perinephric abscess, a mycetoma, urinary obstruction, nephrocalcinosis, ureterocele, and/or hydronephrosis, among others.

Diagnosis is based on the growth of *C. albicans* in urine cultures, and treatment with intravenous antifungal medications is required. In certain cases, depending on clinical presentation of the infection, surgical management may be necessary.

Imaging Findings

Renal ultrasound shows an increase in renal parenchyma echogenicity as well as a well-defined rounded lesion with thick walls and internal echos consistent with a mycetoma (arrows) (Fig. 7.37). An ultrasound image of a renal abscess caused by *C. albicans* is shown (Fig. 7.38). Pyeloureteral dilatation consistent with the patient's history of PUVs is identified (Fig. 7.39). Follow-up studies after antifungal treatment show a decrease in parenchymal echogenicity with persistent pelvicalyceal dilatation (Fig. 7.40).

Figure 7.37
Figure 7.38
Figure 7.39
Figure 7.40

Further Reading

Book

Baert AL (ed) (2008) Encyclopedia of diagnostic imagins. Springer, Berlin/Heidelberg/New York

Davidson A (1994) Radiology of the kidney and genitourinary tract. W.B. Saunders, Washington, DC

Donnelly LF et al, ed. (2005) Diagnostic imaging: Pediatrics. Salt Lake City, AMIRISYS (Philadelphia: Elsevier)

Douglas Stephens F, Durhan Smith E, Hutson JM, Douglas Stephens F, Durhan Smith E, Hutson JM (2002) Congenital anomalies of the kidney, urinary and genital tracts, vol 14, 2nd edn. Martin Dunitz, London, pp 167–307

Murphy WM et al, eds. (2004) Kidney tumors in children. In: Atlas of tumor pathology, 4th Series, Fascicle 1. Armed Forces Institute of Pathology, Washington, DC, pp 47–49

Richardson MD, Warnock DW (2003) Fungal infection: diagnosis and management. Blackwell, Malden

Siegel MJ (1999) The kidney. In: Pediatric body CT. Lippincott Williams & Wilkins, Philadelphia, pp 226–252

Slovis Thomas L. Haller Jack. Caffey's pediatric diagnostic imaging. Part V, Neonatal genitourinary tract, 10th edn. Mosby, Philadelphia

Stephen RE (1992) Handbook of gastrointestinal and genitourinary radiology. Mosby, St. Louis, p 180

Swischuk LE (1997) Imaging of the newborn, infant, and young child, 4th edn. Lippincott Williams & Wilkins, Philadelphia, p 608

Web Link

Hicks J. Review of pediatric renal neoplasms. Renal neoplasms in childhood. http://sup.ultrakohl.com/uscap/abs-1998/hicks98h.htm

Hidalgo J, Vasquez J (2010) Candidiasis. Emedicine: WebMD. http://emedicine.medscape.com/article/213853-overview. Updated June 2010

http://emedicine.medscape.com/

http://emedicine.medscape.com/article/439747-overview

http://emedicine.medscape.com/article/989398-diagnosis

http://emedicine.medscape.com/article/993084-overview

Mesoblastic nephorma: eMedicine radiology. Avalaible in http://emedicine.medscape.com/article/411147-overview

www.emedicine.medscape.com/article/378075

www.sordic.com.ar/casos/2004-08c/pag2.php

Articles

Agrons GA, Kingsman KD, Wagner BJ, Sotelo-Avila C (1997) Rhabdoid tumor of the kidney in children: a comparative study of 21 cases. AJR 168:447–451

Alonso RC, Nacenta SB, Martinez PD, Guerrero AS, Fuentes CG (2009) Kidney in danger: CT findings of blunt and penetrating renal trauma. RadioGraphics 29:2033–2053

Amar AM, Tomlinson G, Green DM, Breslow NE, de Alarcon PA (2001) Clinical presentation of rhabdoid tumors of the kidney. J Pediatr Hematol Oncol 23:105–108

Amoury RA, Fellows RA, Goodwin CD, Hall RT, Holder TM, Ashcraft KW (1977) Megacystis-microcolon-intestinal hypoperistalsis syndrome: a cause of intestinal obstruction in the newborn period. J Pediatr Surg 12:1063–1065

Andres V, Muro D, Sanguesa C, Torres D, Berbel Tornero O (2003) Ecografía en el diagnóstico de la candidiasis renal neonatal. Radiología 45:37–42

Angulo JC, Lopez JI, Ereno C, Unda M, Flores N (1991) Hydrops fetalis and congenital mesoblastic nephroma. Child Nephrol Urol 11:115–116

Avni FE, Nicaise N, Hall M, Janssens F, Collier F, Matos C, Metens T (2001) The role of MR imaging for the assessment of complicated duplex kidneys in children: preliminary report. Pediatr Radiol 31:215–223

Babyn P, Owens C, Gyepes M, D'Angio GJ (1995) Imaging patients with Wilms tumor. Hematol Oncol Clin North Am 9:1217–1252

Berdon WE, Baker DH, Blanc WA, Gay B, Santulli TV, Donovan C (1976) Megacystis-microcolon-intestinal hypoperistalsis syndrome: a new case of intestinal obstruction in a newborn. Report of radiological findings in five newborn girls. AJR 126:957–964

Bisset GS, Strife JL (1987) The duplex collecting system in girls with urinary tract infection: prevalence and significance. AJR 148:497–500

Boldus R, Brown R, Culp D (1972) Fungus balls in the renal pelvis. Radiology 102:555–557

Bravo-Bravo C, Martínez-León MI, Ceres-Ruiz L, Weil-Lara B (2003) Childhood xanthogranulomatous pyelonephritis: an uncommon entity. Radiología 45(5):225–227

Carrico C, Lebowitz RL (1998) Incontinence due to an infrasphincteric ectopic ureter: why the delay in diagnosis and what the radiologist can do about it. Pediatr Radiol 28:942–949

Castell V, Muro MD, Brugger S, Moreno A, Sangüesa C (2004) Radiological manifestations of mesoblastic nephroma. Radiología 46:77–82

Chen CP, Wang TY, Chuang CY (1998) Sonographic findings in a fetus with megacystis-microcolon-intestinal hypoperistalsis syndrome. J Clin Ultrasound 26:217–220

Chung-Pin S, Yiu-Wah L, Yang-Jann L, Cheng-Shen H (1998) Bilateral congenital cysts of the seminal vesicle wiyh bilateral duplex kidneys. J Urol 160:184–185

Ciftci AO, Cook RC, van Velzen D (1996) Megacystis microcolon intestinal hypoperistalsis syndrome: evidency of a primary myocellular defect of contractile fiber synthesis. J Pediatr Surg 31:1706–1711

Craig WD, Wagner BJ, Travis MD (2008) Pyelonephritis: radiologic–pathologic review. RadioGraphics 28:255–277

De Campo JF (1986) Ultrasound of Wilms' tumor. Pediatr Radiol 16:21–24

Eeg KR, Khoury AE, Halachmi S, Braga LH, Farhat WA, Bägli DJ, Pippi Salle JL, Lorenzo AJ (2009) Single center experience with application of the ALARA concept to serial imaging studies after blunt renal trauma in children – is ultrasound enough? J Urol 181:1834–1840

El-Husseini TK, Egail SA, Al-Orf AM, Mostert C (2005) Ossifying renal tumor of infancy. Saudi Med J 26(12):1978–1979

Ellisen LW (2002) Regulation of gene expression by WT1 in development and tumorigenesis. Int J Hematol 76:110–116

Fan CM, Whitman GJ, Chew FS, Chew FS (1995) Xanthogranulomatous pyelonephritis. AJR 165:1008

Fernbach SK, Feinstein KA, Spencer K, Lindstrom CA (1997) Ureteral duplication and its complications. RadioGraphics 17:109–127

Garza S, Keeney SE, Angel CA, Thompson LL, Swischuk LE (2004) Meconium obstruction in the very low birth weight premature infant. Pediatrics 114:285–290

Geller E, Smergel E, Lowry P (1997) Renal neoplasms of childhood. Rad Clin North Am 35:1391–1413

Glick RD, Hicks MJ, Nuchtern JG, Wesson DE, Olutoye OO, Cass DL (2004) Renal tumors in infants less than 6 months of age. J Pediatr Surg 39(4):522–525

Gonzalez F, Canning DA, Hyun G, Casale P (2006) Lower pole pelvi-ureteric junction obstruction in duplicated collecting systems. BUJ Int 97:161–165

Guillén G, Asensio M, Piró C, Martin JA, Pérez M (2007) Five years of renal trauma in a paediatric trauma center: new tools in the diagnostic and therapeutic process. Cir Pediátr 20:209–214

Haas JE, Palmer NF, Weinberg AG, Beckwith JB (1981) Ultrastructure of malignant rhabdoid tumor of the kidney. A distinctive renal tumor of children. Hum Pathol 12(7):646–657

Hallscheidt PJ, Fink C, Haferkamp A, Bock M, Luburic A, Zuna I, Noeldge G, Kauffmann G (2005) Preoperative staging of renal cell carcinoma with inferior vena cava thrombus using multidetector CT and MRI: prospective study with histopathological correlation. J Comput Assist Tomogr 29:64–68

Hammedeh MY, Buik RG, Nicholls G, Calder CJ, Corkery JJ (1994) Xanthogranulomatous pyelonephritis in childhood: preoperative diagnosis is possible. Br J Urol 73:83–86

Han TI, Kim MJ, Yoon HK, Chung JY, Choeh K (2001) Rhabdoid tumour of the kidney: imaging findings. Pediatr Radiol 31:233–237

Harms D, Gutjahr P, Hohenfellner R, Willke E (1980) Fetal rhabdomyomatous nephroblastoma with a renal pelvic mass simulating sarcoma botryoides. Eur J Pediatr 133(2):167–172

Hayes WS, Hartman DS, Sesterbenn IA (1991) Xanthogranulomatous pyelonephritis. RadioGraphics 11:485–498

Hussman DA, Allen TD (1991) Resolution of vesicoureteral reflux in completely duplicated systems: fact or fiction? J Urol 145:1022–1023

Irsutti M, Puget C, Baunin C, Duga I, Sarramon MF, Guitard J (2000) Mesoblastic nephroma: prenatal ultrasonographic and MRI features. Pediatr Radiol 30:147–150

Johnson KC, Barone JG (2006) Management of obstructing fungal pyelonephritis in infants. Urology 67(2):424, e7-424.e9

Joseph JM, Suter OC, Nenadov-Beck M, Gudinchet F, Frey P, Meagher-Villemure K (2003) Repeated surgical excision for an unusual variant of nephroblastoma: case report and review of the literature. J Pediatr Surg 38(4):E13

Karlowicz MG (2003) Candidal renal and urinary tract infection in neonates. Semin Perinatol 27(5):393–400

Kawashima A, Sandler C, Goldman S (1997) CT of renal inflammatory disease. RadioGraphics 17:851–866

Kawashima A, Sandler CM, Corl FM, West OC, Tamm EP, Fishman EK, Goldman SM (2001) Imaging of renal trauma: a comprehensive review. RadioGraphics 21:557–574

Kelner M, Droullé P, Didier F, Hoeffel JC (2003) The vascular "ring" in mesoblastic nephroma: report of two cases. Pediatr Radiol 33:123–128

Körner M, Krötz MM, Degenhart C, Pfeifer KJ, Reiser MF, Linsenmaier U (2008) Current role of emergency US in patients with major trauma. RadioGraphics 28:225–242

Lefi M, Jouini R, Guesmi M, Mekki M, Belghith M, Nouri A (2002) Congenital mesoblastic nephroma. Prog Urol 12:663–665

Leroy S, Vantalon S, Larakeb A (2010) Vesicoureteral reflux in children with urinary tract infection. Radiology 255:890–898

Loffroy R, Guiu B, Watfa J, Michel F, Cercueil JP, Krause D (2007) Xanthogranulomatous pyelonephritis in adults: clinical and radiological findings in difuse and focal forms. Clin Radiol 62:884–890

Lonergan GJ, Martinez-Leon MI, Agrons GA, Montemarano H, Suarez ES (1998) Nephrogenic rest, nephroblastomatosis and associated lesions of the kidney. RadioGraphics 18:947–968

López-Medina A, Ereno MJ, Fernández-Cantón G, Calder CJ, Zuazo A (1995) Focal xanthogranulomatous pyelonephritis simulating malignancy in children. Abdom Imaging 20:270–271

Lougué-Sorgho LC, Lambot K, Gorincour G, Chaumoître K, Chapuy S, Bourlière-Najean B et al (2006) Kidney trauma in children: state of the art medical imaging. J Radiol 87: 275–283

Lowe LH, Isuani BH, Heller RM, Stein SM, Johnson JE, Navarro OM et al (2000a) Pediatric masses: Wilms tumor and beyond. RadioGraphics 20:1585–1603

Lowe LH, Isuani BH, Heller RM, Stein SM, Johnson JE, Navarro OM, Hernanz-Schulman M (2000b) Pediatric renal masses: Wilms tumor and beyond. RadioGraphics 20:1585–1603

Lowe LH, Isuani B, Heller R, Stein S, Johnson J, Navarro O (2000c) Pediatric renal masses: Wilms tumor and beyond. RadioGraphics 20:1585–1603

Maes P, Delemarre J, de Kraker J, Ninane J (1999) Fetal rhabdomyomatous nephroblastoma: a tumour of good prognosis but resistant to chemotherapy. Eur J Cancer 35(9): 1356–1360

McGahan PJ, Richards JR, Bair AE, Rose JS (2005) Ultrasound detection of blunt urological trauma: a 6-year study. Injury 36:762–770

McHugh K (2007) Renal and adrenal tumours in children. Cancer Imaging 7:41–51

Mekki M, Belghith M, Krichène I, Zakhama A, Landolsi A, Chelly S, Nouri A (2002) Fetal rhabdomyomatous nephroblastoma: report of 2 cases and review of the literature. Ann Urol (Paris) 36(4):245–249

Murthi GV, Carachi R, Howatson A (2003) Congenital cystic mesoblastic nephroma. Pediatr Surg Int 19:109–111

Nakagawa T, Misawa H, Nakajima Y, Takaki M (2005) Absence of peristalsis in the ileum of W/W(V) mutant mice that are selectively deficient in myenteric interstitial cells of Cajal. J Smooth Muscle Res 41:141–151

Nguyen MM, Das S (2002) Pediatric renal trauma. Urology 59:762–767

Noyola DE, Fernandez M, Moylett EH, Baker CJ (2001) Ophthalmologic, visceral, and cardiac involvement in neonates with candidemia. Clin Infect Dis 32(7):1018–1023

Pickhardt PJ, Lonergan GJ, Davis CJ, Kashitani N, Eagner BJ (2000a) From the archives of the AFIP. Infiltrative renal lesions: radiologic-pathologic correlation. RadioGraphics 20:215–243

Pickhardt PJ, Lonergan GJ, Kashitani N, Wagner BJ (2000b) Infiltrative renal lesions: radiologic and pathologic correlation. RadioGraphics 20:215–243

Pollono D, Drut R, Tomarchio S, Fontana A, Ibañez O (2003) Fetal rhabdomyomatous nephroblastoma: report of 14 cases confirming chemotherapy resistance. J Pediatr Hematol Oncol 25(8):640–643

Porteus MH, Narkool P, Neuberg D, Guthrie KN, Breslow DM (2000) Characteristics and outcome of children with Beckwith–Wiedemann syndrome and Wilms' tumor: A report from the National Wilms Tumor Study Group. JCO 18:2026–2037

Privett JT, Jeans WD, Roylance J (1976) The incidence and importance of renal duplication. Clin Radiol 4:521–530

Quinn FM, Dick AC, Corbally MT, McDermott MB, Guiney EJ (1999) Xanthogranulomatous pyelonephritis in childhood. Arch Dis Child 81:483–486

Riebel T, Kebelmann-Betzing C, Sarioglu N, Wit J, Seeger K (2003) Unusual mesoblastic nephroma in a young child. Pediatr Radiol 33:62–65

Rite Gracia S, Fernández Álvarez de Sotomayor B, Rebage Moisés V, Marco Tello A, Esteban Ibarz JA et al (2000) Megabladder-microcolon–intestinal hypoperistalsis syndrome. An Esp Pediatr 53(3):253–256

Roberts CW, Biegel JA (2009) The role of SMARCB1/INI1 in development of rhabdoid tumor. Cancer Biol Ther 8:412–416

Rolle U, Piaseczna-Piotrowska A, Puri P (2007) Interstitial cells of Cajal in the normal gut and in intestinal motility disorders of childhood. Pediatr Surg Int 23:1139–1152

Saba LM, de Camargo B, Gabriel-Arana M (1998) Experience with six children with fetal rhabdomyomatous nephroblastoma: review of the clinical, biologic, and pathologic features. Med Pediatr Oncol 30(3):152–155

Samuel M, Duffy P, Capps S, Mouriquand P, Williams D, Ransley P (2001) Xanthogranulomatous pyelonephritis in childhood. J Pediatr Surg 36:598–601

Sato M, Yoshii H (2004) Reevaluation of ultrasonography for solid-organ injury in blunt abdominal trauma. J Ultrasound Med 23:583–596

Schelling J, Schröder A, Stein R, Rösch WH (2007) Ossifying renal tumor of infancy. J Pediatr Urol 3(3):258–261

Schenk JP, Graf N, Günther P, Ley S, Göppl M, Kulozik A, Rohrschneider WK, Tröger J (2008) Role of MRI in the management of patients with nephroblastoma. Eur Radiol 18:683–691

Seixas-Mikelus SA, Khan A, Williot PE, Greenfield SP (2009) Three-month-old boy with juvenile granulosa cell tumor of testis and ossifying renal tumor of infancy. Urology 74(2):311–313

Shinohara N, Koanagi T, Hanioka K (1998) Ossifying renal tumor of infancy: the first Japanese case with long-term follow-up. Patol Int 48:151–159

Siegel MJ, Chung EM (2008) Wilms' tumor and other pediatric renal masses. Magn Reson Imaging Clin N Am 16:479–497

Siomou E, Papadopoulou F, Kollios KD et al (2006) Duplex collecting system diagnosed during the first 6 years of life after a first urinary tract infection: a study of 63 children. J Urol 175:678–681

Sister CL, Siegel MJ (1989) Malignant rhabdoid tumor of the kidney: radiologic features. Radiology 172:211–212

Sotelo-Avila C et al (1995) Ossifying renal tumor of infancy: a clinicopathologic study of nine cases. Pediatr Pathol Lab Med 15:745–762

Steffens J, Kraus J, Misho B, Remberger K (1993) Ossifying renal tumor of infancy. J Urol 149(5):1080–1081

Stokland E, Jodal U, Sixt R, Swerkersson S, Hansson S (2007) Uncomplicated duplex kidney and DMSA scintigraphy in children with urinary tract infection. Pediatr Radiol 37:826–828

Umbreit EC, Routh JC, Husmann DA (2009) Nonoperative management of nonvascular grade IV blunt renal trauma in children: meta-analysis and systematic review. Urology 74: 579–582

Vasquez T (2009) Epidemiología clínica del micetoma renal por Candida. Rev Enfer Infec Pediatr 22(89):6

Vazquez JL, Barnewolt CE, Shamberger RC, Chung T, Perez-Atayde AR (1998) Ossifying renal tumor of infancy presenting as a palpable abdominal mass. Pediatr Radiol 28:454–457

Vázquez O, Campos Rivera T, Jiménez R, Ahumada Mendoza H, Martínez I (2001) Candidiasis renal en pacientes pediátricos. Rev Mex Patol Clin 48(1):17–22

Vicandi B, Picazo ML, González MC, Contreras F (1985) Fetal rhabdomyomatous nephroblastoma: study of 2 cases and review of the literature. An Esp Pediatr 23(3):205–210

Vujanic GM (2006) Renal tumors in early life. Curr Diagn Pathol 12:210–219

Vujanic GM, Charles AK (2008) Renal tumours of childhood: an update. Pathology 40:217–227

Vujanic GM, Sandstedt B, Harms D, Boccon-Gibod L, Delemarre JF (1996) Rhabdoid tumour of the kidney: a clinicopahological study of 22 patiens from the International Society of Paediatric Oncology (SIOP) nephroblastoma file. Histopathology 28:333–340

Weese DL, Applebaum H, Taber P (1991) Mapping intravascular extension of Wilms' tumor with magnetic resonance imaging. J Pediatr Surg 26:64–67

Wigger HJ (1976) Fetal rhabdomyomatous nephroblastoma-a variant of Wilms tumor. Hum Pathol 7(6):613–623

Wimalendra M, Reece A, Nicholl RM (2004) Renal fungal ball. Arch Dis Child Fetal Neonatal Ed 89(4):F376

Winger DI, Buyuk A, Bohrer S, Turi G, Scimeca P, Price A et al (2006) Radiology–pathology conference: rhabdoid tumor of the kidney. Clin Imaging 30:132–136

Winter RM, Knowles SAS (1986) Megacystis-microcolon-intestinal hipoperistalsis syndrome: confirmation of autosomal recessive inheritance. J Med Genet 23:3260–3262

Yigit S, Barlas C, Yurdakok M, Onderoglu L, Zafer Y, Saltik I (1996) The megacystis-microcolon-intestinal hypoperistalsis syndrome: report of a case and review of the literature. Turk J Pediatr 38:137–141

Zarate YA, Mena R, Martin LJ, Steele P, Tinkle BT, Hopkin RJ (2009) Experience with hemihyperplasia and Beckwith–Wiedemann syndrome surveillance protocol. Am J Med Genet A 149:1691–1697

Contents

M.I. Martínez-León et al., *Learning Pediatric Imaging*, Learning Imaging,
DOI: 10.1007/978-3-642-16892-5_8, © Springer-Verlag Berlin Heidelberg 2011

Case 8.1
Legg–Calve–Perthes Disease
■
Ignasi Barber Martínez de la Torre

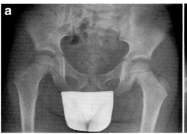
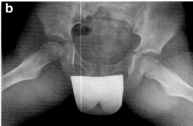

Fig. 8.1

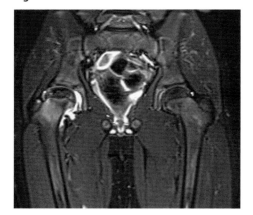

Fig. 8.2

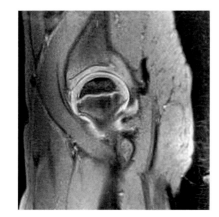

Fig. 8.3

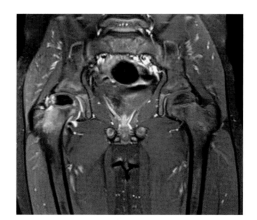

Fig. 8.4

A 6-year-old boy presented a 3-months history of right hip pain. Synovitis of the hip was initially diagnosed, and X-ray were normal. Three months later a slight pain in the hip persisted, and a limitation of joint motion was evident at physical examination. X-ray and MRI at this time revealed evidence of osteonecrosis of the right femoral head.

Comments

Legg–Calvé–Perthes Disease (LCP) is an idiopathic osteonecrosis (or osteochondrosis) of the femoral head. It affects children, especially between 4 and 8 years old, and is four times more common in boys. Both hips are involved in approximately 10–15% of patients, usually not at the same time. The most important clinical signs are pain and limited mobility, and the main duration of symptoms is 4 months.

The lateral pillar classification is the most accepted way to assess severity, based on the loss of height of the lateral third of the femoral head, which is the weight-bearing zone and where revascularization begins. Collapse of the lateral pillar predicts poor outcome. Type A, the full height of the lateral pillar is preserved; Type B, between 50% and 100%; and Type C, more than 50% of the lateral pillar is lost.

Radiography is the primary imaging technique used in patients with suspected or known LCP disease. MR Imaging has been shown to be more accurate in evaluating the extent of epiphyseal necrosis and can be used to stage the hip and identify when the revascularization period begins. The timing of imaging Perthes disease and the treatment options are still controversial. Initial MRI in the acute hip pain phase should include postintravenous contrast dynamic imaging to asses femoral head perfusion. Diffusion-weighted Imaging may be a better indicator of cell damage and necrosis than postcontrast gadolinium Imaging. Recent investigations show that early restricted diffusion is present.

Imaging Findings

X-ray, AP (Fig. 8.1a), and axial (Fig. 8.1b) view of the hips show a slight soft-tissue swelling on the lateral aspect of the right joint and a curvilinear radiolucent shadow beginning in the anterior margin of the epiphysis and extending posteriorly representing a subchondral fracture (radiolucent crescent sign) (Fig. 8.1). Coronal STIR image shows curvilinear subchondral hypointense line in the right proximal femoral epiphysis suggesting subchondral fracture and right hip joint effusion (Fig. 8.2). Sagittal DP weighted image with fat saturation is useful to show the extension of the necrosis (Fig. 8.3). Coronal T1 weighted image with fat saturation obtained immediately after gadolinium administration shows absence of enhancement of the right femoral epiphysis with an incipient revascularization of the lateral pillar (revascularization phase) (Fig. 8.4).

Figure 8.1 (**a**) and (**b**)
Figure 8.2
Figure 8.3
Figure 8.4

Case 8.2
Perisciatic Pyomyositis
■
Héctor Cortina Orts and Naiara Linares Martínez

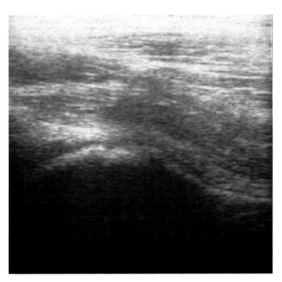

Fig. 8.5

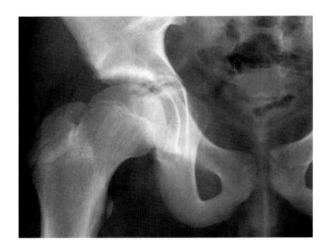

Fig. 8.6

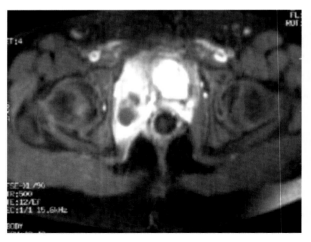

Fig. 8.7

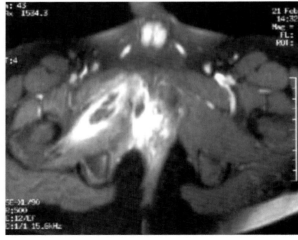

Fig. 8.8

A 13-year-old male presents with a 2-week history of low-grade fever and 5 days of progressive limping on his right leg. Later on, high fever developed and blood work showed leukocytosis with a differential shift to the left.

Pyomyositis is an acute infection of the skeletal muscle. Although generally found in tropical regions, an increased incidence in temperate regions has currently been documented. Blood cultures return positive in approximately 30% of patients, and *Staphylococcus aureus* is the most frequently isolated pathogen. Although it can develop in any anatomical region, it generally occurs in the gluteal muscles, thighs (particularly the quadriceps), and deep pelvis.

Clinical presentation occurring during the subacute phase is common and usually consists of insidious pain and fever. After 1–3 weeks, the suppurative phase ensues with the onset of purulent intramuscular collections, accompanied by high fever, chills, and clinical deterioration. Since conventional radiological studies are often nonspecific during early stages of the disease, diagnosis is sometimes delayed. Subsequently, ultrasound imaging can be decisive as the first diagnostic step.

Pyomyositis of the muscles adjacent to the sciatic nerve causes impaired function that may mimic hip arthritis. The progression of pain and functional limitation can be attributed to irritation of the sciatic nerve and inflammation of the plexus due to the infectious process occurring in neighboring muscles such as the piriformis, obturator internus, and superior and inferior gemelli. The sciatic plexus extends anteriorly to the piriformis muscle, and then the nerve runs through a plane immediately posterior to the gemelli and quadratus femoris muscles.

Since arthritis is a common differential diagnosis to this condition, initial imaging studies usually include hip ultrasound and plain radiography to rule out osteomyelitis (Figs. 8.5 and 8.6). When both return negative, and given the poor visualization of the deep pelvic muscles by US, when septic seeding is suspected, MRI is then performed to detect foci of pyomyositis and/or osteomyelitis. Contrast-enhanced MR T1-weighted images showed enlargement and intense enhancement of the internal and external obturator muscles with abscessed areas within them (Figs. 8.7 and 8.8).

Figure 8.5
Figure 8.6
Figure 8.7
Figure 8.8

Case 8.3
Chronic Recurrent Multifocal Osteomyelitis
■
María I. Martínez León

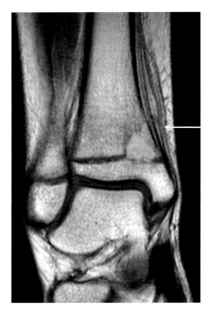

Fig. 8.9

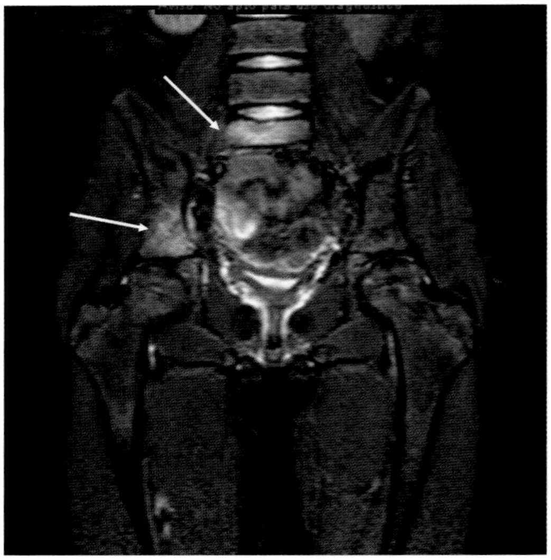

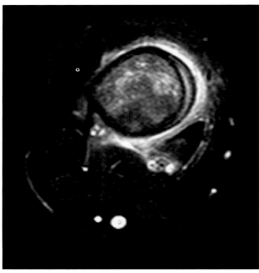

Fig. 8.10

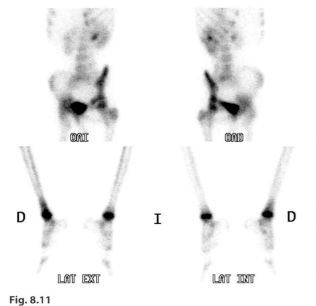

Fig. 8.11

Fig. 8.12

A 10-year-old girl presents with chronic pain in the lumbar region and right ankle, without associated fever.

Chronic recurrent multifocal osteomyelitis (CRMO) is a rare disease that develops in children and is characterized by aseptic inflammation in the metaphyses of long bones. This condition affects fewer than 1 in 200,000 children and manifests with bone or joint pain, swelling, and fever. The etiology is currently unclear, and typically, infectious agents are not isolated from the site of the lesion. CRMO is no longer considered an autoimmune disease, but rather an inherited, auto-inflammatory disease. The term CRMO is self-explanatory of its characteristics:

1. Chronic: characterized by a prolonged, fluctuating clinical course.
2. Recurrent: cycles between painful exacerbations and spontaneous remission.
3. Multifocal: Lesions may affect any location of the skeleton. Each outbreak may develop in a different bone.
4. Osteomyelitis: very similar to this entity, yet no infectious pathogen has been isolated.

Plain radiography shows osteitis, new bone formation, and osteolytic lesions in the metaphysis. Some bones are affected more often than others, including the tibia, femur and clavicle. Bacterial cultures return negative, and biopsies show nonspecific chronic inflammation. CMRO is often diagnosed by the exclusion of its two main differential diagnoses, bacterial infections, and tumors. Diagnosis is established on the basis of characteristic clinical course and findings on conventional radiographs, on occasion supplemented by scintigraphy and MRI. Body-MRI displays the totality of the lesions.

While antibiotic treatment shows poor response, steroidal and nonsteroidal anti-inflammatory drugs may aid in resolving persistent lesions. Radiologists should be familiar with the typical imaging findings of CRMO in order to prevent multiple unnecessary biopsies and long-term antibiotic treatment in children with this condition.

Coronal contrast-enhanced T1-weighted MRI of the right ankle reveals a lytic lesion of the tibial metaphysis with an enhancing physeal base. Periosteal reaction of the internal aspect of the tibia is seen (arrow) (Fig. 8.9). T2-weighted pelvic MRI with fat suppression shows two lesions in body of right ischium and in S1 (arrows) (Fig. 8.10). Scintigraphy displays uptake of three concurrent foci: right ischium, right ankle, and S1 (minimal). There are no other bone lesions (Fig. 8.11). Two months later, a new lesion is detected coinciding with clinical manifestation of contralateral ankle pain. Axial T2-weighted MRI with fat suppression shows the lesion in the left ankle (Fig. 8.12).

Figure 8.9
Figure 8.10
Figure 8.11
Figure 8.12

Case 8.4
Spondylodiscitis
■
María I. Martínez León

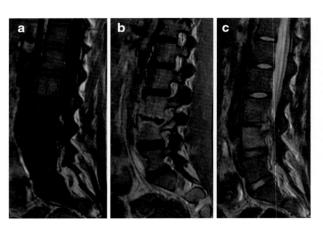

Fig. 8.13

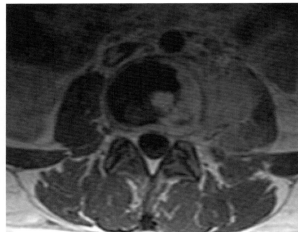

Fig. 8.14

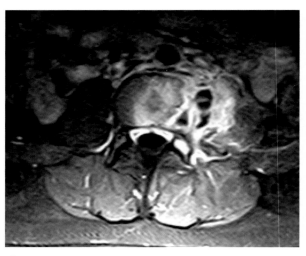

Fig. 8.15

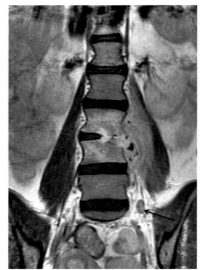

Fig. 8.16

A 9-year-old girl presents pain while in the sitting position and also when walking.

Spondylodiscitis (SD) is the development of an inflammatory process of the intervertebral disk or vertebral plates with a symptomatic decrease in disk space. Clinical presentation tends to be nonspecific and varies according to the patient's age. Laboratory data has also been found to be inconclusive. Song et al. believe the process begins as osteomyelitis of the vertebral metaphysis. The infection then extends through the epiphysis and involves the intervertebral disk. This process could further affect the adjoining vertebral body by following the vascular anastomoses that communicate one vertebra with the other. This vascular network undergoes modifications during the first years of life. A more intricate connection and increased blood flow are present between the disk and vertebral plates, which progressively sustains involution until complete avascularization of the disk is seen in adulthood. The most frequently isolated pathogen is *Staphylococcus aureus*, and the most common location is the lumbar region. Although the clinical course of the condition tends to be favorable, radiologic sequelae may persist. SD may be associated with epidural, paravertebral, and psoas muscle abscesses. Furthermore, non-abscessed inflammatory paravertebral masses have been described in 75% of cases.

Plain radiography is the initial imaging study of choice, although lesions may not appear until up to 2 weeks after onset. Scintigraphy aids in locating the inflammatory process, and CT serves as a guide in diagnostic disk aspiration. MRI is the most accurate study for evaluation, with a sensitivity of 93% and a specificity of 97%. It allows for the assessment of disk and vertebral destruction, spinal edema of the vertebral body, the nature and extension of abscesses with relation to the spinal canal, and differentiation between inflammatory masses and abscesses. Treatment consists of immobilization and antibiotics. Surgical management is reserved for neurologic complications and drainage of abscesses that have not responded to medication.

Sagittal T1-weighted without and with contrast, and T2-weighted MRI reveals involvement of the disk, end plates, and vertebral bodies of L3 and L4. Protrusion of the disk and soft tissues into the spinal canal can also be seen (Fig. 8.13a–c). Axial T1-weighted (Fig. 8.14) and with fat suppression and contrast (Fig. 8.15) MRI shows a left paravertebral abscessed component with necrosis and enhancement. Coronal contrast-enhanced T1-weighted MRI reveals SC with left psoas involvement and an abscessed mass. Locoregional lymphadenopathy (arrow) (Fig. 8.16).

Figure 8.13
Figure 8.14
Figure 8.15
Figure 8.16

Case 8.5
Septic Arthritis of the Hip
■
Luisa Ceres Ruiz

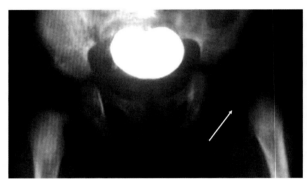

Fig. 8.17

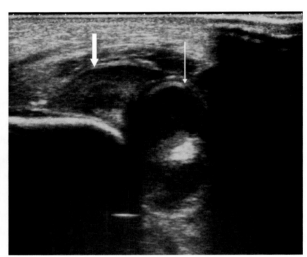

Fig. 8.18

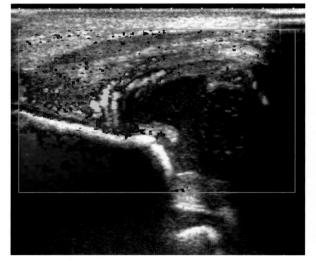

Fig. 8.19

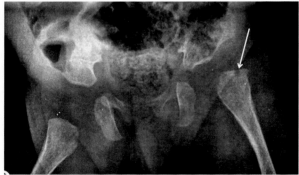

Fig. 8.20

A 15-day-old boy presents with a 3-day history of fever and crying when mobilizing his lower limb, which maintained a flexed position.

Septic arthritis is an acute bacterial infection of the joint, which occurs more frequently in males and in children under the age of 5 years. It generally involves the joints of the lower extremity: knee, ankle, and hip (in the newborn and infant). In neonates, the most commonly isolated pathogens are *Staphylococcus aureus*, group B streptococcus, and enteropathogenic Gram-negative *Bacilli*. An infection that is not controlled by the macrophages of the connective tissue of the synovium produces a severe inflammatory response and purulent joint effusion. In the hip, the joint capsule prevents expansion of the inflammatory process, which may lead to involvement of the vascularization of the femoral head. Since joint cartilage covers the articular surface of the femoral head, the periosteum of the femoral neck comes in close contact with infected fluid, and ultimately osteomyelitis may ensue. In a manner of days, irreversible destructive cartilaginous lesions develop and cause permanent impairment of joint mobility. For these reasons, an early diagnosis and timely drainage of the purulent effusion is essential to a favorable outcome. Clinical presentation usually includes pain associated with joint movement, high fever of rapid onset, and an abduction and external rotation position.

Plain radiography shows an increase in the articular space. Ultrasound reveals fluid within the joint, and hyperemia of the capsule and adjacent soft tissue. It also aids in guiding arthrocentesis, which must be performed immediately after diagnosis is established. Technetium-99 m scintigraphy shows an increased uptake of the affected joint, a finding that is useful in subclinical cases, assessing deep joints, and ruling out associated osteomyelitis. CT and MRI are effective for diagnosis in difficult locations and for determining the extent of involvement (pelvic osteomyelitis).

Pelvic radiography shows a decrease in articular space with femoral displacement and periarticular soft-tissue swelling (Fig. 8.17). Bidimensional ultrasound reveals femoral head luxation (fine arrow) with distension of the joint capsule (thick arrow) due to the accumulation of echogenic fluid (suggests pus) (Fig. 8.18). Power Doppler ultrasound shows significant pericapsular vascularization, which translates to hyperemia of the capsule and of the surrounding soft tissue (Fig. 8.19). 20 days later, necrosis of the femoral epiphysis (the femur is elevated and displaced outside the acetabulum) and an osteolytic femoral neck lesion are seen (arrow) due to contiguous osteomyelitis (Fig. 8.20).

Figure 8.17
Figure 8.18
Figure 8.19
Figure 8.20

Case 8.6

Lipoblastoma
■

María Vidal Denis and María I. Martínez León

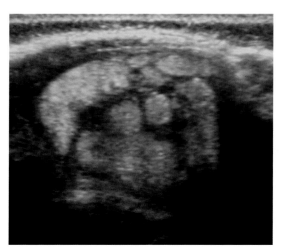

Fig. 8.21

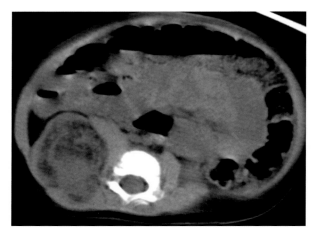

Fig. 8.22

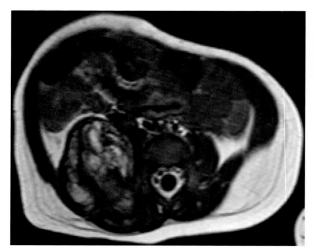

Fig. 8.23

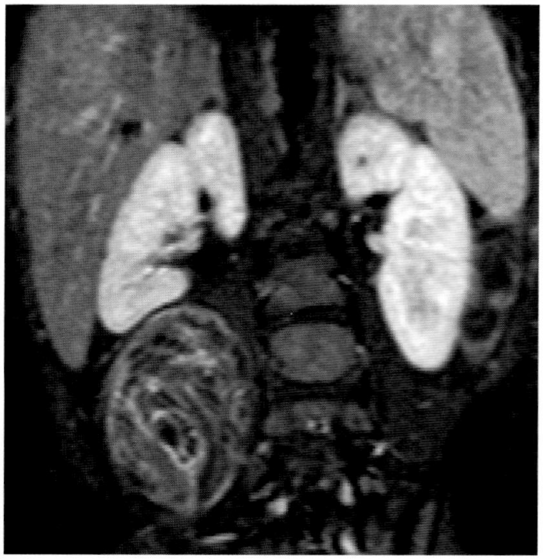

Fig. 8.24

A 1-year-old boy presents with a 3-day history of a right-sided lumbar region mass of elastic consistency, which is painless and does not present adherence to the skin.

The lipoblastoma is a rare, benign mesenchymal tumor that originates from embryonic white adipose tissue. This differentiates it from other tumors such as the hibernoma that arises from brown adipose tissue and the lipoma that derives from mature white fat. Approximately 90% of cases develop in children under 3 years of age.

In 70% of patients, it presents as a partially or completely encapsulated, circumscribed mass that appears in superficial tissue (generally in the extremities but may also develop in the neck and torso). Lipoblastomatosis occurs in 30% of cases and consists of an infiltrative, non-encapsulated lesion that tends to grow in deep tissue (retroperitoneum, mediastinum, and perineum).

Both the lipoblastoma and the lipoblastomatosis are histologically identical and present lobes of immature adipocytes (termed lipoblasts) that are separated by fibrous septations, which contain a myxoid stroma with a rich capillary network. While in small children the myxoid component predominates, the fatty component is greater in older patients. For this reason, in older children, it may easily be confused with lipoma. On the other hand, in younger patients, where the myxoid component is significant, a myxoid liposarcoma may be erroneously diagnosed, although liposarcomas are extremely rare in children under the age of 10 years.

The first line of treatment is complete surgical resection. A recurrence rate of 9–25% has been reported, especially in cases of lipoblastomatosis, given their difficult resectability.

Ultrasound shows a well-defined mass with hyperechogenic areas that correspond to the fatty component of the tumor and lines of lesser echogenicity, which represent the myxoid stromal septations (Fig. 8.21). CT (Fig. 8.22) better locates the lesion and delineates the planes. The two separate components of the tumor are still clearly differentiated: areas of lesser attenuation, fat and denser lines, myxoid stroma. On MRI, the fatty component appears as hyperintense areas of identical signal to that of subcutaneous fat on T1-weighted sequences (Fig. 8.23) and with myxoid septations of low signal on T1 and high signal on T2. These are more evident on fat suppression techniques (not shown). With contrast administration, the myxoid tracts show enhancement (Fig. 8.24).

Figure 8.21
Figure 8.22
Figure 8.23
Figure 8.24

Case 8.7
Osteosarcoma
■
Sara Sirvent Cerdá

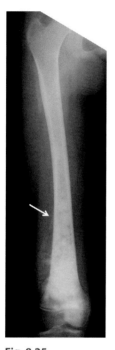

Fig. 8.25

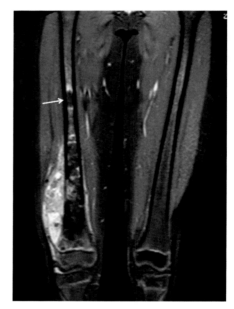

Fig. 8.26

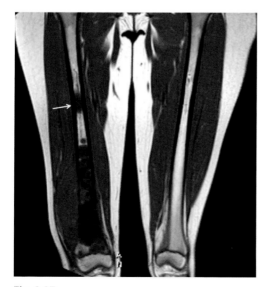

Fig. 8.27

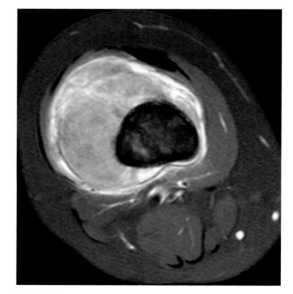

Fig. 8.28

A 9-year-old girl presents with pain and swelling of the right knee.

The osteosarcoma is the most common malignant bone tumor in children and young adults. It characteristically produces immature bone and/or osteoide tumor matrix. Three types of primary osteosarcoma have been described: intramedullary, superficial, and extraosseous. It may also present secondary to an underlying malignancy (fibrous dysplasia, Paget's disease) or to previous radiation therapy. Approximately 80% affect long bones (55% present around the knee) and 20% develop in flat bones or vertebrae. Although initially metaphyseal, up to 80% present epiphyseal infiltration at some point in the course of the disease. Around 7% show distant metastases along the same bone, skip metastases, and 80% develop pulmonary metastases.

Initial treatment consists of neo-adjuvant chemotherapy in order to aid in performing subsequent conservative surgical management. A 5-year 70% survival rate has been described for localized disease. On the other hand, when metastases are documented at onset, the rate drops to 30%.

The intramedullary osteosarcoma is the most frequent subtype (75%). Approximately 90–95% present as a centromedullar and metaphyseal bone lesion with mineralized tumor matrix and associated discontinuous periosteal reaction and soft-tissue mass.

The telangiectatic osteosarcoma is a rare variant (<5%) that presents as an expanding lytic lesion with no mineralized matrix and with internal fluid–fluid levels that appear on MRI.

Osteosarcomas may also affect the surface of long bones. The parosteal osteosarcoma (3%) is the most characteristic type and causes a sclerosing, lobulated, cortical mass that frequently invades bone marrow.

AP plain radiography (Fig. 8.25) shows a mixed metaphyseal-diaphysary lesion of the distal femur with extensive mineralized tumor matrix of cotton-like appearance, associated cortical rupture, and discontinuous periosteal reaction, forming Codman's triangle (arrow). Coronal T2-weighted STIR (Fig. 8.26) and T1-weighted (Fig. 8.27) MR images reveal an extensive, sclerosing, centromedullar lesion with an associated large soft-tissue mass that surrounds the femur and invades the knee joint with a distant metastasis to the middle third of the femoral diaphysis (arrow). With contrast administration and applying fat suppression techniques, the soft-tissue mass displays intense enhancement (Fig. 8.28).

Figure 8.25
Figure 8.26
Figure 8.27
Figure 8.28

Case 8.8
Ewing's Sarcoma
■
Sara Sirvent Cerdá

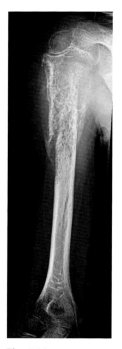

Fig. 8.29

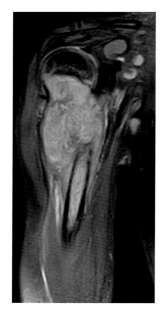

Fig. 8.30

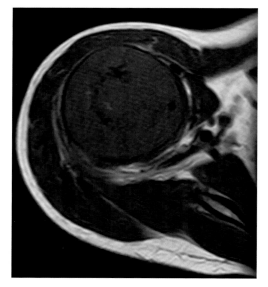

Fig. 8.31

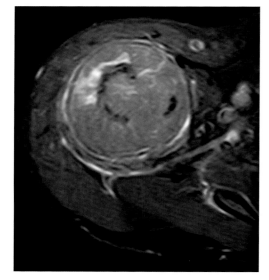

Fig. 8.32

A 10-year-old boy with a history of trauma 6 months prior to diagnosis presents with worsening pain and functional impairment of the right upper extremity.

Ewing's sarcoma (ES) is the second most common primary bone tumor in children after osteosarcoma. It belongs to the Ewing family of tumors, which also includes the extraskeletal ES and the primitive neuroectodermal tumor. The age of onset is usually the first and second decade of life, and it is slightly more prevalent in males. ES may affect both the axial and appendicular skeleton as well as extraosseous structures, yet the most common locations include the long bones (70%), flat bones (25%), and vertebrae (5%). Up to 20–30% of patients present metastases at onset, of which 36% are pulmonary, 32% are osseous, and 21% are both.

The prognosis of localized ES depends on tumor size, location (worse outcome when axial skeleton is affected), and age (the older the patient the poorer the prognosis). A 5-year 70% survival rate has been reported. On the other hand, when metastases are documented at onset, the rate drops to 30%.

Diagnostic imaging in this condition includes conventional radiography, that characterizes bone lesion, and MRI, which evaluates its extension.

AP radiograph of the right arm (Fig. 8.29) shows a lytic bone lesion (moth-eaten appearance) of the proximal metaphyseal-diaphysis of the humerus with associated cortical erosion and disruption, and spiculated periosteal reaction. A metaphyseal, spiral, pathological fracture with thickened, continuous periosteal reaction can also be seen.

Coronal T2-weighted MRI with fat suppression reveals an extensive, hyperintense centromedullar lesion associated with a large, hyperintense, heterogeneous perilesional soft-tissue mass (Fig. 8.30). Axial T1-weighted MRI (Fig. 8.31) shows cortical rupture and a large hypointense soft-tissue mass surrounding the humerus. With contrast administration and fat suppression (Fig. 8.32), the lesion presents an intense heterogeneous enhancement, surrounds the tendon of the long head of the biceps brachii muscle, and infiltrates the deltoid, infraspinatus, subscapularis, and coracobrachialis muscles.

Figure 8.29
Figure 8.30
Figure 8.31
Figure 8.32

Case 8.9

Lumbar Ewing's Sarcoma

Juan E. Gutiérrez and L. Santiago Medina

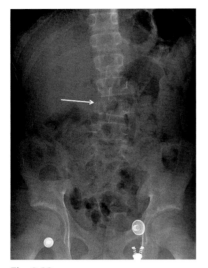

Fig. 8.33

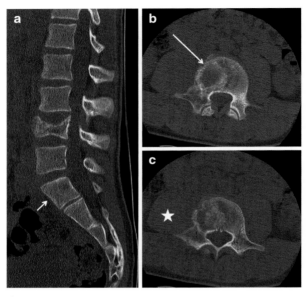

Fig. 8.34

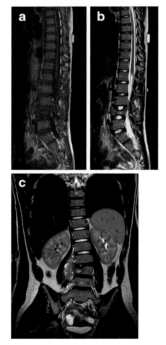

Fig. 8.35

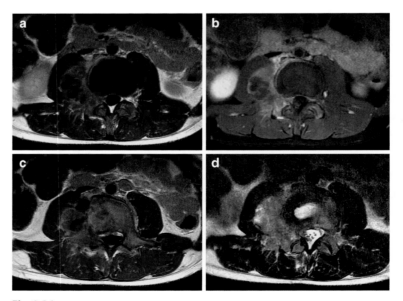

Fig. 8.36

A 13-year-old male presents with severe lower back pain with no apparent cause.

ES is the second most common primary pediatric bone tumor. It most commonly presents between the ages of 4 and 15 years old. Most often, it begins as a primary bone tumor from elsewhere that affects the spine, although it may also occur as a primary osseous and infrequently extraosseous spinal tumor. Extraosseous spinal tumors are referred to as peripheral primitive neuroectodermal tumors (PNET). 25% of ES tumors occur in or near the femur, 14% in or near the ilium, and others may occur in the humerus, ribs, or other locations.

Patients often present with severe pain, soft-tissue mass, pathologic fracture, fever, and/or leukocytosis. Lytic lesions with poor demarcation and a "moth-eaten" appearance are visible on plain radiograph and CT. In long bones, there is commonly an "onionskin" appearance due to the periosteal reaction. T1-weighted MR images exhibit hypointense bone signal, while T2-weighted MR images of Ewing sarcoma vary between hypo- and hyperintense signals.

The differential diagnosis for ES includes osseous leukemia, metastatic neuroblastoma, lymphoma, Langerhans' cell histiocytosis, and infection. Treatment includes the combination of chemotherapy, surgery, and/or radiation. Staging and follow-up are guided by imaging studies. Often a hypointense T2-weighted MRI signal posttreatment may indicate a successful therapeutic effect.

High loss of L3, more severe on the right superior endplate (arrow) with misalignment of the spinal column to the right can been seen (Fig. 8.33). Pathological compression of L3 with a biconcave defect, apparent lytic lesion on the right suprachondral superior edge (long arrow), and lateral displacement of the right psoas muscle (asterisk) are suggestive of paravertebral compromise (Fig. 8.34a–c). Sagittal T1-weighted and coronal and sagittal T2-weighted images exhibiting lytic lesions on L3 with paravertebral mass on the right (Fig. 8.35a–c). Axial MR images (T1w w/wo contrast and FS, T2w) showing compromise of the vertebral body, a paravertebral mass involving the adjacent psoas muscle and the right lateral foramen, and compromise of the right vertebral facet are observed (Fig. 8.36a–d).

Figure 8.33
Figure 8.34
Figure 8.35
Figure 8.36

Acknowledgment Acknowledgment to Dr. Raj Palani and Sara Koenig for their help on the preparation of this case.

Case 8.10

Granulocytic Sarcoma
■

Roberto Llorens Salvador and Héctor Cortina Orts

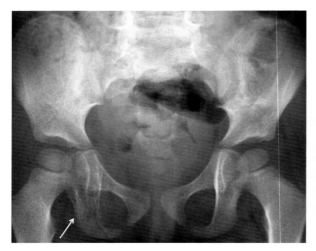

Fig. 8.37

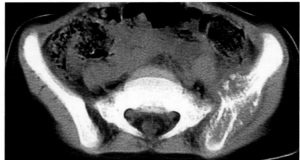

Fig. 8.38

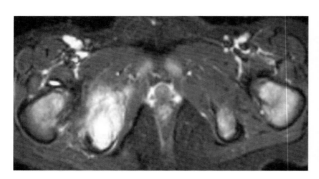

Fig. 8.39

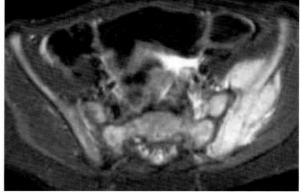

Fig. 8.40

A 2-year-old girl presented with acute right groin pain without fever or other symptomology associated. Eight months earlier, the patient had complained of similar intermittent episodes in the left hip.

Granulocytic sarcoma (GS) or myeloid sarcoma is a rare solid tumor originating from immature myeloid cells of the granulocytic series of white blood cells. In the past, the term "chloroma" was used for this kind of tumor. The growth of immature cells at an extramedullary site is secondary to acute or chronic myeloid leukemia or other myeloproliferative disorders. Although very unusual, it may precede leukemia.

Clinical presentation of GS is generally related to its anatomic location. Nevertheless, it may also be asymptomatic and be discovered incidentally in the monitoring of a child with acute myeloid leukemia. Although GS has been found to develop anywhere in the body, the most common sites are the orbit and subcutaneous tissue followed by paranasal sinuses, lymph nodes, and bone. Bone GS arises from the bone marrow, extends through the Haversian canals, reaches the periosteum, and ultimately affects the surrounding soft tissue.

The most common radiographic findings are osteolysis and rarefaction with ill-defined margins. Differential diagnoses include osteomyelitis, Langerhans cell histiocytosis, neuroblastoma metastases, ES, and lymphoma.

A lytic, permeative tumor in the right ischium (arrow) is seen on pelvic radiography (Fig. 8.37). On pelvic CT (Fig. 8.38), another lesion expanding the left iliac bone with associated periosteal reaction is shown. On postcontrast MR images (Figs. 8.39 and 8.40), bone marrow infiltration and soft-tissue involvement are revealed.

In this rare case of GS, where two pelvic bone lesions appeared before leukemia was diagnosed, a biopsy was necessary. However, currently, immunohistochemical stains using monoclonal antibodies and flow cytometry are the mainstay of diagnosis.

Figure 8.38
Figure 8.39
Figure 8.40
Figure 8.37

Further Reading

Book

Barkovich JA (2005) Pediatric neuroimaging. Lippincott Williams & Wilkins, Philadelphia

Labrune M, Kalifa G (2000) Diagnóstico por imagen de la columna vertebral en la infancia. Colección de diagnóstico por imagen. Ed Masson SA, Barcelona

Parizel PM, Vanhoenacker FM (2006) Imaging of soft tissue tumors, 3rd edn. Springer, New York, p 227

Resnick D (2001a) Bone and joint imaging, vol II. W.B. Saunders, Philadelphia, p 667

Resnick D (2001b) Bone and joint imaging, 2nd edn. W.B. Saunders, Philadelphia

Resnick D. (2005) Diagnosis of bone and joint disorders, vol 5, 3rd edn. W.B. Saunders, Philadelphia, Chapter 81, pp 3559–3610

Resnick D. (2005) Diagnosis of bone and joint disorders, 3rd edn. W.B. Saunders, Philadelphia

Silverman FN, Kuhn JP (1993) Caffey's pediatric X-ray diagnosis. An integrated imaging approach, 9th edn. Mosby, St. Louis, p 1850

Stoller DW, Tirman PF, Bredella MA, Beltrán S, Branstetter RM, Blease SC (2004) Diagnostic imaging, vol 8. Amirsys, pp 14–17, Salt Lake City, Utah: Amirsys

Stoller DW, Tirman PFJ, Bredella MA, Beltrán S, Branstetter RM, Blease SC (2004) Diagnostic imaging. Orthopedics. Amirsys, pp 814–817, Salt Lake City, Utah: Amirsys

Web Link

http://emedicine.medscape.com/article/826935-overview

http://journals.lww.com/spinejournal/pages/default.aspx

http://www.ich.ucl.ac.uk/gosh/clinicalservices/Rheumatology/MedicalConditions/#H2_1834

http://www.nlm.nih.gov/medlineplus/ency/article/001302.htm

http://www.revistapediatria.cl/vol3num2/pdf/8_Lipoblastoma.pdf

http://www.uptodate.com/home/index.html

www.bonetumor.org

www.emedicine.medscape-com/article/1259337overview

Articles

Anik Y, Corapcioglu F, Yildiz DK (2008) Radiological findins of atypical extraskeletal Ewing sarcoma. Pediatr Hematol Oncol 25:469–471

Averill LW, Hernandez A, Gonzalez L, Peña AH (2009) Jaramillo D Diagnosis of osteomyelitis in children: utility of fat-suppressed contrast-enhanced MRI. AJR 192:1232–1238

Baleato Gonzalez S, Vilanova JC, García Figueras R (2008) The role of MRI in the early diagnosis of pyomyositis in children. Radiología 50:495–501

Bansal M, Bhaliak V, Bruce CE (2008) Obturator internus muscle abscess in a child. A case report. J Pediatr Orthop B 17:223–224

Benesch M, Christian U, Herwig L, Reinhold K, Wolfgang S, Christine B-S et al (1999) Typical extraosseous Ewing sarcoma of the spinal canal with bone marrow involvement in a two-month-old boy. Med Pediatr Oncol 32(6):471

Bestic JM, Peterson JJ, Bancroft LW (2009) Use of FDG PET in staging, restaging, and assessment of therapy response in Ewing sarcoma. RadioGraphics 29:1487–1500

Bodart E, Motte F, Michel M (2008) Limp with fever in adolescent: about 2 cases of pyomyositis. Arch Pediatr 15:1304–1307

Brown R, Hussain M, McHugh K, Novelli V, Jones D (2001) Discitis in young children. J Bone Joint Surg Am 83:106–111

Browne LP, Mason EO, Kaplan SL (2008) Optimal imaging strategy for community-adquired *Staphylococcus aureus* musculoskeletal infections in children. Pediatr Radiol 38:841–847

Buchmann RF, Jaramillo D (2004) Imaging of articular disorders in children. Radiol Clin North Am 42:151–168

Campidelli C, Agostinelli C, Stitson R, Pileri SA (2009) Myeloid sarcoma: extramedullary manifestation of myeloid disorders. Am J Clin Pathol 132(3):426–437

Carr AJ, Cole WG, Roberton DM, Chow CW (1993) Chronic multifocal osteomyelitis. J Bone Joint Surg Br 75:582–591

Chan LL, Czerniak BA, Ginsberg LE (2000) Radiation-induced osteosarcoma after bilateral childhood retinoblastoma. AJR 174:1288

Chantal JD, Krebs S, Kahan A (2001) Chronic recurrent multifocal osteomielitis: five-year outocomes in 14 pediatric cases. Joint Bone Spine 68:242–251

Choi EK, Ha HK, Park SH, Lee SJ, Jung SE, Kim KW, Lee SS (2007) Granulocytic sarcoma of bowel: CT findings. Radiology 243(3):752–759

David Pienkowski et al (2009) Novel three-dimensional MRI technique for study of cartilaginous hip surfaces in Legg–Calvé–Perthes disease. J Orthop Res 27(8):981–988

De Boeck H (2005) Osteomyelitis and septic arthritis in children. Acta Orthop Belg 71:505–515

Demharter J, Bhondorf K, Milch W, Vogt H (1997) Chronic recurrent multifocal osteomyelitis: a radiological and clinical investigation of five cases. Skeletal Radiol 26:579–588

Dillman JR, Hernandez RJ (2009) MRI of Legg–Calve–Perthes disease. AJR 193(5):1394–1407

Dobbs MB, Sheridan JJ, Gordon JE, Corley CL, Szymanski DA, Schoenecker PL (2003) Septic arthritis of the hip in infancy: long-term follow-up. J Pediatr Orthop 23:162–168

Doria AS et al (2008) Legg–Calvé–Perthes disease: multipositional power Doppler sonography of the proximal femoral vascularity. Pediatr Radiol 38(4):392–402

Downey Carmona FJ, Farrington Rueda D (2006) Pyomiositis of hip obturator muscles. Cir Pediátr 19:241–243

Drevelegas A, Pilavaki M, Chourmouzi D (2004) Lipomatous tumors of soft tissue: MR appearance with histological correlation. Eur J Radiol 50:257–267

Dwek JR (2009) The hip: MR imaging of uniquely pediatric disorders. Magn Reson Imaging Clin N Am 17(3):509–520

Fabry G (2010) Clinical practice: the hip from birth to adolescence. Eur J Pediatr 169(2):143–148

Fink LH, Meriweather MW (1979) Primary epidural Ewing's sarcoma presenting as a lumbar disc protrusion case report. J Neurosurg 51(1):120–123

Forlin E, Milani C (2008) Seqelae of septic arthritis of the hip in children: a new classification and a review of 41 hips. J Pediatr Orthop 28:524–528

Galant J, Martí-Bonmatí L, Sáez F, Soler R, Alcalá-Santaella R, Navarro M (2003) The value of fat-suppressed T2 or STIR sequences in distinguishing lipoma from well-differentiated liposarcoma. Eur Radiol 13:337–343

Gamble JG, Rinsky LA (1986) Chronic recurrent multifocal osteomielitis: distinct clinical entity. J Pediatr Orthop 6:579–584

Garner HW, Kransdorf MJ et al (2009) Benign and malignant soft-tissue tumors: post-treatment MR imaging. RadioGraphics 29:119–134

Girschick HJ, Zimmer C, Klaus G, Darge K, Dick A, Morbach H (2007) Chronic recurrent multifocal osteomyelitis: what is it and how should it be treated? Nat Clin Pract Rheumatol 3(12):733–738

Gutierrez K (2005) Bone and joint infections in children. Pediatr Clin North Am 52:779–794

Ha TV, Kleinman PK, Fraire A, Speavak MR, Nimkin K, Cohen IT et al (1994) MR Imaging of benign fatty tumours in children: report of four cases and review of the literature. Skeletal Radiol 25:361–367

Ha AS, Wells L, Jaramillo D (2008) Importance of sagittal MR imaging in nontraumatic femoral head osteonecrosis in children. Pediatr Radiol 38(11):1195–1200

Haresh KP, Joshi N, Gupta C, Prabhakar R, Sharma DN, Julka PK, Rath GK (2008) Granulocytic sarcoma masquerading as Ewing's sarcoma: a diagnostic dilemma. J Cancer Res Ther 4(3):137–139

Hernández R, Strouse PJ (2002) Focal pyomyositis of the perisciatic muscles in children. AJR 179:1267–1271

Hernández F, Nistal, Encinas JL (2004) Lipoblastoma: el menos conocido de los tumores adiposos. Cir Pediátr 17:175–178

Herring JA (1994) The treatment of Legg–Calve–Perthes disease. A critical review of the literature. J Bone Joint Surg Am 76: 448–458

Hoffer FA, Nikanorov AY, Reddick WE (2000) Accuarcy on MR imaging for detecting epiphyseal extension of osteosarcoma. Pediatr Radiol 30:289–298

Jagodzinski NA, Kanwar R, Graham K, Bache CE (2009) Prospective evaluation of a shortened regimen of treatment for acute osteomyelitis and septic arthritis in children. J Pediatr Orthop 29:518–525

Jansen BR, Hart W, Schreuder O (1993) Discitis in childhood. 12–35-year follow up of 35 patients. Acta Orthop Scand 64:33–36

Jaramillo D (2009) What is the optimal imaging of osteonecrosis, Perthes, and bone infarcts? Pediatr Radiol 39:216–219

Jordanov MI, Block JJ, Gonzalez AL, Green NE (2009) Transarticular spread of Ewing sarcoma mimicking septic arthritis. Pediatr Radiol 39:381–384

Jurik AG (2004) Chronic recurrent multifocal osteomyelitis. Semin Mucsuloskelet Radiol 8(3):243–253

Karmazyn B, Loder RT, Kleiman MB (2007) The role of pelvic MRI in evaluating nonhip sources of infection in children with acute nontraumatic hip pain. J Pediatr Orthop 27: 158–164

Kayser R, Mahlfeld K, Greulich M, Grasshoff H (2005) Spondylodiscitis in childhood: results of a long-term study. Spine 30:318–323

Khanna G, Sato TS, Ferguson P (2009) Imaging of chronic recurrent multifocal osteomyelitis. RadioGraphics 29(4): 1159–1177

Klimo P Jr, Codd PJ, Grier H, Goumnerova LC (2009) Primary pediatric intraspinal sarcomas. J Neurosurg 4(3):222–229

Krandorf MJ (1995) Benigg soft-tissue tumors in a large referral population: distribution of specific diagnosis by age, sex and location. AJR 164:395–402

Lan TY, Lin DT, Tien HF, Yang RS, Chen CY, Wu K (2009) Prognostic factors of treatment outcomes in patients with granulocytic sarcoma. Acta Haematol 122(4):238–246

Li W, Brock P, Saunders DE (2005) Imaging characteristics of primary cranial Ewing sarcoma. Pediatr Radiol 35(6): 612–618

Llorente Otones L, Vázquez Román S (2007) Piomiositis en los niños. No sólo una enfermedad tropical. An Pediatr 67:568–571

Ludwig JA (2008) Ewnig sarcoma: historical perspectives, current state-of-art, and opportunities for targeted therapy in the future. Curr Opin Oncol 20:412–418

Mar WA, Taljanovic MS, Bagatell R, Graham AR, Speer DP, Hunter TB et al (2008) Update on imaging and treatment of Ewing's sarcoma family tumors: what the radiologist needs to know? J Comput Assist Tomogr 32:108–118

Merlini L et al (2010) Diffusion-weighted imaging findings in Perthes disease with dynamic gadolinium-enhanced subtracted (DGS) MR correlation: a preliminary study. Pediatr Radiol 40(3):318–325

Miller TT (2008) Bone tumors and tumorlike conditions: analysis with conventional radiography. Radiology 246:662–674

Mitsionis GI, Manoudis GN, Lykissas MG (2009) Pyomyositis in children. Early diagnosis and treatment. J Pediatr Surg 44:2173–2178

Mortenson W, Edeburn G, Fiers M, Nilsson R (1988) Chronic recurrent multifocal osteomyelitis in children. Acta Radiol 29:565–570

Murphey MD, Robbin MR, McRae GA, Flemming DJ, Temple HT, Kransdorf MJ (1997) The many faces of ostesarcoma. RadioGraphics 17:1205–1231

Murphey MD, Carroll JF, Flemming DJ (2004a) From de archives of the AFIP: benign musculoskeletal lipomatous lesions. RadioGraphics 24:1433–1466

Murphey MD, Jelinek JS, Temple HT, Flemming DJ, Gannon FH (2004b) Imaging of periosteal ostesarcoma: radiologic–pathologic comparison. Radiology 233:129–138

Neiman RS, Barcos M, Berard C et al (1981) Granulocytic sarcoma: a clinicopathologic study of 61 biopsied cases. Cancer 48:1426–1437

O'Keeffe F, Lorigan JG, Wallace S (1990) Radiological features of extraskeletal Ewing sarcoma. Br J Radiol 63:456–460

Paydas S, Zorludemir S, Ergin M (2006) Leuk granulocytic sarcoma: 32 cases and review of the literature. Leuk Lymphoma 47(12):2527–2541

Pekala JS, Gururangan S, Provenzale JM, Mukundan S Jr (2006) Central nervous system extraosseous Ewing sarcoma: radiologic manifestations of this newly defined pathologic entity. Am J Neuroradiol 27:580–583

Perlis CS, Collins MH, Honig PJ, Low DW (2000) Forehead lipoblastoma mimicking a hemangioma. Pediatrics 105:123–128

Pileri Sa, Ascani S, Cox MC, Campidelli C, Bacci et al (2007) Myeloid sarcoma: clinico-pathologic, phenotypic and cytogenetic analysis of 92 adult patients. Leukemia 21:340–350

Post MJ, Bowen BC, Sze G (1991) Magnetic resonance imaging of spinal infection. Rheum Dis Clin Norh Am 17:773–794

Pretorius ES, Hruban RH, Fishman EK (1996) Tropical pyomyositis:imaging findings and a review of the literature. Skeletal Radiol 25:576–579

Pui M, Fletcher B, Langston J (1994) Granulocytic sarcoma in childhood leukemia: imaging features. Radiology 190: 698–702

Quan GM, Slavin JL, Schlicht SM, Smith PJ, Powell GJ, Choong PF (2005) Osteosarcoma near joints: assessment and implications. J Surg Oncol 91:159–166

Ranson M (2009) Imaging of pediatric musculoskeletal infection. Semin Musculoskelet Radiol 13:277–299

Regueras Santos L, Ledesma Benítez I, Regueras Santos L, Ledesma Benítez I, de la Mano LJ Ferrero, Del Río González E, Fernández Castaño MT (2007) Chronic recurrent multifocal osteomyelitis. Our experience. Bol Pediatr 47:136–141

Reiseter T, Nordushus T, Borthne A, Roald B, Naess P, Schistad O (1999) Lipoblastoma: MRI appearances of a rare paediatric soft tissue tumour. Pediatr Radiol 29:542–545

Rodriguez DP, Poussaint TY (2010) Imaging of back pain in children. Am J Neuroradiol 31(5):787–802

Sabourin SM, Jayashankar A, Mullins ME (2008) Imaging of osteosarcoma after irradiation: self-assessment module. AJR 191:S28–S30

Schultz E, Rosenblatt R, Mitsudo S, Weinberg G (1993) Detection of a deep lipoblastoma by MRI and ultrasound. Pediatr Radiol 23:409–410

Shapeero LG, Vanel D, Sundaram M, Ackerman VL, Wuisman P, Bauer TW et al (1994) Periosteal Ewing sarcoma. Radiology 191:825–831

Shin JH, Lee HK, Rhim SC, Cho KJ, Choi CG, Suh DC (2001a) Spinal epidural extraskeletal Ewing sarcoma: MR findings in two cases. AJNR 22:795–798

Shin JH, Lee HK, Rhim SC, Cho K, Choi CG, Suh DC (2001b) Spinal epidural extraskeletal ewing sarcoma: MR findings in two cases. Am J Neuroradiol 22:795–798

Smith AS, Blaser SI (1991) Infectious and inflammatory processes of the spine. Rad Clin Norh Am 29:809–827

Song KS, Ogden JA, Ganey T, Guidera KJ (1997) Contiguous discitis and osteomyelitis in children. J Pediatr Orthop 14:470–477

Song HR et al (2000) Classification of metaphyseal change with magnetic resonance imaging in Legg–Calvé–Perthes disease. J Pediatr Orthop 20(5):557–561

Song J, Letts M, Monson R (2001) Differentiation of psoas muscle abscess from septic arthritis of the hip in children. Clin Orthop Relat Res 391:258–265

Song X, Choi J, Rao C (2008) Primary Ewing sarcoma of lumbar spine with massive intraspinal extension. Pediatr Neurol 38(1):58–60

Spiegel PG, Kengla KW, Isaacson AS, Wilson JC (1972) Intervertebral disc-space inflammation in children. J Bone Joint Surg Am 54:284–296

Stacy GS, Ravinder SM, Peabody TD (2006) Staging of bone tumors: a review with illustrative examples. AJR 186:967–976

Stein-Wexler R (2009) MR imaging of soft tissue masses in children. Radiol Clin North Am 47(6):977–995

Strouse PJ, DiPietro MA, Adler RS (1998) Pediatric hip effusions: evaluation withpower Doppler sonography. Radiology 206:731–735

Suresh S, Saifuddin A (2007) Radiological appereances of appendicular osteosarcoma: a comprehansive pictorial review. Clin Radiol 62:314–323

Tapia Moreno R, Espinosa Fernández MG, Martínez León MI, González Gómez JM, Moreno Pascual P (2009) Spondylodiscitis: diagnosis and medium-long term follow up of 18 cases. An Pediatr (Barc) 71(5):391–399

Tlougan BE, Podjasek JO, O'Haver J, Cordova KB, Nguyen XH, Tee R et al (2009) Chronic recurrent multifocal osteomyelitis (CRMO) and synovitis, acne, pustulosis, hyperostosis, and osteitis (SAPHO) syndrome with associated neutrophilic dermatoses: a report of seven cases and review of the literature. Pediatr Dermatol 26(5):497–505

Uhl M, Saueressig U, Van Buiren M, Kontny U, Niemeyer C, Köhler G et al (2006) Osteosarcoma: preliminary results in vivo assessment of tumor necrosis after chemotherapy with diffusion- and perfusion-weigthed magnetic resonance imaging. Invest Radiol 41:618–623

Vogel G, Gane A, Salai M (2001) Lipoblastoma in an infant's foot. Isr Med Assoc J 3:540–541

Wenger DR, Bobechko WP, Gilday DL (1978) The spectrum of intervertebral disc-space infection in children. J Bone Joint Surg Am 60:100–108

Wootton-Gorges SL (2009) MR imaging of primary bone tumors and tumor-like conditions in children. MRI Clin North Am 17:469–487

Worch J, Ritter J, Frühwald MC (2008) Presentation of acute promyelocytic leukemia as granulocytic sarcoma. Blood Cancer 50(3):657–660

Zawin JK, Hoffer FA, Rand FF, Teele RL (1993) Joint effusion in children with an irritable hip US diagnosis and aspiration. Radiology 187:459–463

Zwaga T, Boveé JV, Kroon HM (2008) Osteosarcoma of the femur with skip, lymph node, and lung metastases. RadioGraphics 28:277–283

Contents

M.I. Martínez-León et al., *Learning Pediatric Imaging*, Learning Imaging,
DOI: 10.1007/978-3-642-16892-5_9, © Springer-Verlag Berlin Heidelberg 2011

Case 9.1
Surfactant Deficiency Disease
■
Carmen Gallego Herrero

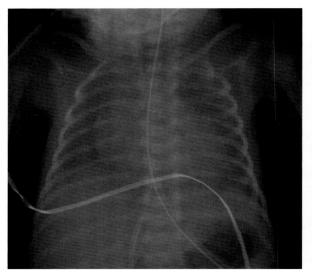

Fig. 9.1

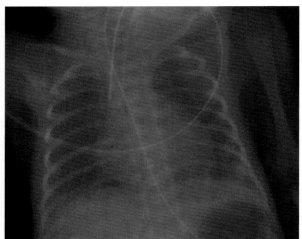

Fig. 9.2

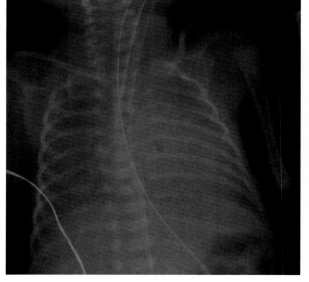

Fig. 9.3

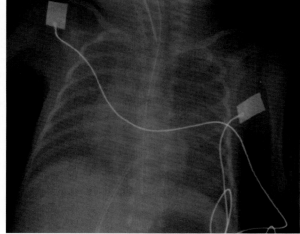

Fig. 9.4

Immediate respiratory distress in a 29-week-gestational-age preterm infant that required endotracheal surfactant administration. On the third day of life, a sudden increase in respiratory work is appreciated.

Surfactant Deficiency Disease (SDD) reflects the pulmonary immaturity and deficiency of surfactant phospholipids covering the alveoli. SDD leads to respiratory distress syndrome (RDS) clinically and hyaline membrane disease pathologically in neonates less than 36 weeks of gestational age. Despite the many complications associated to prematurity, lung disease remains the leading cause of neonatal morbidity.

SDD courses with tachypnea, expiratory grunting, retractions, and some degree of cyanosis within the first 8 h of life. In the absence of surfactant, the alveolar surface tension is increased, with the resultant collapse of alveoli and subsequent poor gas exchange, hypoxia, hypercarbia, increased pulmonary resistance, and ventilation perfusion imbalance. The advent of technical innovations in therapy that include antenatal corticoid administration, postnatal surfactant instillation, and more gentle mechanical ventilation have modified both the radiological appearance and clinical evolution of SDD. Surfactant administration may result in a rapid clinical improvement with a more variable radiological response ranging from complete to partial or less frequently non-clearance of the lungs. With the progressive recruitment of ventilated alveoli, a decrease in pulmonary vascular resistance may lead to a hemodinamically significant left-to-right shunt via a patent ductus arteriosus (PDA) that puts the patient in pulmonary vascular congestion and edema. Mechanical ventilation and oxygen are responsible for the air block complications in SDD that include interstitial emphysema, pneumomediastinum, pneumothorax, and pneumopericardium.

The most common radiological manifestation in SDD is a reticulogranular lung pattern secondary to alveolar collapse, interstitial fluid, and overdistension of bronchioles (Fig. 9.1). More severe involvement of the lungs correlates with increased opacification of the lungs and air bronchograms. Clearance of reticulogranular opacities is seen in up to 35% after surfactant instillation (Fig. 9.2). An increase in heart size and pulmonary density with effacement of pulmonary borders suggests the presence of PDA (Fig. 9.3) with a significant left-to-right shunting that leads to pulmonary edema. Closure of the PDA is accomplished with indomethacin therapy – if not contraindicated – with the subsequent disappearance of pulmonary edema and reduction in heart size (Fig. 9.4).

Figure 9.1
Figure 9.2
Figure 9.3
Figure 9.4

Case 9.2
Bronchogenic Cyst
■

Elisa Cuartero Martínez and María I. Martínez León

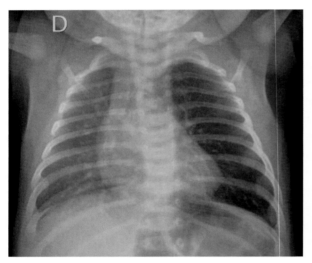

Fig. 9.5

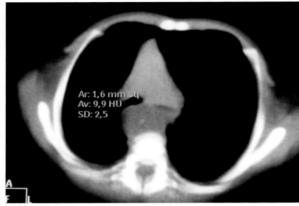

Fig. 9.6

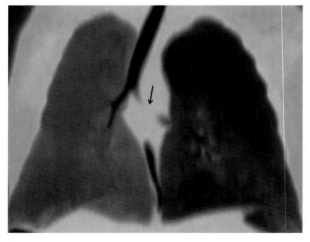

Fig. 9.7

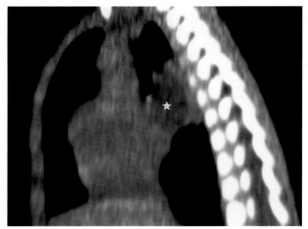

Fig. 9.8

A 1-month-old boy is brought to the emergency department with tachypnea, moderate subcostal retractions, and decreased breath sounds on the left.

Comments

Bronchogenic cysts (BCs) are congenital malformations of the bronchial tree caused by abnormal budding of the tracheal diverticulum in the ventral foregut between weeks 5 and 16 of fetal age. Histologically, BC is a closed sac composed of a ciliary or columnar epithelial membrane filled with fluid or mucus material.

According to their location, BCs can be divided into intrapulmonary or mediastinal. Other, less frequent locations include the neck, pericardium, abdomen, and subcutaneous cellular tissue. The mediastinal or central form is more frequent. In this variant, the cyst is generally located at the distal trachea or the proximal main bronchus. Three subtypes for mediastinal BC have been described: paratracheal (usually right-sided), carinal, and hilar, the carinal subtype being the most common.

On the other hand, intrapulmonary cysts are usually located in the inferior lobes. Cysts may vary in size, be single or multiple, and/or present with multiloculation. Furthermore, some show communication with adjacent airways, a feature that predisposes them to infection.

Although the vast majority of BCs are asymptomatic, clinical presentation may vary according to the size and location of the mass. Mediastinal cysts may compress the trachea or bronchi causing cough, dyspnea, chest pain, hemoptysis, and air entrapment due to an associated valve effect.

On the other hand, the intrapulmonary form presents clinically with respiratory tract infections. This complication is usually seen in BCs that show communication with the tracheobronchial tree. In these cases, air or air–fluid levels can be seen within the cyst itself. Spontaneous rupture of these structures is a rare finding.

The treatment of choice for symptomatic BC is surgical resection. A complete removal decreases the incidence of recurrences.

Imaging Findings

AP chest radiograph shows hyperinflation of the left hemithorax in comparison to the right (Fig. 9.5). Low radiation-dose axial CT image without contrast shows a thin-walled nodular lesion containing material with fluid attenuation (9.9 HU) located in the posterior mediastinum (Fig. 9.6). Coronal CT MIP image depicts a mass compressing over 50% of the lumen of the left main bronchus (arrow) (Fig. 9.7). Hyperlucency of the left lung can be seen due to the valvular mechanism caused by the cyst. Sagittal CT MIP image exhibits a cystic mass in the posterior mediastinum (asterisk) (Fig. 9.8).

Figure 9.5
Figure 9.6
Figure 9.7
Figure 9.8

Case 9.3
Localized Persistent Pulmonary Interstitial Emphysema
■

María I. Martínez León

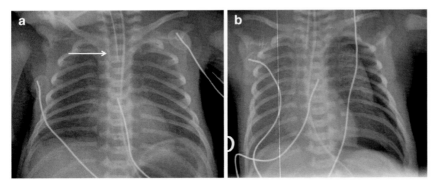

Fig. 9.9

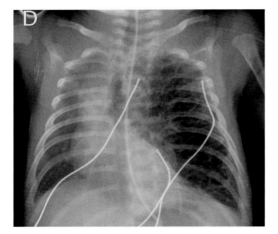

Fig. 9.10

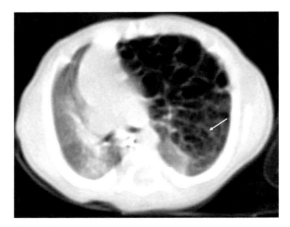

Fig. 9.11

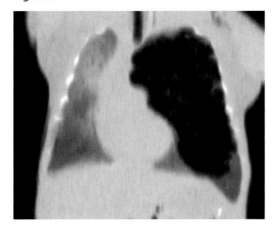

Fig. 9.12

Premature (36 weeks), male newborn, product of twin pregnancy, weighing in at 1,550 g presents with respiratory distress since birth.

Localized persistent pulmonary interstitial emphysema (LPPIE) is a syndrome character-ized by air-leakage in the perivascular tissues of the lung. It generally presents during ini-tial hospitalization of premature newborns due to clinical distress and immaturity. History of mechanical ventilation is common, although cases of LPPIE have been reported in full-term neonates without mechanical ventilation. Typically, development of hyperinflated radiolucent lobar lung lesions appear after radiologic findings of pulmonary interstitial emphysema have been documented.

The difference with interstitial emphysema (IE) is that LPPIE is localized (usually lobar, but can be multilobular or less frequently, bilateral), persistent on time, and expanding, causing mass effect and progressive respiratory distress. The first line of treatment for LPPIE is surgical resection, although there are cases where conservative nonsurgical meth-ods (decubitus positioning, selective intubation) may apply. Differential diagnoses include other radiolucent congenital lung lesions such as congenital cystic adenomatoid malfor-mation and congenital lobar emphysema. Differentiating between them is essential in establishing an adequate treatment plan.

Radiography appearance of LPPIE is similar to IE except for that it is localized and pres-ents associated mass effect. CT findings are different to that of IE because it characteristi-cally shows solid linear or punctiform structures within air-filled cysts, consistent with bronchovascular bundles surrounded by interstitial gas ("line-and-dot pattern"). The final diagnosis is confirmed histologically when surgical resection is performed.

Chest radiography shows a mechanically ventilated neonate (arrow) with light diffuse opacities consistent with surfactant deficiency disease (Fig. 9.9a). Two days later, chest radi-ography reveals a left-sided pneumothorax (Fig. 9.9b). Ten days later, chest radiography displays findings consistent with left LPPIE (Fig. 9.10). Axial CT MIP reconstruction image with lung window shows localized involvement of the left lung with irregular cystic air spaces and elongated solid components surrounded by smaller air spaces, line-and-dot pattern (arrow) (Fig. 9.11). Coronal CT miniMIP reconstruction image reveals a localized expansive cystic lesion of the upper lobe with mass effect and secondary mediastinal con-tralateral shift (Fig. 9.12). The patient underwent surgical lobectomy and there was histo-logical diagnostic confirmation.

Figure 9.9a, b
Figure 9.10
Figure 9.11
Figure 9.12

Case 9.4

Posthemorrhagic Hydrocephalus in the Preterm Infant

Cristina Bravo Bravo and Pascual García-Herrera Taillefer

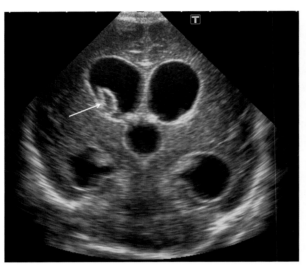

Fig. 9.13

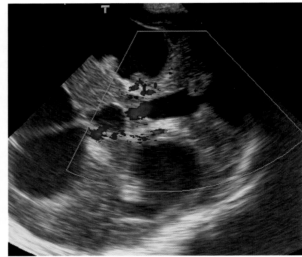

Fig. 9.14

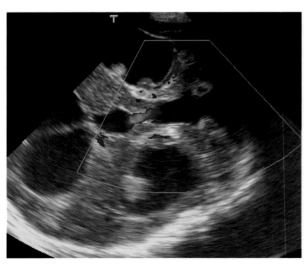

Fig. 9.15

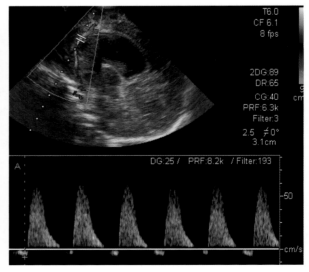

Fig. 9.16

Preterm newborn presents severe intraventricular hemorrhage, increased cephalic perimeter, and progressive dilatation of the ventricular system.

Posthemorrhagic hydrocephalus consists of a progressive dilatation of the ventricular system due to obstruction of the circulatory pathways and CSF reabsorption secondary to hemorrhage in the ventricular system and spaces containing CSF. It is considered a severe complication of intraventricular bleeding in the preterm neonate. Ultrasound is the preferred imaging modality in the evaluation of this condition. The progressive enlargement of the ventricular system can be quantified by the measurement of ventricular size on serial studies. Findings that aid in diagnosing hydrocephalus and differentiate it from ex-vacuo ventriculomegaly include rounding of the frontal horns, dilatation of the temporal horns, and bulging of the third ventricle. The morphological characteristics of the dilatation indicate the level of obstruction, which may have therapeutic implications. In intraventricular hydrocephalus (noncommunicating) the obstruction occurs in the Sylvian aqueduct (in which case the fourth ventricle is normal) or in the openings that drain the fourth ventricle (the ventricle would appear dilated and the cisterna magna, small). In extraventricular hydrocephalus (communicating), the entire ventricular system is dilated and the cisterna magna is either normal or enlarged. Exploration through the mastoid fontanelle allows for adequate assessment of the posterior fossa. In cases where blood particles or detritus are present in CSF, color Doppler may aid in evaluating the permeability of the Sylvian aqueduct or of the foramen of Luschka or Magendie. An increase in intracranial pressure is reflected on the resistance index (RI) of the intracranial vessels. Compression of the anterior fontanelle increases the sensitivity of the RI for the detection of intracranial compliance abnormalities.

Coronal view US of the anterior fontanelle (Fig. 9.13) shows ventricular dilatation with thickening and hyperechogenicity of the ependyma (chemical ependymitis) and a blood clot in the right ventricle (arrow). Axial US images obtained through the mastoid fontanelle (Figs. 9.14 and 9.15) reveal extraventricular hydrocephalus with dilatation of the fourth ventricle and the cisterna magna, as well as permeability of the Sylvian aqueduct, which shows color signal in its interior due to the presence of mobile blood particles in the CSF. Also, diastole inversion and an RI increase (>1) of the anterior cerebral artery (Fig. 9.16) can be seen, which indicate elevated intracranial pressure.

Figure 9.13
Figure 9.14
Figure 9.15
Figure 9.16

Case 9.5

Hypoxic–Ischemic Encephalopathy in the Full-Term Neonate

Eva Gómez Roselló

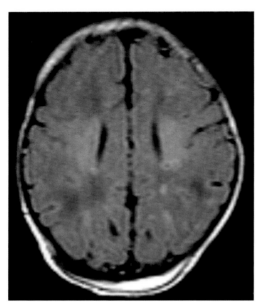

Fig. 9.17

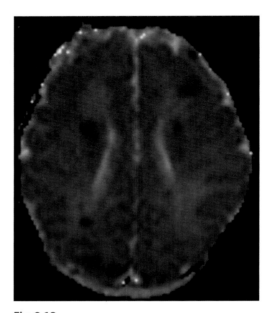

Fig. 9.18

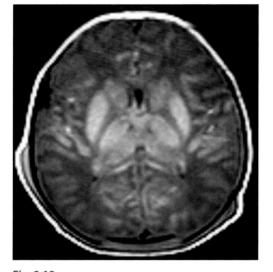

Fig. 9.19

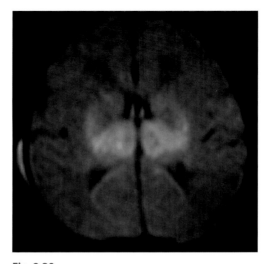

Fig. 9.20

Case 9.5a: Woman with a 41-week gestation with labor dystocia. The newborn presented epileptic seizures 24 h after birth.

Case 9.5b: Woman with a 40-week gestation with history of cesarean section presents uterine rupture. Neonate is born by urgent c-section with a low Apgar score.

Hypoxic–ischemic injury is an important cause of morbidity and mortality in the neonate and produces cerebral paralysis as a possible sequela. Imaging findings are unique to the newborn, with different patterns appearing according to cerebral maturity and the severity and duration of the ischemic insult. Moderate damage refers to sustained yet incomplete deficit, which causes redistribution to hypermetabolic areas and in turn, damage to intervascular watershed territories. Severe damage consists of a sudden and complete hypoxia that predominantly affects deep gray matter and myelinated fibers. While mild hypotension produces parasagittal cortical and subcortical white matter lesions, severe hypotension affects the posterior putamen, hippocampus, lateral aspect of the thalamus, corticospinal tract, and the sensitive and motor cortex.

Conventional, diffusion (DWI), and spectroscopy MRI are the most sensitive modalities used to detect patterns of ischemic damage. A combination of T1-, T2-, and DWI is recommended for evaluating hypoxic–ischemic lesions during the early neonatal period in the full-term newborn. Certain signs have been described as indicative of hypoxic injury, including an increased signal of the basal ganglia and thalami on T1, loss of hypersignal of the posterior limb of the internal capsule, and diffusion restriction of the injured areas. An earlier diffusion is seen between 24 h and 8 days after birth and it is more sensitive to cytotoxic edema, an important indicator of outcome. Spectroscopy may also be useful in providing information used to determine prognosis.

Case 9.5a: Ultrasound performed at 24 h was normal. MRI 5 days later revealed multiple cortical and subcortical lesions in watershed territory that are hyperintense on T2-weighted/FLAIR MR images (Fig. 9.17) and show restricted diffusion on the ADC map without hemorrhagic transformation (Fig. 9.18).

Figure 9.17
Figure 9.18

Case 9.5b: MRI performed 4 days after the ischemic event revealed severe ischemic damage. T1-weighted MR image shows bilateral hyperintensity of the basal ganglia, mesencephalon, and precentral cortex (Fig. 9.19). The lesions display restricted diffusion (Fig. 9.20).

Figure 9.19
Figure 9.20

Case 9.6
Cerebral Sinovenous Thrombosis in Neonates
■
Cristina Bravo Bravo and
Pascual García-Herrera Taillefer

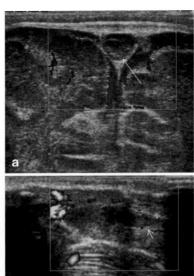

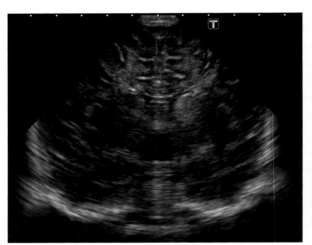

Fig. 9.21

Fig. 9.22

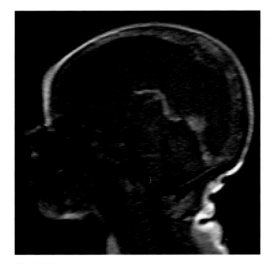

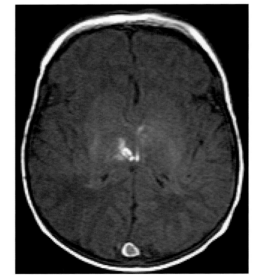

Fig. 9.23

Fig. 9.24

A 7-day-old full-term neonate presents with seizures.

Cerebral sinovenous thrombosis (CSVT) is a relatively uncommon disorder in children and it occurs most commonly in neonates. Signs and symptoms are nonspecific and the diagnosis can be delayed or easily misdiagnosed. Seizures are the presenting feature in 71% of neonates. Less common manifestations include lethargy, respiratory distress, irritability, macrocephaly, and a bulging fontanelle. The main risk factors are perinatal complications, dehydration, and sepsis. Often a prothrombotic state is associated. In some cases the etiology remains unknown. The thrombosis can affect the superficial system, the deep system or both, and one or multiple sinuses. The most commonly involved sinuses are the transverse sinuses, the superior sagittal sinus (SSS), and the straight sinus. Focal brain abnormalities have been identified in approximately 50–60% of patients, and often are hemorrhagic. US Doppler is a useful tool for the initial diagnosis and monitoring of neonatal sinovenous thrombosis. Color Doppler and power Doppler techniques can image the major portions of the deep and superficial venous pathways. The diagnosis is established when an enlarged sinus with reduced or absent blood flow is observed. MRI and MR venography are the imaging studies of choice. The absence of a flow void and the presence of altered signal intensity in the sinus is a primary finding of sinus thrombosis. The signal intensity varies according to the interval between the onset of thrombus formation and the time of imaging. Parenchymal lesions (venous congestion, edema, infarct) are better depicted and identified with MRI than with US or CT. On non-enhanced CT, a thrombosed dural sinus typically has homogeneous hyperdensity, which produces a filling defect on enhanced CT ("delta sign"). Another classical sign is the "cord sing" (cortical hyperdense vein). Infarcts are a predictor for unfavorable neurological outcome.

US reveals diffuse white matter echogenicity and bilateral lesions in the thalami (not shown) and left basal ganglia. The ventricular system is collapsed (Fig. 9.21). Coronal view color Doppler through the anterior fontanelle (Fig. 9.22 a) and power Doppler axial image through the posterolateral fontanelle (Fig. 9.22 b) show an enlarged SSS (arrow) and transverse sinus (arrowhead), with thrombi and absent blood flow (asterisk: cerebellum). Sagittal T1-weighted MR image shows the SSS, internal cerebral veins, Galen vein, straight sinus, and a torcular thrombosis in the subacute stage (Fig. 9.23). Axial T1-weighted MR image reveals a small hemorrhagic venous infarct in the right thalamus (Fig. 9.24).

Figure 9.21
Figure 9.22a, b
Figure 9.23
Figure 9.24

Case 9.7
Disseminated Cerebral Candidiasis in Preterm Infants
Cristina Bravo Bravo and Pascual García-Herrera Taillefer

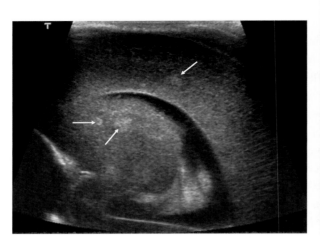

Fig. 9.25

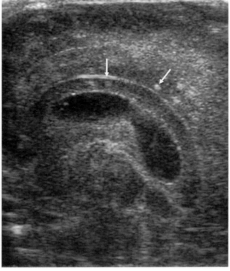

Fig. 9.26

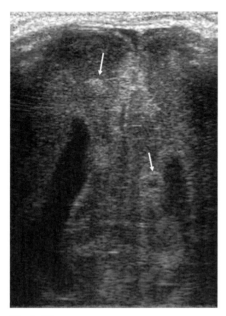

Fig. 9.27

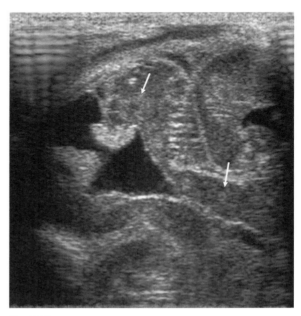

Fig. 9.28

Extremely low-birth-weight neonate, born at 26 weeks of gestation with a birth weight of 736 g. She was mechanically ventilated and required antibiotic treatment for high infection risk and sepsis. On day 14, her clinical condition deteriorated and she developed new signs of infection. Brain US revealed disseminated brain microabscesses. Blood culture was positive for *C. albicans*. Patient died on day 40.

Systemic candidiasis is a frequently clinical problem in neonatal intensive care units. It occurs in 3–5% of very low-birth-weight neonates. Premature infants have a high risk for systemic fungal infection: prematurity, low birth weight, prolonged intubation, in-dwelling catheters, central lines, parenteral feeding, prior cutaneous colonization, and prolonged use of broad-spectrum antibiotics.

After the kidneys, the brain has been reported to be the second most commonly involved organ. Central nervous system (CNS) candidiasis is a serious complication of a candidemia in preterm infants, and is associated with high mortality and morbidity. Symptoms and signs are often nonspecific and subtle, with CSF findings variables, even can be normal.

A high clinical suspicion and appropriate imaging study findings permit the early diagnosis, that is, essential to choose the correct antifungal therapy and its duration.

The most common imaging findings in brain candidiasis are multiple microabscesses (<3 mm), distributed in the subcortical and periventricular regions, thalami, basal ganglia, brain stem, and cerebellum. Other findings in CNS candidiasis are meningitis, ventriculitis, and ventricular dilatation, or macroabscesses. Ultrasound should be the preferred initial imaging method, given its portability, lack of required sedation, avoidance of radiation, and easy follow-up. At US the microabscesses are small, echogenic rimlike lesion with hypoecoic centers scattered in the brain parenchyma. MRI is best to depict infratentorial lesions. Contrast-enhanced MRI shows enhancing-ring lesion and DW-MR shows restricted diffusion lesions.

Parasagital image through anterior fontanelle (Fig. 9.25) shows small hyperchoic nodules in basal ganglia and periventricular white matter. Seven days later, US shows more numerous nodules, some of them with rimlike appearance. Midline image (Fig. 9.26): lesions in corpus callosum and brain parenchyma. Posterior, angled, coronal image (Fig. 9.27): periventricular and subcortical lesions. Coronal image through posterolateral fontanelle (Fig. 9.28): lesions in brain stem and cerebellum.

Figure 9.25
Figure 9.26
Figure 9.27
Figure 9.28

Case 9.8
Necrotizing Enterocolitis
■
Amparo Moreno Flores and Roberto Llorens Salvador

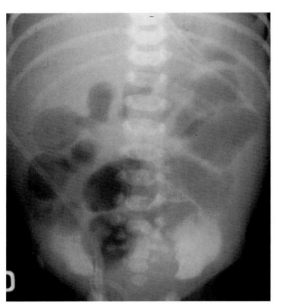

Fig. 9.29

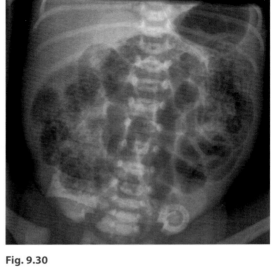

Fig. 9.30

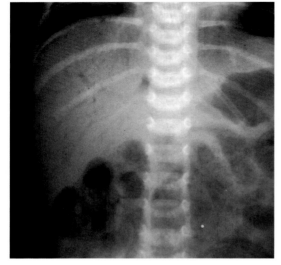

Fig. 9.31

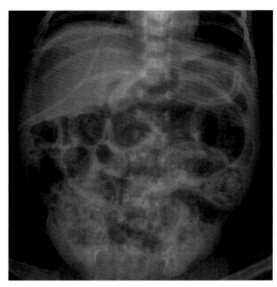

Fig. 9.32

A 29-week premature newborn weighing 1,100 g at birth presents with abdominal distention and increased gastric aspirates. A day later, he presents bloody stools.

Necrotizing enterocolitis (NEC) remains a major cause of neonatal morbidity and mortality, yet its pathogenesis is poorly understood. A multifactorial theory suggests that four key risk factors including prematurity, intestinal ischemia, bacterial colonization and formula feeding, are involved in the development of an intestinal injury characterized by coagulative and hemorrhagic necrosis of portions of intestine in newborns. NEC is the cause of approximately 1–5% of neonatal care unit admissions and over 90% of patients are born preterm (risk is inversely related to birth weight and gestational age). Since more preterm infants of very low birth weight (less than 1,500 g) survive the early neonatal period, the population at risk for developing NEC increases.

NEC typically presents with both gastrointestinal and systemic manifestations. Abdominal distension, bloody stools, diarrhea, feeding intolerance, sepsis, apnea–bradycardia, and lethargy are commonly seen. Many infants with NEC recover with medical therapy (bowel rest with placement of a nasogastric tube, total parenteral nutrition, fluid therapy, antibiotics) and have long-term outcomes similar to unaffected infants of matched gestational age. Plain abdominal radiography (AbXR) is the imaging modality of choice for evaluation of NEC. Serial abdominal X-ray films are recommended. Findings range from normal to suggestive to diagnostic, according to the presence, amount, and distribution of abdominal gas.

Ultrasound can provide useful information such as the presence of free intraabdominal fluid, bowel wall thickness, air porthogram, and perfusion abnormalities.

Suggestive findings of NEC in AbXR are asymmetric bowel loop dilatation with loss of the mosaic pattern and development of elongated or rounded loops (Fig. 9.29). The degree and pattern of bowel dilatation are the most important signs for early diagnosis and follow-up because they usually correlate well with clinical severity and subsequent response to medical therapy. Definitive findings are related to pneumatosis intestinalis (Fig. 9.30) as submucosal (bubble-like) or serosal (curvilinear) patterns. Occasionally, it may mimic stool or meconium. Advanced disease is suspected when portal venous gas (Fig. 9.31), persistent loop sign or free intraperitoneal air are seen (Fig. 9.32), the latter being the most frequent indication for surgery in patients with NEC.

Figure 9.29
Figure 9.30
Figure 9.31
Figure 9.32

Case 9.9
Midgut Volvulus
■

Pascual García-Herrera Taillefer and Cristina Bravo Bravo

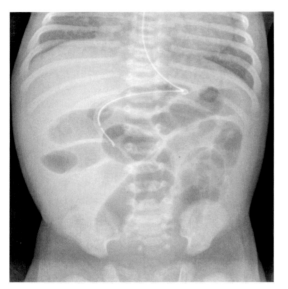

Fig. 9.33

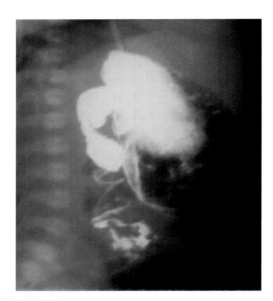

Fig. 9.34

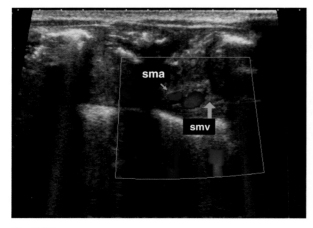

Fig. 9.35

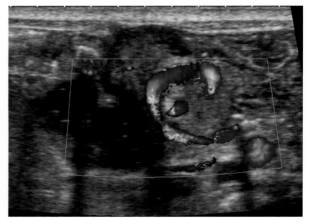

Fig. 9.36

A 6-day-old boy presents with continuous crying, abdominal distension, and bilious vomiting.

The rotation and subsequent fixation of the intestine occurs between the fourth and tenth week of embryonic development. The proximal section then situates itself posteriorly to the mesenteric vessels and the distal portion, anteriorly. With the mesenteric fixation from the duodenojejunal junction to the cecal base, the bowel adopts a fan-like configuration. Abnormal rotation of the intestine and fixation to the mesointestine may cause various consequences, the most serious one being a midgut volvulus. This condition occurs more frequently in the neonatal period (75%), when the mesentery and bowel rotate clockwise with the superior mesenteric artery as their axis. Since the final consequence of this condition may be extensive intestinal necrosis, a timely and accurate diagnosis is essential in order to determine prompt surgical treatment.

A normal plain abdominal radiograph does not exclude the presence of volvulus. This modality is especially effective at evaluating intestinal obstruction (Fig. 9.33) and pneumoperitoneum. The gastrointestinal study with oral contrast is considered the technique of choice for determining the location of the duodenojejunal junction and for assessing the corkscrew-like arrangement of the proximal intestine in these patients (Fig. 9.34). Barium enemas have been used to identify the location of the cecum, yet this is the most variable of the radiologic findings. Sonographic findings include gastric and duodenal distention, thickened bowel wall in the right upper quadrant, and an abnormal layout of the mesenteric vein (smv) and artery (sma) in their initial portion (Fig. 9.35). Currently, a spiral whirpool sign consisting of curving vessels on the superior mesenteric artery (Fig. 9.36) has a sensitivity of 83–92% and a specificity of 100% for the diagnosis of midgut volvulus. The rotation observed must be clockwise (only one case of counterclockwise volvulus rotation has been reported). CT allows for the evaluation of the mesenteric vessels in the characteristic whirpool sign arrangement, as well as the presence of ischemic bowel.

Figure 9.33
Figure 9.34
Figure 9.35
Figure 9.36

Case 9.10
Portal Calcification Secondary to Umbilical Vein Catheterization
Cristina Serrano García

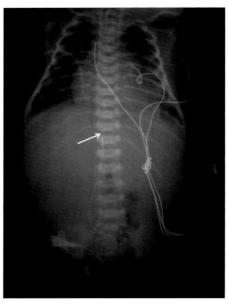

Fig. 9.37

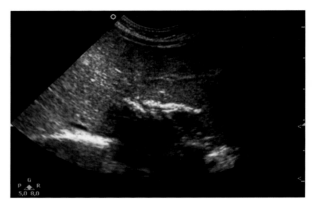

Fig. 9.38

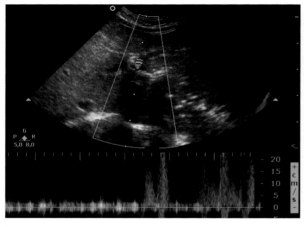

Fig. 9.39

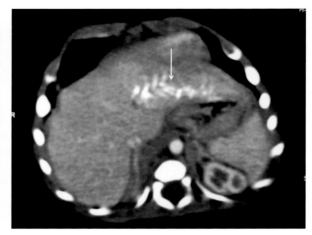

Fig. 9.40

Neonate born at 36 weeks of gestation is admitted to the neonatal intensive care unit (NICU) due to respiratory distress. During the patient's hospitalization, an umbilical venous line is placed.

Umbilical vein catheters are routinely placed in the NICU. The main indications for its use include monitorization, venous access in low-birth-weight premature newborns, analytic extractions, parenteral nutrition, IV medication, and fluid therapy.

The distal end of the catheter should be located at the most cranial portion of the inferior vena cava (IVC), at the junction of the IVC with the right atrium or at the distal portion of the right atrium.

It is considered inadequate positioning of the umbilical vein catheter when it has been placed in the foramen ovale, left atrium, superior vena cava (SVC), internal jugular vein, right ventricle through the tricuspid valve, umbilical recess, trunk and branches of the portal vein, splenic vein, or superior mesenteric vein. The main complications derived from umbilical vein catheter placement include:

- Portal thrombosis (most common cause of extrahepatic portal hypertension), cavernomatosis, portal pneumatosis, and hepatic hematomas
- Vascular calcifications
- Hemorrhage and extravasation due to catheter rupture

Plain abdominal films are used as a routine technique to confirm the placement of umbilical vein catheters. By means of B-mode ultrasound and Doppler, certain vascular complications such as calcifications, thrombosis, and aneurysms can be detected, as well as secondary visceral involvement. CT studies are not commonly used, nevertheless they may aid in diagnosing vascular calcifications, evaluating the integrity of abdominal viscera, and determining vascular permeability.

Plain abdominal films identify the distal end of the umbilical vein catheter ill-positioned within the umbilical recess (arrow) (Fig. 9.37). Abdominal ultrasound detects linear calcifications in the wall of the left portal vein (Fig. 9.38). Doppler ultrasound shows predominant arterial blood flow in the left lobe, while minimal portal flow is evident (Fig. 9.39). Abdominal contrast-enhanced CT confirms the presence of complete calcification of the left portal vein branch (arrow) (Fig. 9.40).

Figure 9.37
Figure 9.38
Figure 9.39
Figure 9.40

Further Reading

Books

Donnelly L et al (2005) Diagnostic imaging. Pediatrics, vol 4. Amirsys, Salt Lake City, UT, pp 4–36

Gomella T, Cunningham M, Eyal F (2009) Neonatology: management, procedures, on-call problems, diseases, and drugs, 6th edn. McGraw-Hill, New York

Leonard E (2005) Swischuck. Radiología el niño y en el recién nacido. Editorial Marbán, SL

Lucaya J, Strife JL (eds) (2002) Pediatric chest imaging. Chest imaging in infants and children. Springer-Verlag, Berlín

Osborn AG (2007) Diagnostic imaging: Brain. Salt Lake City: Ed Amirsis

Swischuk LE. (2004) Trombosis venosa profunda. Cabeza, cerebroy meninges. En: Radiología en el niño y en el recién nacido. Ed. Marban

Siegel MJ (2004) Hemorragia intracraneal. En: Siegel MJ (ed) Ecografía Pediátrica, Philadelphia: Lippincott Williams and Wilkins, 2nd edn, pp 58–72

Siegel MJ (2004) Infeccion intracraneal. En: Siegel MJ (ed) Ecografía Pediátrica, Philadelphia: Lippincott Williams and Wilkins, 2nd edn, pp 104–110

Sivit CJ, Siegel MJ (2004) Malrotación intestinal. En: Siegel MJ, ed. Ecografía Pediátrica, Philadelphia: Lippincott Williams and Wilkins, 2nd edn, pp 352–355

Spitzer AR (1996) Intensive care of the fetus and neonate, vol 34. Mosby Year Book, St. Louis, MO, pp 345–400

Web Links

http://emedicine.medscape.com/article/409409-overview

http://rad.usuhs.edu/medpix/new_topic.html?mode=single&recnum=3518&table=card&srchstr=bronchogeniccyst&search=bronchogeniccyst#top. Accessed October 2009

http://www.springer.com/medicine/radiology/journal/247

www.neonatology.org

http://www.ajnr.org/

http://emedicine.medscape.com

www.neonatology.org

http://www.uptodate.com/home/index.html

www.emedicine.medscape.com/article/930576-overview

http://www.adhb.govt.nz/newborn/Guidelines/VascularCatheters/UmbilicalCatheters.htm

Articles

Agrons GA, Courtney SE, Stocker JT, Markowitz RI (2005) Lung disease in premature neonates: radiologic-pathologic correlation. Radiographics 25:1047–1073

Aidlen J, Anupindi SA, Jaramillo D, Doody DP (2005) Malrotation wirth midgut volvulus: CT findings on bowel infarction. Pediatr Radiol 35:529–531

Applegate KE (2009) Evidence-based diagnosis of malrotation and volvulus. Pediatr Radiol 39(Suppl 2):S161–S163

Applegate KE, Anderson JM, Klatte EC (2006) Intestinal malrotation in children: a problem-resolving approach to the upper gastrointestinal series. Radiographics 26:1485–1500

Barkovich AJ, Westmark K, Partidge C, Sola A, Ferreiro DM (1995) Perinatal asphyxia: MR findings in the first 10 days. AJNR Am J Neuroradiol 16:427–438

Barnacle A, Arthurs OJ, Roebuck D, Hiorns MP (2008) Malfunctioning central venous catheters in children: a diagnostic approach. Pediatr Radiol 38:363–378

Belcher E, Abbasi MA, Hansell DM, Ffolkes L, Nicholson AG, Goldstraw P (2009) Persistent interstitial pulmonary emphusema requirirng penumonectomy. J Thorac Cardiovasc Surg 138(1):237–239

Benjamin D, Poole C, Steinbach W, Rowen J, Walsh T (2003) Neonatal candidemia an end-organ damage: a critical appraisal of the literature using Meta-analytic techniques. Pediatrics 112:634–640

Berrocal T, Madrid C, Novo S, Gutiérrez J, Arjonilla A, Gómez-León N (2000) Congenital anomalies of the tracheobronchial tree, lung, and mediastinum: embryology, radiology, and pathology. Radiographics 24:e17

Blankenberg FG, Loh NN, Bracci P, D´Arceuil HE, Thine WD, Norbash AM et al (2000) Sonography, CT and MR imaging: a prospective comparison of neonates with suspected intracranial ischemia and hemorrhage. AJNR Am J Neuroradiol 21:213–218

Buonomo C (1999) The radiology of necrotizing enterocolitis. Radiol Clin North Am 37(6):1187–1198, vii

Chao CP, Zaleski CG, Patton AC (2006) Neonatal hypoxic-ischemic encephalopathy: multimodality imaging findings. Radiographics 26:S159–S172

Cioffi U, De Simone M, Ciulla MM (2008) Computed tomography and endoscopic ultrasound in detection and characterization of mediastinal masses. J Thorac Cardiovasc Surg 136(6):1606

Cleveland RH (1995) A radiologic update on medical diseases of the newborn chest. Pediatr Radiol 25:631–637

Coursey CA, Hollingsworth CL, Wriston C, Beam C, Rice H, Bisset G 3rd (2009) Radiographic predictors of disease severity in neonates and infants with necrotizing enterocolitis. AJR Am J Roentgenol 193:1408–1413

Couture A, Veyrac C, Baud C, Saguintaah M, Ferran JL (2001) Advanced cranial ultrasound: transfontanellar doppler imaging in neonates. Eur Radiol 11:2399–2410

Dean LM, Taylor GA (1995) The intracranial venous system in infants: normal and abnormal findings on duplex and color doppler sonography. AJR Am J Roentgenol 164:151–156

Demura Y, Ishizaki T, Nakanishi M, Ameshima S, Itoh H (2007) Persistent diffuse pulmonary interstitial emphysema mimicking pulmonary emphysema. Thorax 62(7):652

DeVeber G, Andrew M, Adams C, Bjornson B, Booth F, Buckley D et al (2001) Cerebral sinovenous thrombosis in children. N Engl J Med 345:417–423

Dinger J, Schwarze R, Rupprecht E (1997) Radiological changes after therapeutic use of surfactant in infants with respiratory distress syndrome. Pediatr Radiol 27:26–31

Donnelly LF, Frush DP (1999) Localized radiolucent chest lesions in neonates: causes and differentiation. AJR Am J Roentgenol 172:1651–1658

Donnelly LF, Lucaya J, Ozelame V, Frush DP, Strouse PJ, Sumner TE et al (2003) CT findings and temporal course of persistent pulmonary interstitial emphysema in neonates: a multiinstitutional study. AJR Am J Roentgenol 180:1129–1133

du Plessis AJ (1998) Posthemorrhagic hydrocephalus and brain injury in the preterm infant: dilemas in diagnosis and management. Semin Pediatr Neurol 5:161–179

Enriquez G, Correa F, Aso C, Carreño JC, Gonzalez R, Padilla NF, Vazquez E (2006a) Mastoid fontanelle approach for sonography imaging of the neonatal brain. Pediatr Radiol 36: 532–540

Enriquez G, Correa F, Aso C, Carreño JC, Gonzalez R, Padilla NF, Vazquez E (2006b) Mastoid fontanelle approach for sonographic imaging of the neonatal brain. Pediatr Radiol 36:532–540

Epelman M (2006) The whirlpool sing. Radiology 240:910–911

Epelman M, Daneman A, Navarro OM, Morag I, Moore AM, Kim JH, Faingold R, Taylor G, Gerstle JT (2007) Necrotizing enterocolitis: review of state-of-the-art imaging findings with pathologic correlation. Radiographics 27:285–305

Faix RG, Chapman RL (2003) Central nervous system candidiasis in the high-risk neonate. Semin Perinatol 27:384–392

Govaert P (2009) Sonographic stroke templates. Semin Fetal Neonatal Med 14:284–298

Gursoy S, Ucvet A, Ozturk AA, Erbaycu AE, Basok O, Yucel N (2009) Seven years experience of bronchogenic cysts. Saudi Med J 30:238–242

Hantous-Zannad S, Charrada L, Mestiri I, Fennira H, Horchani H, Kammoun N et al (2000) Radiological and clinical aspects of bronchogenic lung cysts: 4 case reports. Rev Pneumol Clin 56:249–254

Heinz ER, Provenzale JM (2009) Imaging findings in neonatal hypoxia: a practical review. AJR Am J Roentgenol 192:41–47

Helbich TH, Popow C, Dobner M et al (1998) New-born infants with severe hyaline membrane disease: radiological evaluation during high frequency oscillatory versus conventional ventilation. Eur J Radiol 28:243–249

Henesh SM, Nance ML, Jaramillo D (2006) Enhanced CT perfusion cutt-off sing in midgut volvulus. Pediatr Radiol 36: 355–357

Henry MC, Moss RL (2008) Neonatal necrotizing enterocolitis. Semin Pediatr Surg 17:98–109

Huang BY, Castillo M (2008) Continuing medical education: hypoxic-ischemis brain injury: imaging findings from birth to adulthood. Radiographics 28:417–439

Huang C, Chen C, Yang H, Wang S, Chang Y, Liu C (1998) Central nervous system candidiasis in very low-birth-weight premature neonates and infants: US characteristics and histhopatologic and MR imaging correlates in five patients. Radiology 209:49–56

Jabra AA, Fishman EK, Shehata BM, Perlman EJ (1997) Localized persistent pulmonary interstitial emphysema: CT findings with radiographic-pathologic correlation. AJR Am J Roentgenol 169:1381–1384

Jassal MS, Benson JE, Mogayzel PJ Jr (2008) Spontaneous resolution of diffuse persistent pulmonary interstitial emphysema. Pediatr Pulmonol 43(6):615–619

Kattwinkel J, Bloom BT, Delmore P et al (2000) High-versus low-threshold surfactant retreatment for neonatal respiratory distress syndrome. Pediatrics 106:282–288

Khemiri M, Ouederni M, Ben Mansour F, Barsaoui S (2008) Bronchogenic cyst: an uncommon cause of congenital lobar emphysema. Respir Med 102:1663–1666, Epub 2008 Aug 28

Kim JH, Lee YS, Kim SH, Lee SK, Lim MK, Kim HS (2001) Does umbilical vein catheterization lead to portal venous thrombosis? Prospective US evaluation in 100 neonates. Radiology 219:645–650

Kim WY, Kim WS, Kim IO, Kwon TH, Chang W, Lee EK (2005) Sonographic evaluation of neonates with early-stage necrotizing enterocolitis. Pediatr Radiol 35(11):1056–1561

Kimchi TJ, Lee SK, Agid R, Shroff M, Ter Brugge KG (2007) Cerebral sinovenous thrombosis in children. Neuroimaging Clin N Am 17(2):239–244

Konen O, Daneman A, Traubici J, Epelman M (2004) Intravascular linear thrombus after catheter removal: sonographic appearance mimicking retained catheter fragment. Pediatr Radiol 34:125–129

Lai P, Lin S, Pan H, Yan C (1997) Disseminated miliary cerebral candidiasis. AJNR Am J Neuroradiol 18:1303–1306

Lanza C, Russo M, Fabrizzi G (2006) Central venous cannulation: are routine chest radiographs necessary after B-mode and colour Doppler sonography check? Pediatr Radiol 36:1252–1256

Leach JL, Fortuna RB, Jones BV, Gaskill-Shipley MF (2006) Imaging of cerebral venous thrombosis: current techniques, spectrum of findings and diagnostic pitfalls. Radiographics 26:S19–S41

Leonidas JC, Magid N, Soberman N, Glass TS (1991) Midgut volvulus in infants: diagnosis with US. Radiology 179:491–493

Liauw L, Palm-Meinders IH, van der Grond J, Leijser LM, le Cessie S, Laan LA et al (2007) Differentiating normal myelination from hypoxic-ischemic encephalopathy on T1-weighted MR Images: a new approach. AJNR Am J Neuroradiol 28: 660–665

Liauw L, van der Grond J, van den Berg-Huysmans AA, Laan LA, van Buchem MA, van Wezel-Meijler G (2008a) Is there a way to predict outcome in (near) term neonates with hypoxic-ischemic encephalopathy based on MR imaging? AJNR Am J Neuroradiol 29:1789–1794

Liauw L, van der Grond J, van den Berg-Huysmans AA, Palm-Meinders IH, van Buchem MA, van Wezel-Meijler G (2008b) Hypoxic-ischemic encephalopathy: diagnostic value of conventional MR imaging pulse sequences in term-born neonates. Radiology 247:204–212

Lima M, Gargano T, Ruggeri G, Manuele R, Gentili A, Pilu G et al (2008) Clinical spectrum and management of congenital pulmonary cystic lesions. N Pediatr Med Chir 30:79–88

Lin PW, Stoll BJ (2006) Necrotising enterocolitis. Lancet 368:1271–1283

Lin PW, Nasr TR, Stoll BJ (2008) Necrotizing enterocolitis: recent scientific advances in pathophysiology and prevention. Semin Perinatol 32:70–82

Long FR, Kramer SS, Markowitz RI, Taylor GE (1996) Radiographic patterns of intestinal malrotation in children. Radiographics 16:547–556

Maertzdorf WJ, Vles JS, Beuls E, Mulder AL, Blanco CE (2002) Intracranial pressure and cerebral blood flow velocity in preterm infants with posthaemorrhagic ventricular dilatation. Arch Dis Child Fetal Neonotal Ed 87:185–188

Magilner AD, Capitanio MA, Wertheimer I, Burko H (1974) Persistent localized intrapulmonary interstitl emphysema: an observation in three infants. Radiology 111:379–384

Marcinkowski M, Bauer K, Stoltenburg-Didinger G, Versmold H (2001) Fungal brain abscesses in neonates: sonographics appaerances and corresponding histopathologic findings. J Clin Ultrasound 29:417–421

Mata M, Pino A, Santos JG, Oyágüez P, Aragón MP (2003) Candidiasis cerebral en un recién nacido. An Pediatr 58:194–194

McAdams P, Kirejczyk WM, Rosado-de- Christenson ML, Matsumoto S (2000) Bronchogenic cyst: imaging features with clical and histopathologic correlation. Radiology 217:441–446

Narla LD, Hom M, Lofland GK, Moskowitz WB (1991) Evaluation of umbilical catheter and tube placement in premature infants. Radiographics 11:849–863

Newman B (1999) Imaging of medical disease of the newborn lung. Radiol Clin North Am 37:1049–1065

Nishimaki S, Iwasaki Y, Akamatsu H (2004) Cerebral blood flow velocity before and after cerebrospinal fluid drainage in infants with posthemorrhagic hydrocephalus. J Ultrasound Med 23:1315–1319

Oppenheimer DA, Carroll BA, Garth KE (1982) Ultrasonic detection of complications following umbilical arterial catheterization in the neonate. Radiology 145:667–672

Pahud BA, Greenhow TL, Piecuch B, Weintrub PS (2009) Preterm neonates with candidal brain microabscesses: a case series. J Perinatol 29:323–326

Pierro A, Hall N (2003) Surgical treatments of infants with necrotizing enterocolitis. Semin Neonatol 8:223–232

Pracros JP, Sann L, Genin G et al (1992) Ultrasound diagnosis of midgut volvulus: the "whirpool" sing. Pediatr Radiol 22:18–20

Puig J, Pedraza S, Mendez J, Trujillo A (2006) Neonatal cerebral venous thrombosis: diagnosis by magnetic resonance angiography. Radiología 48:169–171

Rao P (2006) Neonatal gastrointestinal imaging. Eur J Radiol 60(2):171–186

Rao S, Ali U (2005) Systemic fungal infections in neonates. J Postgrad Med 51(Suppl 1):S27–S29

Rao J, Hochman MI, Miller GG (2006) Localized persistent pulmonary interstitital emphysema. J Pediatr Surg 41(6):1191–1193

Rutherford M, Martinez Biarge M, Allsop J, Counsell S, Cowan F (2010) MRI of perinatal brain injury. Pediatr Radiol 40:819–833

Sanchez-Portocarrero J, Pérez-Cecilia E, Corral O, Romero-Vivas J, Picazo JJ (2000) The central nervous system and infection by *Candida* species. Diagn Microbiol Infect Dis 37:169–179

Satoh K, Kobayashi T, Kawase Y et al (1996) CT appearance of interstitial pulmonay emphysema. J Thorac Imaging 11:153–154

Schlesinger AE, Braverman RM, DiPietro MA (2003) Neonates and umbilical venous catheters: normal appearance, anomalous positions, complications, and potential aid to diagnosis. AJR Am J Roentgenol 180:1147–1153

Sébire G, Tabarki B, Saunders E, Leroy I, Liesner R, Saint-Martin C et al (2005) Cerebral venous sinus thrombosis in children: risk factors, presentation, diagnosis and outcome. Brain 128:477–489

Seibert JJ, Northington FJ, Miers JF, Taylor BJ (1991) Aortic thrombosis after umbilical artery catheterization in neonates: prevalence of complications on long-term follow-up. AJR Am J Roentgenol 156:567–569

Shew SB (2009) Surgical concerns in malrotation and midgut volvulus. Pediatr Radiol 39(Suppl 2):S167–S171

Shimanuki Y, Aihara T, Takano H et al (1996) Clockwise whirlpool sing at color Doppler US: an objetive and definite sing of midgut volvulus. Radiology 199:261–264

Slovis TL, Shankaran S (1980) Patent ductus arteriosus in hyaline membrane disease: chest radiography. AJR Am J Roentgenol 135:307–309

Srinivasan PS, Brandler MD, D'Souza A (2008) Necrotizing enterocolitis. Clin Perinatol 35(1):251–272, x

Stoker JT, Madewell JE (1977) Persistent interstitial emphysema: another complication of the respiratory distress syndrome. Pediatrics 59:847–857

Sundaramoorthi T, Mahadevan R, Nedumaran K, Jayaraman S, Vaidyanathan KR (2009) Intrabronchial rupture of bronchogenic cyst. Ann Thorac Surg 87:1919–1920

Swischuk LE (1977) Bubbles in hyaline membrane disease. Differentiation of three types. Radiology 122:417–426

Swischuk LE, John SD (1996) Immature lung problems: can our nomenclature be more specific? AJR Am J Roentgenol 166: 917–918

Taylor GA (2001) Sonography assessment of posthemorrhagic ventricular dilatation. Radiol Clin North Am 39: 541–551

Taylor GA, Madsen J (1996) Neonatal hydrocephalus: hemodynamic response to fontanelle compression. Correlation with intracranial pressure and need for shunt placement. Radiology 201:685–689

Taylor GA, Phillips MD, Ichord RN, Carson BS, Gates JA, James CS (1994) Intracranial compliance in infants: evaluation with Doppler US. Radiology 191:787–791

Teele SA, Emani SM, Thiagarajan RR, Teele RL (2008) Catheters, wires, tubes and drains on postoperative radiographs of pediatric cardiac patients: the whys and wherefores. Pediatr Radiol 38:1041–1053

Teissier N, Elmaleh-Bergès M, Ferkdadji L, François M, Van den Abbeele T (2008) Arch cervical bronchogenic cysts: usual and unusual clinical presentations. Otolaryngol Head Neck Surg 134:1165–1169

Teksam O, Kale G (2009) The effects of surfactant and antenatal corticosteroid treatment on the pulmonary pathology of preterm infants with respiratory distress syndrome. Pathol Res Pract 205:35–41

Teksam M, Moharir M, Deveber G, Shroff M (2008) Frecuency and topographic distribution of brain lesions in pediatric cerebral venous thrombosis. AJNR Am J Neuroradiol 29:1961–1965

Tsao PN, Lee WT, Peng SF, Lin JH, Yau KI (1999) Power doppler ultrasound imaging in neonatal cerebral venous sinus thrombosis. Pediatr Neurol 21:652–655

Valk JW, Plötz FB, Schuerman FA, van Vught H, Kramer PP, Beek EJ (2001) The value of routine chest radiographs in a paediatric intensive care unit: a prospective study. Pediatr Radiol 31:343–347

Vermeulen RJ, van Schie PE, Hendrikx L, Barkhof F, van Weissenbruch M, Knol DL et al (2008) Diffusion-weighted and conventional MR imaging in neonatal hypoxic ischemia: two-year follow-up study. Radiology 249:631–639

Veyrac C, Couture A, Saguintaah M, Baud C (2006) Brain ultrasonography in the premature infant. Pediatr Radiol 36: 626–635

Whitelaw A, Thoresen M, Pople I (2002) Posthaemorrhagic ventricular dilatation. Arch Dis Child Fetal Neonatal Ed 86:72–74

Wong K, Gruenewald S, Larcos G, Jamali M (2006) Neonatal fungal ventriculitis. J Clin Ultrasound 34:402–406

Wright CD (2009) Mediastinal tumors and cysts in the pediatric population. Thorac Surg Clin 19:47–61

Contents

M.I. Martínez-León et al., *Learning Pediatric Imaging*, Learning Imaging,
DOI: 10.1007/978-3-642-16892-5_10, © Springer-Verlag Berlin Heidelberg 2011

Case 10.1
Fetal Open-Lip Schizencephaly
■
María I. Martínez León

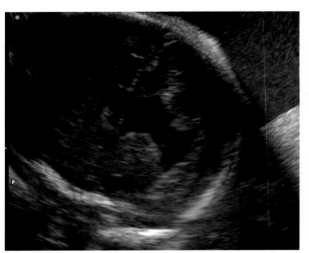

Fig. 10.1

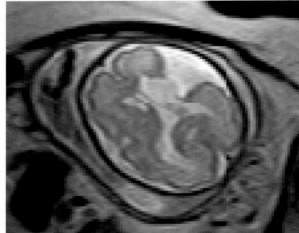

Fig. 10.2

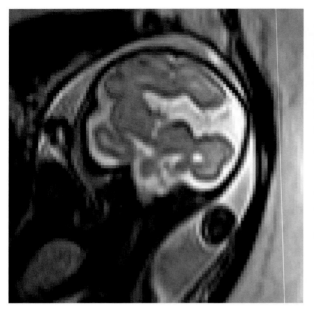

Fig. 10.3

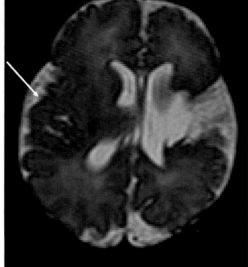

Fig. 10.4

A 29-week fetus is referred to MRI for asymmetric ventriculomegaly.

Comments

Schizencephaly (SchC) is the most frequent neuronal migration disorder consistent in a cerebrum spinal fluid–filled cleft, lined by gray matter. The clefts may extend through the hemisphere from the ependymal lining of the lateral ventricles to the pial surface of the hemisphere. The cleft can be uni- or bilateral and are commonly located near the pre- or postcentral gyry. It develops between the third and fifth gestational months. There are two types: closed-lip SchC, characterized by gray matter-lined lips that are in contact with each other (type 1), and open-lip SchC, which has separated lips and a cleft of CSF that is lined by gray matter and extending to the underlying ventricle (type 2). Prenatal imaging allows detection and characterization of open-lip Sch; there are no reported cases prenatally diagnosed of close-lip SchC. Additional abnormalities, such as polymicrogyria, gray matter heterotopia, absence of the septum pellucidum, may also be demonstrated.

The etiology is unclear, genetic (EMX2 gen), vascular, and infectious (cytomegalovirus) theories have been described.

The severity of the motor and mental impairment is directly related to the extent of the anatomic defect. Treatment should be symptomatic and multidisciplinary.

The differential diagnosis for a CSF-containing abnormality of the fetal brain includes both developmental (arachnoid cyst, ventriculomegaly, monoventricle in holoprosencephaly, agenesis of the corpus callosum with and interhemispheric cyst) and destructive lesions (poroencephalic cyst, ventriculomegaly after infection or bleeding, hydranencephaly).

Imaging Findings

Transvaginal sonography of the head fetus shows unilateral parenchymal defect (Fig. 10.1).

Fetal MR, axial T2, left pre-central open-lip SchC (Fig. 10.2). Fetal MR, coronal T2, large cleft in continuity with the lateral ventricle. Continuity of gray matter lining the cleft is clearly seen, which is the pathognomonic finding of SchC (Fig. 10.3). Newborn, head MR axial T2, confirmation of open-lip SchC with gray matter lining the defect. Presence of associated structural abnormality, contralateral polymicrogyria (arrow) (Fig. 10.4).

Figure 10.1
Figure 10.2
Figure 10.3
Figure 10.4

Case 10.2
Classic Lissencephaly
■
Ignacio Alonso Usabiaga

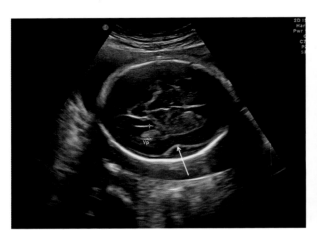

Fig. 10.5

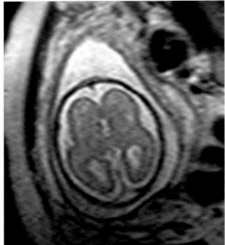

Fig. 10.6

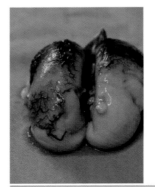

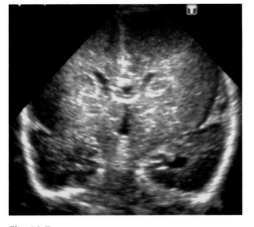

Fig. 10.7

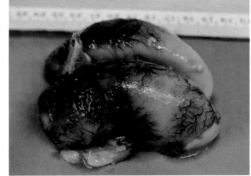

Fig. 10.8

Fetal CNS ultrasound performed at 27 weeks of gestation.

Classic lissencephaly is one of the multiple forms of presentation of genetic malformations of the cerebral cortex (GMCCs). Classification systems for these conditions are constantly being updated because of technological advances in MRI and the discovery of new genetic abnormalities related to these disorders. The way GMCCs present depends on the developmental period in which the abnormality occurs (proliferation, migration, or cortical organization) and associated abnormalities. Different gene mutations and deletions are continuously being discovered in relation to these malformations, and they lead to multiple syndromes with distinctive clinical manifestations and imaging findings.

    Classic lissencephaly, according to the most recent classification (Barkovich 2005), belongs to group II and is characterized by a defective development of cerebral sulci and circumvolutions due to an incomplete neuronal migration. This agyria or pachygyria may be an isolated finding or be accompanied by other malformations such as in Miller–Dieker syndrome, where there is a deletion of the 17p13.3 locus that causes facial dysmorphism, mental retardation, and occasionally cardiac, gastrointestinal, or genitourinary malformations.

Comments

Cerebral US shows poor development of cerebral sulci for the gestational age. Progressive microcephaly and mild dilatation of the lateral ventricles may also develop, yet they are not seen in this particular case. The Sylvian fissure is superficial and maintains a rounded morphology due to a delayed insular operculation, which should be evident after week 25 of gestation (Fig. 10.5). On MRI, the same findings are also observed (Fig. 10.6). On postnatal US obtained on a coronal plane, the poor development of the Sylvian fissure is seen, as well as in the sulci that originate from the interhemispheric fissure (Fig. 10.7). The macroscopic specimen obtained by autopsy shows a smooth brain surface because of the underdeveloped cerebral sulci and circumvolutions (Fig. 10.8).

Imaging Findings

Figure 10.5
Figure 10.6
Figure 10.7
Figure 10.8

Case 10.3
Fetal Thyrocervical Teratoma
■

María I. Martínez León

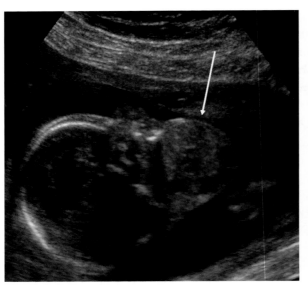

Fig. 10.9

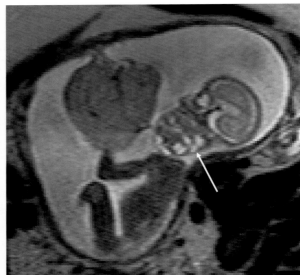

Fig. 10.10

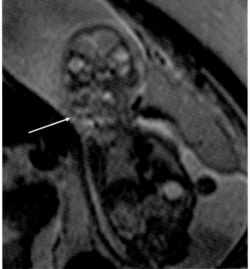

Fig. 10.11

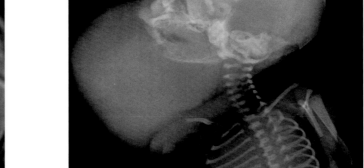

Fig. 10.12

MRI is performed on a 19-week-old fetus due to a mass seen on routine prenatal US.

Fetal teratomas are rare tumors that contain components of all embryonic germ layers. Cervical teratomas are infrequent and account for only a small portion of all teratomas. Teratomas of the head and neck region may be localized around the thyrocervical area, palate, or nasopharynx. They are often large, mobile, bulky masses containing both cystic and solid elements. Although calcifications are virtually diagnostic for teratomas, they are only present in 50% of cases. There is no definitive theory about the etiology or pathogenesis of anterior cervical teratomas, yet they are not thought to originate directly from thyroid tissue.

These tumors are frequently large and usually arise from the anterior and lateral aspect of the neck, and may extend posteriorly to the trapezius muscle, superiorly to the mastoid, and inferiorly to the clavicle or even into the mediastinum. For this reason, it is sometimes difficult to determine the original site of the tumor.

Cystic malformation, "hygroma," is the primary differential diagnosis for a large neck mass, yet these generally appear as septated fluid-filled collections rarely with solid components. While cervical teratomas are located anteriorly, cystic malformations arise more posteriorly. Other differential diagnoses include goiter, hemangioma, neuroblastoma, branchial cleft cyst, macerated twin fetus, and other soft-tissue tumors.

Polyhydramnios is a common and important associated finding and is caused by a direct mass effect that interferes with swallowing and ultimately leads to an accumulation of amniotic fluid.

It is important a careful delivery is planned, with a close and coordinated management among the perinatal team because reported mortality from lack of airway control is high. A substantial improvement in survival rates can be achieved by using the ex-utero intrapartum treatment (EXIT) procedure. In the EXIT procedure, the fetus is partially delivered by cesarean section while the placenta and umbilical cord remain intact.

Prenatal ultrasound shows a large solid and cystic cervical mass (arrow) (Fig. 10.9). Sagittal T2-weighted MR image shows a large anterior mixed-signal-intensity mass within the soft tissues of the fetal neck (arrow). Moderate fetal polyhydramnios is observed (Fig. 10.10). Coronal T2-weighted MR image shows right lateralization of the mass (arrow) (Fig. 10.11). Plain X-ray of the fetus after intrauterine death shows that the head is being deviated and hyperextended to the side by the anterior neck mass. No calcification of the mass is seen (Fig. 10.12).

Figure 10.9
Figure 10.10
Figure 10.11
Figure 10.12

Case 10.4
Congenital Cystic Adenomatoid Malformation, Type II
■
César Martín Martínez

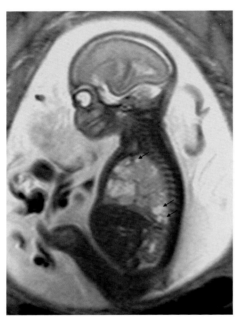

Fig. 10.13

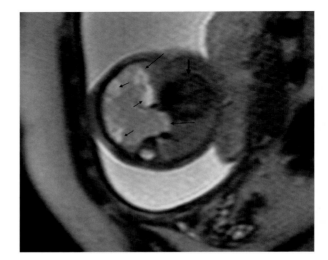

Fig. 10.14

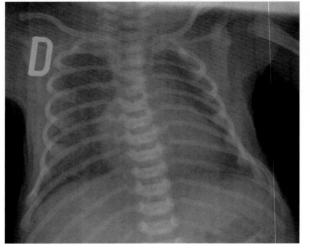

Fig. 10.15

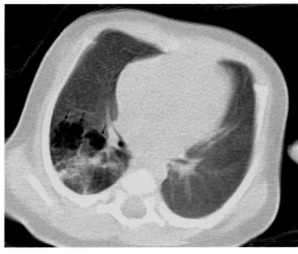

Fig. 10.16

After routine sonographic screening at 20 weeks' gestation detected a fetal lung anomaly in a woman with no relevant history, MRI was performed to characterize the anomaly. The child was born asymptomatic, but underwent plain-film chest X-ray on the first day of life and CT at 30 days to confirm the prenatal findings. He was operated on at the age of 9 months.

Congenital cystic adenomatoid malformation (CCAM) is characterized by a multicystic mass of pulmonary tissue with abnormal proliferation of bronchial structures. Its incidence is unknown, as many neonates with CCAM are asymptomatic at birth. It is thought to be caused by an embryogenetic alteration in lung development in the first 8–9 weeks of gestation. CCAM can affect a single lobe or an entire lung, but it rarely affects both lungs. Stockes suggested three types of CCAM: Type I (macrocystic), with cysts between 2 and 10 cm; type II (macrocystic with a microcystic component), with cysts less than 2 cm; and type III (microcystic) with cysts less than 0.5 cm. The appearance of the lesion depends on the type of CCAM.

In the absence of hydrops, the prognosis is very good, with survival rates practically 100%. CCAM rarely enlarges after diagnosis; in fact, most lesions become smaller with increasing gestational age, sometimes to the point of being imperceptible on X-rays after birth. However, the lesion does not disappear and CT is necessary to detect it. CCAM must be differentiated from lung sequestration, hybrid malformation (sequestration and CCAM), diaphragmatic hernia, neurenteric cyst, and teratoma. Other, less likely, diagnoses include congenital lobar emphysema, bronchial atresia, or bronchogenic cyst. CCAM is not usually associated to extrapulmonary or chromosomal anomalies. After birth, although most patients are asymptomatic, the treatment of choice is surgical resection of the mass.

Sonography showed a hyperechogenic solid lesion with cysts inside it in the base of the right lung (not shown).

Sagittal (Fig. 10.13) and axial (Fig. 10.14) HASTE images at 22 weeks' gestation show a hyperintense lesion (long arrows) with some small cysts inside (short arrows). The heart is displaced to the left (thick arrow). No pleural effusion or hydrops fetalis is evident. Findings at chest X-ray after birth (Fig. 10.15) are normal. CT 30 days later (Fig. 10.16) shows cystic lesions in the lower lobe of the right lung (arrows). The lesion is proportionately much smaller than in the fetal study.

Figure 10.13
Figure 10.14
Figure 10.15
Figure 10.16

Case 10.5
Congenital Diaphragmatic Hernia

Ignacio Alonso Usabiaga

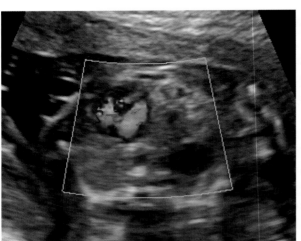
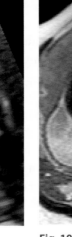

Fig. 10.17

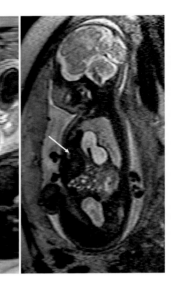

Fig. 10.18

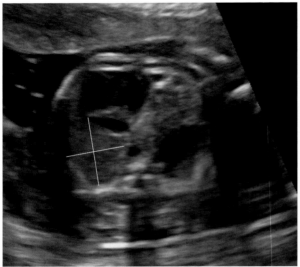

Fig. 10.19

Fig. 10.20

Diaphragmatic hernias consist of the displacement of abdominal content through an opening in the diaphragm into the chest cavity. In 80% of cases the diaphragmatic defect is located in the posterolateral region of the left hemidiaphragm (Bochdalek hernia). Its relation with chromosome disorders is frequent, and in approximately half of patients other associated abnormalities are detected.

The earlier the condition is diagnosed, the worse the prognosis. Outcome depends on the degree of secondary pulmonary hypoplasia and the presence of pulmonary hypertension in the neonatal period.

The response to treatment of diaphragmatic hernias by tracheal occlusion during the prenatal period is currently controversial.

Comments

Diagnosis is established by US, and the characteristic finding is the presence of a predominantly cystic heterogeneous mass located in the chest with associated displacement of the heart to one side (Fig. 10.17).

The absence of the stomach in the abdominal cavity and the visualization of peristaltic waves within the intrathoracic mass are pathognomonic signs of diaphragmatic hernias.

MRI may aid in confirming the diagnosis by analyzing the signal from intrathoracic bowel or by identifying the presence of liver within the herniated mass (arrow) (Fig. 10.18). The lung to head ratio (LHR) can be determined by MRI or US by dividing the area of the lung contralateral to the hernia (the multiplication of both diameters measured on the axial plane) by the fetal head circumference. A LHR of less than one indicates a worse prognosis (Fig. 10.19).

Differential diagnosis includes cystic adenomatoid malformation (CAM type I or II), although in the latter the presence of an intra-abdominal stomach (arrow) and the visualization of the integrity of the diaphragm with a caudal displacement rule out the presence of diaphragmatic hernia (Fig. 10.20).

Imaging Findings

Figure 10.17
Figure 10.18
Figure 10.19
Figure 10.20

Case 10.6

Multicystic Dysplasia of the Kidney
■

Ignacio Alonso Usabiaga

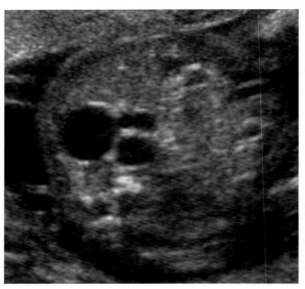

Fig. 10.21

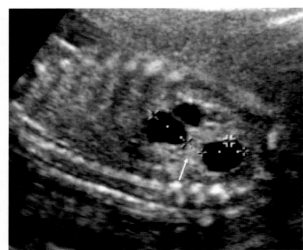

Fig. 10.22

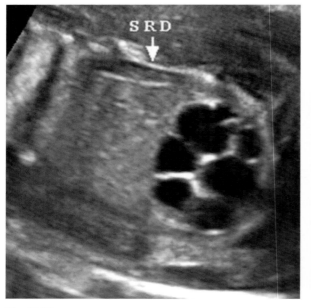

Fig. 10.23

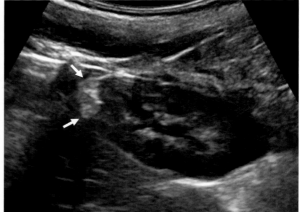

Fig. 10.24

Transabdominal prenatal ultrasound is performed at 19 weeks of gestation.

Multicystic dysplasia of the kidney (MCDK) corresponds to a type II kidney dysplasia according to Potter's classification system. The incidence among live births is 1 in 4,300. MCDK is characteristically unilateral (80%), predominantly left-sided, and more prevalent in males. Its pathogenesis consists of a rapid and complete obstruction of the pyeloureteral junction, which leads to poor differentiation of the metanephros and a subsequent inability to develop mature nephrons. A segmental variation has been described, which consists of a dysplastic transformation of the superior system when a double collecting system is present.

The prognosis of unilateral MCDK is excellent when there are no associated abnormalities (30% in the contralateral kidney and 5% extrarenal). No oligoamnios is detected, and fetal development is normal. The typical clinical course of the condition tends toward involution, and in approximately half of patients there are no apparent findings after the age of 3–4 years. Neoplastic transformation of residual dysplastic tissue is uncommon.

Differential diagnosis includes severe hydronephrosis with stenosis of the pyeloureteral junction; but in this case the cystic lesions are connected because they represent dilated calyces, and although the renal parenchymal thickness is reduced, an area of parenchyma of normal echogenicity is always present.

Autosomal recessive dysplasia (type I) is bilateral and is associated with oligoamnios. The cysts that develop in this subtype are so small that they cannot be visualized as separate structures, and therefore appear as two large masses of increased echogenicity within the fetal abdomen. The autosomal dominant form of the condition (type III) does not tend to manifest during fetal life, and an evident positive family history is present.

Prenatal fetal US reveals a large multicystic mass toward one side of the abdominal cavity (Fig. 10.21). Within the cysts, which tend to be of different sizes, dysplastic tissue of increased echogenicity is seen (arrow), but normal parenchyma is never present (Fig. 10.22). The multicystic kidney may frequently be located ectopically, usually in the pelvis (the arrow indicated the adrenal gland) (Fig. 10.23). Normal renal parenchyma is seen exclusively in the segmental variant. US of a different patient shows the evolution of a segmental multicystic kidney at 3 years, with the multicystic segment folding over the normal inferior renal pole (Fig. 10.24).

Figure 10.21
Figure 10.22
Figure 10.23
Figure 10.24

Case 10.7

Fetal Posterior Urethral Valves

Luisa Ceres Ruiz

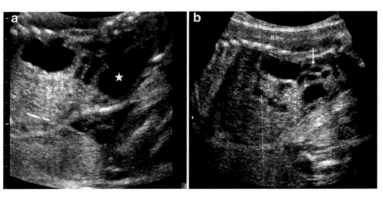

Fig. 10.25

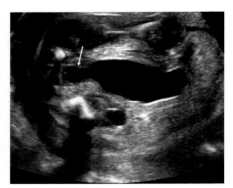

Fig. 10.26

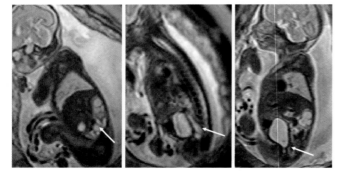

Fig. 10.27

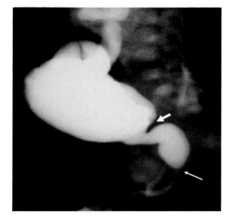

Fig. 10.28

A male fetus of 22 weeks gestation shows bilateral ureteropyelocalycial ectasia and a distended bladder on serial studies.

Posterior urethral valves (PUVs) in males are remnants of the urethrovaginal folds or "plicae colliculi" (from the Wolfian duct), that remain fixed anteroinferiorly to the "veru montanum" and cause obstruction of the urethra with dilatation of its posterior portion. Around 30% of PUVs result in terminal renal insufficiency, which is why an opportune diagnosis is essential. Currently, diagnosis is established in the prenatal period.

When fetal hydronephrosis is detected, one must consider the following: (a) whether it is uni- or bilateral, (b) if there is contralateral renal involvement, (c) whether there is evidence of mega ureter on the side of the hydronephrosis, (d) bladder studies that evaluate distension, thickness, and voiding, (e) gestational age and fetal gender, (f) associated fetal abnormalities, (g) amniotic fluid volume. And when oligoamnios is detected, whether there is renal dysplasia and pulmonary hypoplasia.

The bladder may either be distended or may show a decrease in size with wall thickening due to "hostile bladder." Although prenatal US is a sensitive and specific method of diagnosis, MRI further evaluates hydronephrosis and pulmonary hypoplasia. Severe forms of the condition are detected at 15 weeks and findings include bilateral ureterohydronephrosis of varying degrees, dilated bladder with thickened walls, dilated posterior ureter ("keyhole sign"), fetal ascitis, and oligoamnios. In approximately 50% of cases, PUVs may be associated with vesicoureteral reflux and would then be termed VURD syndrome (vesicoureteral reflux and dysplasia). Patients with severe oligoamnios almost always show pulmonary hypoplasia and renal dysplasia with a poor prognosis. Differential diagnoses include prune belly syndrome, urethral atresia, massive vesicoureteral reflux, and certain rare abnormalities. Diagnosis is confirmed by performing a voiding cystourethrogram (VCUG) on the newborn.

Sagittal fetal US: (a) Dilated left ureteropyelocalycial system with thin renal parenchyma. Distended bladder (asterisk). (b) Dilated right excretory system with a tortuous ureter (arrow) (Fig. 10.25). Sagittal image of the fetal bladder shows elongation with posterior urethral dilatation (arrow) ("keyhole sign") (Fig. 10.26). Fetal MRI: (a) Dilated and tortuous ureter. (b) Dilated left ureter. (c) Distended bladder (Fig. 10.27). VCUG reveals proximal dilatation of the urethra due to obstruction by PUVs (long arrow). Hypertrophy of the posterior lip of the internal sphincter (short arrow). Large bladder capacity. Grade IV right vesicoureteral reflux (Fig. 10.28).

Figure 10.25 (**a, b**)
Figure 10.26
Figure 10.27 (**a–c**)
Figure 10.28

Case 10.8
Fetal Jejunal Atresia

Roberto Llorens Salvador and Amparo Moreno Flores

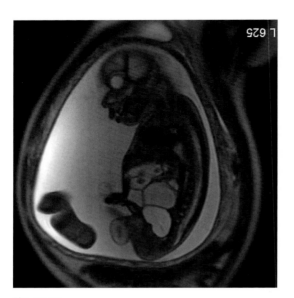

Fig. 10.29

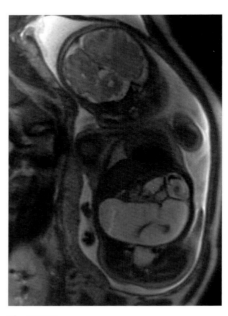

Fig. 10.30

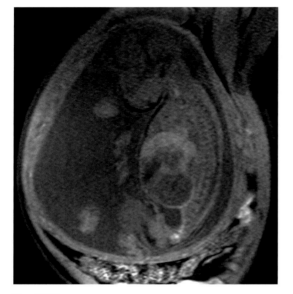

Fig. 10.31

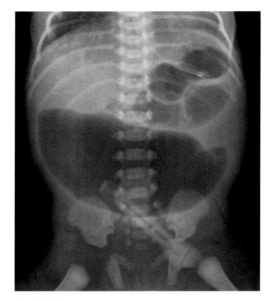

Fig. 10.32

A 34-week fetus is referred for dilated bowel loop seen on routine prenatal sonography.

Intestinal atresia is one of the most common causes of bowel obstruction in the newborn and can occur at any point in the gastrointestinal tract. Jejunal atresia (JA) is usually an isolated anomaly (only 10% associate other malformations) and comprises approximately 50% of small bowel atresias and may be associated with other jejunal and ileal atresias. (In about 10% of cases, multiple atresia is seen.)

To date, the most accepted theory regarding the etiology of JA is that of an intrauterine vascular accident resulting in necrosis of the affected segment, with subsequent resorption. The atresia has been classified into four types based upon their anatomic characteristics representing a spectrum of severity, from a simple web to full atresia with loss of bowel length.

JA is normally detected by prenatal ultrasound because of the presence of dilated bowel loops, hyperechogenic bowel, ascites, and maternal polyhydramnios. Fetal MR can be used to improve antenatal detection of surgically correctable anomalies allowing a planned delivery with prompt surgical intervention. Affected infants typically develop abdominal distension and bilious emesis within the first 2 days. Meconium could be passed initially in high intestinal obstruction. Postnatal imaging should start with plain-film evaluation. Resection of the proximal dilated bowel with primary anastomosis with or without tapering of the proximal bowel is commonly performed.

Several dilated small bowel loops in a sagittal T2 fetal MR (Fig. 10.29). In patients with JA, a proximal segment of bowel usually becomes markedly dilated due to continuing peristalsis proximal to the obstruction as it is shown in a coronal T2 (Fig. 10.30). Fat saturation T1 MR is used to identify meconium distribution in fetal gastrointestinal tract normally seen in the colon beyond 24 weeks' gestation. Sagittal T1 with linear high signal intensity related to a small abnormal quantity of meconium in fetal rectum (Fig. 10.31). Postnatal abdominal radiograph (Fig. 10.32) showing a big dilated bowel loop and no distal gas in JA. Number of dilated loops reflects level of obstruction (few loops implies upper obstruction like JA and many loops implies distal ileal or colonic atresia).

Figure 10.29
Figure 10.30
Figure 10.31
Figure 10.32

Case 10.9
Prune Belly Syndrome (Eagle–Barrett Syndrome)
Ignacio Alonso Usabiaga

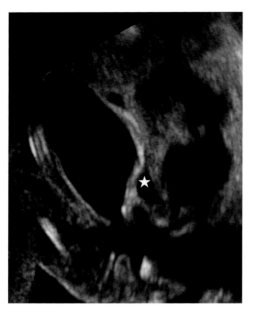

Fig. 10.33

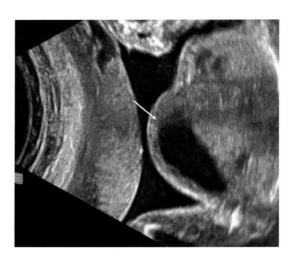

Fig. 10.34

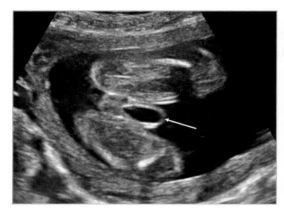

Fig. 10.35

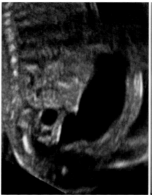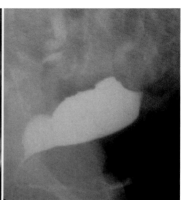

Fig. 10.36

Prenatal ultrasound performed at 20 weeks of gestation.

Prune belly syndrome (PBS) is a rare condition (1/35–1/50,000 live births) characterized by a defective development of the abdominal musculature with a significant dilatation of the urinary tract (ureters and bladder) and cryptorchidism (triad syndrome). It is very uncommon in females. The etiology of PBS is poorly understood, and although the most accepted theory is a primary abnormality of the mesodermal tissue, some authors believe in a multifactorial origin due to an early ureteral obstruction and a poor development of the embryonic prostate. Furthermore, a primary genetic disorder has also been proposed as a possible cause.

Prognosis is generally poor because of the associated severe renal insufficiency caused by renal tissue dysplasia due to abnormalities present in the urinary tract. Early oligoamnios indicates a worse clinical outcome.

The external appearance of the newborn is characterized by a prune-like flaccid and wrinkled abdomen due to an absence of abdominal musculature, which gives the condition its name. Apart from the classic triad, PBS may manifest itself in association with other malformations, commonly gastrointestinal and cardiac (10%). The degree of pulmonary hypoplasia and limb deformity depends on the severity of the oligoamnios.

A differential diagnosis includes megacystis-microcolon-hypoperistalsis syndrome, which is much more frequent in females and presents ureterohydronephrosis without associated oligoamnios. PUVs may also present similar manifestation, although in this case the bladder–urethra complex tends to develop the typical keyhole-like appearance, unlike the "beak" morphology acquired in PBS, which indicates a functional obstruction.

Fetal US reveals significant ureteral dilatation (asterisk) and a large bladder, whose dome appears as if adhered to the anterior wall of the abdomen in the umbilical region (arrow) (Figs. 10.33 and 10.34). The sonographic renal pattern is abnormal, and the kidneys are small and present some cysts within, which indicate the dysplastic transformation of the renal tissue (hypodysplastic kidneys) (not shown). A mild dilatation of the pyelocalycial system is seen, which is disproportionate to the large dilatation of the ureters and bladder. Occasionally, dilatation of the entire urethra (megalourethra, arrow) due to cavernous body agenesis, which is considered a typical sign of the condition, is seen (Fig. 10.35). The beak-like morphology of the bladder–urethra complex correlates between the fetal US and postnatal voiding cystourethrogram (Fig. 10.36).

Figure 10.33
Figure 10.34
Figure 10.35
Figure 10.36

Case 10.10
Gastroschisis
■

María I. Martínez León

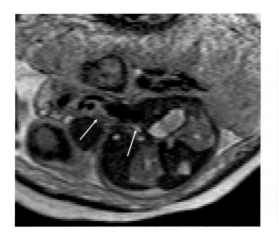

Fig. 10.37

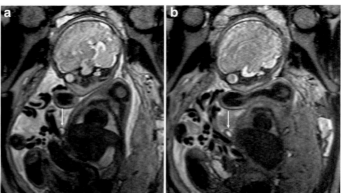

Fig. 10.38

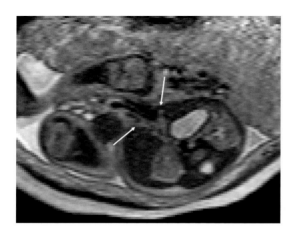

Fig. 10.39

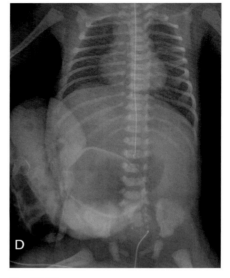

Fig. 10.40

A 28-year-old woman with an estimated 32 weeks of pregnancy was referred to MRI for evaluation of fetal extra-abdominal bowel loops seen on prenatal ultrasound.

Gastroschisis is a congenital abdominal wall defect in which the abdominal organs, generally the small intestines, herniate into the amniotic cavity. The herniation is usually to the right of the umbilical cord. The small bowel eviscerates through the defect and is nonrotated and lacking secondary fixation to the posterior abdominal wall. The loops of bowel in this condition are never covered by a membrane.

Three theories have been suggested to explain the pathogenesis of gastroschisis: abnormal involution of the umbilical vein, intravascular event of the omphalomesenteric artery, and early intrauterine rupture of an omphalocele with complete resorption of the sac. The abdominal wall does not close until week 6–10 of fetal development; this leaves an opening on the right side of the umbilical cord, allowing the intestines to protrude through the abdomen and float freely in the amniotic fluid.

Almost all cases are diagnosed during the prenatal period by ultrasound and there is also an elevation of alpha-fetoprotein (AFP) levels in maternal serum and amniotic fluid. (Open fetal defect allows diffusion of AFP from the fetal circulation into amniotic fluid.)

The main differential diagnosis is omphalocele, another more frequent abdominal fusion defect that differs because the herniated organs remain enclosed in visceral peritoneum. Also, omphalocele is more frequently associated with other malformations than gastroschisis. Other abdominal wall defects such as bladder exstrophy, body stalk anomalies, and amniotic band syndrome may resemble gastroschisis.

Gastroschisis requires surgical management after delivery to return the exposed viscera to the abdominal cavity. Also, parenteral nutrition until bowel motility permits oral feedings and evaluation for coexisting malformations must also be performed.

Axial T2-weighted MR image of the fetal abdomen shows the right paraumbilical herniation of bowel (arrows) (Fig. 10.37). Sagittal paramedian T2-weighted MRI of the abdomen reveals herniated bowel without dilatation (arrows), the walls are not thickened nor distended, which indicates that there is no obstruction (Fig. 10.38a, b). Axial T2-weighted MRI shows the small abdominal wall defect (usually measuring 2–4 cm) (arrows) (Fig. 10.39). Abdominal plain X-ray of the 38-week newborn shows periumbilical loop distention related to gastroschisis and obstruction, which was confirmed during surgery (Fig. 10.40).

Figure 10.37
Figure 10.38
Figure 10.39
Figure 10.40

Further Reading

Books

Avni F et al (2002) Perinatal imaging: from ultrasound to MR imaging. Springer-Verlag, Berlin

Barkovich AJ (2000) Pediatric neuroimaging, 3rd edn. Lippincott Williams & Wilkins, Philadelphia, pp 289–291

Callen PW (1994) Ultrasonography in obstetrics and gynecology, 3rd edn. W.B. Saunders, Philadelphia, pp 373–376

Diamond DA et al (1999) Perinatal urology. In: Martin Barrett T (ed) Pediatric nephrology, 4th ed, vol 56. Lippincott Williams & Wilkins, Philadelphia, pp 897–912

Goldstein RB (2003) The thorax. In: Nyberg DA, McGahan JP, Pretorius DH, Pilu G (eds) Diagnostic imaging of fetal anomalies. Lippincott Williams & Wilkins, Philadelphia, pp 381–420

Gratacós E et al (2007) Medicina fetal, 1st edn. Editorial Médica Panamericana, Argentina

Isaacs H (1997) Germ cell tumors. In: Isaacs H (ed) Tumors of the fetus and newborn. W.B. Saunders, Philadelphia, pp 1–38

Woodward PJ (2005) Diagnostic imaging obstetrics. Amirsys, Manitoba

Web Links

http://www.thefetus.net/page.php?id=1784

http://www.ninds.nih.gov/disorders/lissencephaly/lissencephaly.htm

http://www.thefetus.net/page.php?id=217

http//www.thefetus.net/index.php

http://emedicine.medscape.com/article/978118-overview

http://emedicine.medscape.com/article/411365-overview

http://emedicine.medscape.com/article/412226

www.thefetus.net

http://www.prunebelly.org/

http://emedicine.medscape.com/article/403800-overview

Articles

Adzick N, Harrison M, Glick P et al (1985) Diaphragmatic hernia in the fetus: prenatal diagnosis and outcome in 94 cases. J Pediatr Surg 20:357–361

Agarwal R (2005) Prenatal diagnosis of anterior abdominal wall defects: Pictorial essay. Indian J Radiol Imaging 15:361–372

Al-Khaldi N, Watson AR, Zuccollo J, Twining P, Rose DH (1994) Outcome of antenatally detected cystic dysplastic kidney disease. Arch Dis Child 70:520–522

Aslam M, Watson AR (2006) Unilateral multicystic dysplastic kidney: long term outcome. Arch Dis Child 91:820–823

Barkovich AJ, Kjos BO (1992) Shizencephaly: correlation of clinical findings with MR characteristics. AJNR 13:85–94

Barkovich AJ, Kuzniecky RI, Jackson GD, Guerrini R, Dobyns WB (2005) A developmental and genetic classification for malformations of cortical development. Neurology 65:1873–1887

Benacerraf B, Adzick N (1987) Fetal diaphragmatic hernia: Ultrasound diagnosis and clinical outcome in 19 cases. Am J Obstet Gynecol 156:573–576

Bendersky M, Musolino P, Rugilo C, Shuster G, Sica R (2006) Normal anatomy of the developing fetal brain. Ex vivo anatomical-magnetic resonance imaging correlation. J Neurol Sci 250:20–26

Berrocal T, Lamas M, Gutieérrez J et al (1999) Congenital anomalies of the small intestine, colon, and rectum. Radiographics 19:1219–1236

Berrocal T, Lopez-Pereira P, Arjonilla A, Gutierrez J (2002) Anomalies of the distal ureter, bladder and urethra in children: embryologic, radiologic and pathologic features. Radiographics 22:1139–1164

Bouchard S, Johnson MP, Flake AW, Howell LJ, Adzick NS, Crombleholme TM et al (2002) The EXIT procedure: experience and outcome in 31 cases. J Pediatr Surg 37:418–426

Buonomo C (1997) Neonatal gastrointestinal emergencies. Radiol Clin North Am 35:845–864

Ceccherini A, Twining P, Variend S (1999) Schizencephaly: antenatal detection using ultrasound. Clin Radiol 59:620–622

Cohen HL, Zinn HL, Patel A, Zinn DL, Haller JO (1998) Prenatal sonographic diagnosis of posterior urethral valves: identification of valves and thickening of the posterior urethral wall. J Clin Ultrasound 26(7):366–370

Cohen-Sacher B, Lerman-Sagie T, Lev D, Malinger G (2006) Sonographic development milestones of the fetal cerebral cortex: a longitudinal study. Ultrasound Obstet Gynecol 27:494–502

Dalla Vecchia LK, Grosfeld JL, West KW, Rescorla FJ, Scherer LR, Engum SA (1998) Intestinal atresia and stenosis: a 25-year experience with 277 cases. Arch Surg 133:490–496

Denis D, Maugey-Laulom B, Carles D, Pedespan J, Brun M, Chateil J (2001) Prenatal diagnosis of schizencephaly by fetal magnetic resonance imaging. Fetal Diagn Ther 16:354–359

Eagle JF, Barret GS (1950) Congenital deficiency of abdominal musculature with associated genitourinary abnormalities: syndrome report of nine cases. Pediatrics 6:721–736

Eckoldt F, Woderich R, Wolke S, Heling K, Stöver B, Tennstedt C (2003) Follow-up of unilateral multicystic kidney dysplasia after prenatal diagnosis. J Matern Fetal Neonatal Med 14(3):177–186

Emanuel PG, Garcia GI, Angtuaco TL (1995) Prenatal detection of anterior abdominal wall defects with US. Radiographics 15:517–530

Ertl-Wagner B, Lienemann A, Strauss A et al (2002) Fetal magnetic resonance imaging: indications, technique, anatomical considerations and a review of fetal abnormalities. Eur Radiol 12:1931–1940

Estroff JA, Mandell J, Benacerraf BR (1991) Increased renal parenchymal echogenicity in the fetus: importance and clinical outcome. Radiology 181:135–139

Fernbach SK, Maizels M, Conway JJ (1993) Ultrasound grading of hydronephrosis: introduction to the system used by the Society for fetal Urology. Pediatr Radiol 23:478–480

Fisk NM, Dhillon HK, Ellis CE, Nicolini U, Tannirandorn Y, Rodeck CH (1990) Antenatal diagnosis of megalourethra in a fetus with the prune belly syndrome. J Clin Ultrasound 18(2):124–128

Fong KW, Ghai S, Toi A, Blaser S, Winsor EJT, Chitayat D (2004) Prenatal ultrasound findings of lissencephaly associated with Miller-Dieker syndrome and comparison with pre- and postnatal magnetic resonance imaging. Ultrasound Obstet Gynecol 24:716–723

Ghai S, Fong KW, Toi A, Chitayat D, Pantazi S, Blaser S (2006) Prenatal US and MR imaging findings of lissencephaly: review of fetal cerebral sulcal development. Radiographics 26:389–405

Grahan G, Connor P (2005) Antenatal diagnosis of congenital diaphragmatic hernia. Sem Perinatol 29:69–76

Granata T, Freri E, Caccia C, Setola V, Taroni F, Battaglia G (2005) Schizencephaly: clinical spectrum, epilepsy, and pathogenesis. J Child Neurol 20:313–318

Greco P, Resta M, Vimercati A, Dicuonzo F, LoverroG VicinoM, Selvaggi L (1998) Antenatal diagnosis of isolated lissencephaly by ultrasound and magnetic resonance imaging. Ultrasound Obstet Gynecol 12:276–279

Greskovich FJ, Nyberg LM (1988) The prune-belly syndrome: a review of its etiology, defects, treatment and prognosis. J Urol 140:707–712

Harrison MR, Albanese CT, Hawgood SB, Farmer DL, Farrell JA, Sandberg PL, Filly RA (2001) Fetoscopic temporary tracheal occlusion by means of detachable balloon for congenital diaphragmatic hernia. Am J Obstet Gynecol 185:730–733

Hayashi N, Tsutsumi Y, Barkovich AJ (2002) Morphological features and associated anomalies of schizencephaly in the clinical propulation: detailed analysis of MR images. Neuroradiology 44:418–427

Heling KS, Wauer RR, Bollmann R, Chaoui R (2005) Reliability of the lung-to-head ratio in predicting outcome and neonatal ventilation parameters in fetuses with congenital diaphragmatic hernia. Ultrasound Obstet Gynecol 25(2):112–118

Herndon CD, McKenna P, Kolon Th et al (1999) A multicenter outcomes analysis of patients with neonatal reflux presnting with prenatal hydronephrosis. J Urol 162:1203–1208

Hill B, Joe B, Qayyum A, Yeh B, Goldstein R (2005) Supplemental Value of MRI in Fetal Abdominal Disease Detected on Prenatal Sonography: Preliminary Experience. AJR 184:993–998

Hirose S, Farmer DL, Lee H, Nobuhara KK, Harrison MR (2004) The ex utero intrapartum treatment procedure: looking back at the EXIT. J Pediatr Surg 39:375–380

Hitchcock A, Sears RT, O'Neill T (1987) Immature cervical teratoma arising in one fetus of a twin pregnancy. Case report and review of the literature. Acta Obstet Gynecol Scand 66:377–379

Holmdahl G (1997) Bladder dysfunction in boys with posterior urethral valves. Scand J Urol Nephrol Suppl 188:1–36

Holmes N, Harrison MR, Baskin LS et al (2001) Fetal surgery for posterior urethral valves: long-term postnatal outcomes. Pediatrics 108: E

Hubbard AM (2001) Magnetic resonance imaging of fetal thoracic abnormalities. Top Magn Reson Imaging 12(1):18–24

Hubbard AM, Adzick N, Crombleholme T, Coleman B, Howel L, Haselgrove J et al (1999) Congenital chest lesions: diagnosis and characterization with prenatal MR imaging. Radiology 212:43–48

Inyard P, Chitty L (2001) Dysplastic and polycystic kidney: diagnosis, associations and management. Prenat Diagn 21:924–935

Jaureguizar E, López-Pereira P, Martinez-Urrutia MJ (2002) The valve bladder: etiology and outcome. Curr Urol Rep 3(2):115–120

Jeon A, Cramer BC, Walsh E, Pushpanathan C (1999) A spectrum of segmental multicystic renal disease. Pediatr Radiol 29:309–315

Kajbafzadeh A (2005) Congenital urethral anomalies in boys. Part I: posterior urethral valves. Urol J 2:59–78

Kajbafzadeh AM, Payabvash S, Sadeghi Z, Elmi A, Jamal A, Hantoshzadeh Z, Eslami L, Mehdizadeh M (2008) Comparison of magnetic resonance urography with ultrasound studies in detection of fetal urogenital anomalies. J Pediatr Urol 4:32–39

Katz AL, Wiswell TE, Baumgart S (1998) Contemporary controversies in the management of congenital diaphragmatic hernia. Clin Perinatol 25(1):219–248

Kener B, Flaum E, Mathews H, Carlson DE, Pepkowitz SH, Hixon H et al (1998) Cervical teratoma: prenatal diagnosis and long-term follow up. Prenat Diagn 18:51–59

Khemiri M, Khaldi F, Hamzaoui A, Chaouachi B, Hamzaoui M, Ben Becher S et al (2009) Cystic pulmonary malformations: clinical and radiological polymorphism. A report on 30 cases. Rev Pneumol Clin 65(6):333–340

King J, Askin DF (2003) Gastroschisis: etiology, diagnosis, delivery options, and care. Neonatal Netw 22(4):7–12

Komarniski CA, Cyr DR, Mack LA, Weinberger E (1990) Prenatal diagnosis of schizencephaly. J Ultrasound Med 9:305–307

Kuzniecky RI (2006) Malformation of cortical development and epilepsy, part 1: diagnosis and classification scheme. Rev Neurol Dis 59:471–476

Lazebnik N, Bellinger MF, Ferguson JE, Hogge JS, Hogge WA (1999) Insights into the pathogenesis and natural history of fetuses with multicystic dysplastic kidney disease. Prenat Diagn 19:418–423

Levine D, Barnewolt C, Mehta T, Trop I, Estroff J, Wong G (2003) Tetal thoracic abnormalities: MR imaging. Radiology 228:379–388

Lipshutz G, Albanese C, Harrison M et al (1997) Prospective analysis of lung to head ratio predicts survival for patiens with prenatally diagnosed congenital diaphragmatic hernia. J Pediatr Surg 32:1634–1636

Loder RT, Guiboux JP, Bloom DA, Hensinger RN (1992) Musculoskeletal aspects of prunne-belly syndrome: description and pathogenesis. Am J Dis Child 146:1224–1229

Matsushita M, Ishii K, Tamura M, Takahashi Y, Kamura T, Takakuwa K et al (2008) Perinatal magnetic resonance fetal lung volumetry and fetal lung-to-liver signal intensity ratio for predicting short outcome in isolated congenital diaphragmatic hernia and cystic adenomatoid malformation of the lung. J Obstet Gynecol Res 34(2):162–167

Monteagudo A, Timor-Tritsch I (1997) Development of fetal gyri, sulci and fissures: a transvaginal sonographic study. Ultrasound Obstet Gynecol 9:222–228

Morof D, Levine D, Grable I, Barnewolt C, Estroff J, Fishman S et al (2004) Oropharyngeal teratoma: prenatal diagnosis and assessment using sonography, MRI, and CT with management by ex utero intrapartum treatment procedure. AJR 183:493–496

Nakayama DK, Harrison MR, Chin DH, de Lorimier AA (1984) The pathogenesis of prune-belly. Am J Dis Child 138:834–836

Narchi H (2005) Risk of Wilms´tumour with multicystic kidney disease: a systematic review. Arch Dis Child 90:147–149

Narla LD, Doberty RD, Hingsbergen EA, Fullcher AS (1998) Pediatric case of the day (Eagle-Barrett syndrome, triad syndrome). Radiographics 18:1318–1322

Nunn IN, Stephens FD (1961) The triad syndrome: a composite anomaly of the abdominal wall, urinary system and testes. J Urol 86:782–794

Oh KY, Kennedy AM, Frias AE, Byrne JLB (2005) Fetal Schizencephaly: pre- and postnatal imaging with a review of the clinical manifestations. Radiographics 25:647–657

Ono K, Kikuchi A, Takikawa KM, Hiroma T, Yoshizawa K, Sunagawa S et al (2009) Hernia of the umbilical cord and associated ileal prolapse through a patent omphalomesenteric duct: prenatal ultrasound and MRI findings. Fetal Diagn Ther 25:72–75

Pagon RA, Smith DW, Shepard TH (1979) Urethral obstruction malformation complex: a cause of abdominal muscle deficiency and the "Prunne-Belly". J Pediatr 94:900–906

Perella RR, Ragavendra N, Tessler FN, Boechat I, Crandall B, Grant EG (1991) Fetal abdominal wall mass detected on prenatal sonography: gastroschisis vs omphalocele. AJR 157:1065–1068

Phelps S, Fisher R, Partington A, Dykes E (1997) Prenatal ultrasound diagnosis of gastrointestinal malformations. J Pediatr Surg 32:438

Quarello E, Strinemann J, Ville Y, Guibaud L (2008) Assessment of fetal Sylvian fissure operculization between 22 and 32 weeks: a subjective approach. Ultrasound Obstet Gynecol 32:44–49

Quintero RA, Morales WJ, Bornick PW, Johnson PK (2000) Minimally invasive intraluminal tracheal occlusion in a human fetus with left congenital diaphragmatic hernia at 27 weeks' gestation via direct fetal laryngoscopy. Prenatal Neonatal Med 3:13

Ramsden WH, Arthur RJ, Martinez D (1997) Gastroschisis: a radiological and clinical review. Pediatr Radiol 27(2):166–169

Rempen A, Feige A (1985) Differential diagnosis of sonographically detected tumours in the fetal cervical region. Eur J Obstet Gynecol Reprod Biol 20:89–105

Richard M, Stocker JT (1999) Extralobar sequestration with frequently associated congenital cystic adenomatoid malformation, Type 2: report of 50 cases. Pediatr Dev Pathol 2:454–463

Robson WLM, Leung AKC, Thomason MA (1995) Multicystic dysplasia of the kidney. Clin Pediatr 34:32–40

Ruano R, Joubin L, Sonigo P, Benachi P, Aubry MC et al (2004) Fetal lung volume estimated by 3-dimensional ultrasonography and magnetic resonance imaging in cases with isolated congenital diaphragmatic hernia. J Ultrasound Med 23(3):353–358

Saguintaah M, Couture A, Veyrac C, Baud C, Quere MP (2002) MRI of the fetal gastrointestinal tract. Pediatr Radiol 32(6):395–404

Salzman DH, Krauss CM, Goldman JM, Benacerraf BR (1991) Prenatal diagnosis of lissencephaly. Prenat Diagn 11:139–143

Sarhan O, Zaccaria I, Macher MA, Muller F, Vuillard E et al (2008) A Long-term outcome of prenatally detected posterior urethral valves: single center study of 65 cases managed by primary valve ablation. J Urol 179:307–312

Sasaki Y, Miyamoto T, Hidaka Y, Satoh H, Takuma N, Sengoku K et al (2006) Three-dimensional magnetic resonance imaging after ultrasonography for assessment of fetal gastroschisis. Magn Reson Imaging 24(2):201–203

Schott S, Mackensen-Haen S, Wallwierner M, Meyberg-Solomayer G, Kagan KO (2009) Cystic adenomatoid malformation of the lung causing hydrops fetalis: case report and review of the literature. Arch Gynecol Obstet 280:293–296

Schreuder MF, Westland R, Van Wijk JAE (2009) Unilateral multicystic dysplastic kidney: a meta-analysis of observational studies on the incidence, associated urinary tract malformations and the contralateral kidney. Nephrol Dial Transplant 24:1810–1818

Shawis R, Antao B (2006) Prenatal bowel dilatation and the subsequent postnatal management. Eary Hum Dev 82:297–303

Sherer DM, Woods JR Jr, Abramowicz JS et al (1993) Prenatal sonographic assessment of early, rapidly frowing fetal cervical teratoma. Prenat Diagn 13:1079–1084

Shinmoto H, Kashima K, Yuasa Y et al (2000a) MR imaging of non-CNS fetal abnormalities: a pectoral essay. Radiographics 20:1227–1243

Shinmoto H, Kashima K, Yuasa Y, Tanimoto A, Morikawa Y, Ishimoto H, Yoshimura Y, Hiramatsu K (2000b) MR imaging of non-CNS fetal abnormalities: a pictorial essay. Radiographics 20:1227–1243

Simonovský V, Lisý J (2007) Meconium pseudocyst secondary to ileal atresia complicated by volvulus: antenatal MR demonstration. Pediatr Radiol 37:305–309

Skari H, Bjornland K, Haugen G, Egeland T, Emblem R (2000) Congenital Diaphragmatic hernia: a meta-analysis of mortality factors. J Pediatr Surg 35:1187–1195

Stanton M, Njere I, Ade-Ajayi N, Pastel S, Davenport M (2009) Systematic review and meta-analysis of the postnatal management of congenital cystic lung lesions. J Pediatr Surg 44(5):1027–1033

Stocker JT, Madewill JE, Drake RM (1977) Congenital cystic adenomatoid malformation of the lung: classification and morphologic spectrum. Hum Pathol 8:155–171

Sukthankar S, Watson AR (2000) Unilateral multicystic dysplastic kidney disease:defining the natural history. Acta Paediatr 89(7):811–813

Toi A, Lister WS, Fong KW (2004) How early are fetal cerebral sulci visible at prenatal ultrasound and what is the normal pattern of early fetal sulcal development? Ultrasound Obstet Gynecol 24:706–715

Tower C, Ong SS, Ewer AK, Khan K, Kilby MD (2009) Prognosis in isolated gastroschisis with bowel dilatation: a systematic review. Arch Dis Child Fetal Neonatal Ed 94(4):268–274

Vachharajani AJ, Dillon PA, Mathur AM (2007) Outcomes in neonatal gastroschisis: an institutional experience. Am J Perinatol 24(8):461–465

Veyrac C, Couture A, Saguintaah M, Baud C (2004) MRI of fetal GI tract abnormalities. Abdom Imaging 29:411–420

Wagner W, Harrison MR (2002) Fetal operations in the head and neck area: current state. Head Neck 24:482–490

Waszak P, Claris O, Lapillone A, Picaud JC, Basson E (1999) Cystic adenomatoid malformation of the lung: neonatal management of 21 cases. Pediatr Surg Int 15:326–331

Winters W, Effmann E, Nghiem H, Nyberg D (1997) Disappearing fetal lung masses: importance of postnatal imaging studies. Pediatr Radiol 27:535–539

Woodward PJ, Sohaey R, Kennedy A, Koeller KK (2005) From the archives od the AFIP: a comprehensive review of fetal tumors with pathologic correlation. Radiographics 25:215–242

Yakovlev PI, Wadsworth RC (1946a) Schizencephalies: a study of the congenital clefts in the cerebral mantle. Clefts with fused lips. J Neuropathol Exp Neurol 5:116–130

Yakovlev PI, Wadsworth RC (1946b) Schizencephalies: a study of the congenital clefts in the cerebral mantle. Clefts with hydo-cephalus and lips separeted. J Neuropathol Exp Neurol 5: 169–206

Zizka J, Elias P, Hodik K, Tintera J, Juttnerova V, Belobradek Z, Klzo L (2006) Liver, meconium, haemorrhage: the value of T1-weighted images in fetal MRI. Pediatr Radiol 36:792–801

Printing and Binding: Stürtz GmbH, Würzburg